Emerging Infectious Diseases of the 21st Century

***Series Editor:* I.W. Fong**
Professor of Medicine, University of Toronto
Infectious Diseases, St. Michael's Hospital

For further volumes:
http://www.springer.com/series/5903

I.W. Fong
Editor

Challenges in Infectious Diseases

Springer

Editor
I.W. Fong
Department of Medicine
University of Toronto
Toronto, ON, Canada

Division of Infectious Diseases
St. Michael's Hospital
Toronto, ON, Canada

ISBN 978-1-4614-4495-4 ISBN 978-1-4614-4496-1 (eBook)
DOI 10.1007/978-1-4614-4496-1
Springer New York Heidelberg Dordrecht London

Library of Congress Control Number: 2012944990

Printed on acid-free paper

Springer is part of Springer Science+Business Media (www.springer.com)

Preface

Infectious diseases continue to pose serious threat to the world's population with no foreseeable solutions in the near future. In fact as the planet faces new challenges with global climate changes and international urbanization, it is predictable that patterns of infectious diseases will change and will be harder to manage than ever before.

Health care persons in the field of infectious disease, microbiology, infection control, and public health and government need to prepare for the future by becoming familiar not only with current demands but possible pending challenges. To control and eradicate present infectious diseases that are posing serious threat to large segments of the world's population represent daunting goals. The ease of international travel since the advent of the "jet age" has simplified the global spread of contagious diseases across the world in a matter of hours or a few days. This has been exemplified by the previous SARS pandemic and the recent H1N1 ["swine flu"] influenza pandemic. Thus, health care professionals, in particular those in the field of infectious diseases and public health, as well as first-line contacts for ill patients, such as emergency physicians and family physicians, should remain cognizant of outbreaks of infectious diseases occurring outside their hemisphere. These diseases are of constant reminder that no country, and its citizens, can survive as an island by itself and remain untouched by diseases ravaging other nations in distant areas of the world.

In the past 50 years, great strides have been made against some crippling and deadly infectious diseases. The world is now free of smallpox, and we are on the verge of conquering or eradicating polio, with only a few countries remaining with active cases. However, many infectious diseases still result in the loss of tens of millions of lives each year and cause severe chronic disability in large proportions of the world's population. These diseases present enormous challenges to control and eventually eradicate from the world.

This new volume *Challenges in Infectious Diseases* is a continuation of the series *Emerging Infectious Diseases of the 21st Century* and aims to address demands and challenges that various infections present to the world at large ("global challenges"), such as the HIV pandemic, continuous threat of spreading common multiresistant pathogenic bacteria, multidrug and extensive drug-resistant tuberculosis, and the influence we can expect on these epidemics with global climate change and international urbanization. Developing countries in tropical and subtropical regions of the world face different problems with infections unique to the underdeveloped and developing nations. Beside HIV and tuberculosis (dealt with under global challenges), there are millions of lives lost each year to malaria and cholera, and even more become afflicted by dengue, typhoid fever, filariasis, chronic schistosomiasis, and others. Chapters on these various topics authored by world-renowned experts on these areas provide state-of-the-art reviews on epidemiology, biology, clinical aspects, prevention, current approaches to control, and prevention such as new vaccines, and reassessment of past and present methods are discussed.

Toronto, Ontario, Canada I.W. Fong

Acknowledgements

I am indebted to Carolyn Ziegler for her invaluable literature searches for references and to Debbie Reid-Marsden for her administration assistance.

Contents

Contributors

Roy Ahn M.P.H. Sc.D. Division of Global Health, Department of Emergency Medicine, Massachusetts General Hospital, Boston, MA, USA

Luther A. Bartelt, M.D., D.T.M. & H. Division of Infectious Diseases and Gastroenterology and the Center for Global Health, University of Virginia, Charlottesville, VA, USA

Robert Bergquist WHO Special Program for Research & Training in Tropical Diseases, IngerodBrastad, Sweden

Thomas F. Burke, M.D. Division of Global Health, Department of Emergency Medicine, Massachusetts General Hospital, Boston, MA, USA

Jaya Chakravarty, M.D. Department of Medicine, Institute of Medical Sciences, Banaras Hindu University, Varanasi, India

Ignatius W. Fong, M.B.B.S., F.R.C.P.C. Department of Medicine, University of Toronto, Toronto, ON, Canada

Division of Infectious Diseases, St. Michael's Hospital, Toronto, ON, Canada

Robert Gaynes, M.D. Division of Infectious Diseases, Department of Medicine, Emory School of Medicine, Atlanta, GA, USA

Atlanta VA Medical Center, Atlanta, GA, USA

Darren J. Gray Molecular Parasitology Laboratory, Infectious Diseases Division, Queensland Institute of Medical Research, Brisbane, QLD, Australia

School of Population Health, University of Queensland, Brisbane, QLD, Australia

School of Public Health, Griffith University, Meadowbrook, QLD, Australia

Richard L. Guerrant, M.D. The Center for Global Health, University of Virginia, Charlottesville, VA, USA

Yuesheng Li Molecular Parasitology Laboratory, Infectious Diseases Division, Queensland Institute of Medical Research, Brisbane, QLD, Australia

Hunan Institute of Parasitic Diseases, WHO Collaborating Centre for Research and Control on Schistosomiasis in Lake Region, Yueyang, People's Republic of China

Daniel Livorsi, M.D. Division of Infectious Diseases, Department of Medicine, Emory University School of Medicine, Atlanta, GA, USA

Atlanta VA Medical Center, Atlanta, GA, USA

Donald P. McManus Molecular Parasitology Laboratory, Infectious Diseases Division, Queensland Institute of Medical Research, Brisbane, QLD, Australia

Thomas B. Nutman, M.D. Helminth Immunology Section, Laboratory of Parasitic Diseases, National Institute of Allergy & Infectious Diseases, Bethesda, MD, USA

Clinical Parasitology Section, National Institutes of Health, Bethesda, MD, USA

Raquel Reyes, M.D., M.P.A. Division of Global Health, Department of Emergency Medicine, Massachusetts General Hospital, Boston, MA, USA

Harvard MGH Medicine & Pediatrics Program, Departments of Internal Medicine and Pediatrics, Massachusetts General Hospital, Boston, MA, USA

Edward Stenehjem, M.D. Division of Infectious Diseases, Department of Medicine, Emory University School of Medicine, Atlanta, GA, USA

Atlanta VA Medical Center, Atlanta, GA, USA

Shyam Sundar, M.D. Department of Medicine, Institute of Medical Sciences, Banaras Hindu University, Varanasi, India

Katherine Thurber, A.B. Division of Global Health, Department of Emergency Medicine, Massachusetts General Hospital, Boston, MA, USA

Sten H. Vermund, M.D., Ph.D. Vanderbilt Institute of Global Health, Vanderbilt University School of Medicine, Nashville, TN, USA

Annelies Wilder-Smith, M.D., Ph.D., MIH Institute of Public Health, University of Heidelberg, Heidelberg, Germany

Gail M. Williams School of Population Health, University of Queensland, Brisbane, QLD, Australia

Part I
Global Challenges

Chapter 1
HIV Epidemic

Sten H. Vermund

1.1 Current Status of Epidemic

The global pandemic of human immunodeficiency virus (HIV) infection is unprecedented in human history. While the bubonic plague in fourteenth-century Europe is estimated to have killed a quarter of the population, the epidemic of 1347–1350 was self-limited once a vast pool of susceptible humans and rodents were killed and persons who recovered were rendered immune [1, 2]. Plague reemerged periodically, but infrequently and with less intensity than the original devastating disease, and was not reported in Europe in epidemic form after the eighteenth century. In contrast, HIV emerged as a global pandemic in the 1980s and is now endemic throughout the world, declining only slightly in the first decade of the twenty-first century [3, 4]. HIV is a sexually transmitted infection (STI) and is propagated by human behavior. Without successful control by biological and behavioral means, HIV will not be so readily controlled as was *Yersinia pestis*, the plague bacterium that was controllable with improved sanitation and rodent control well before the era of antibiotics.

An analogous global pandemic threat is that of influenza; its challenges in viral mutation and recombination and the risk of poor vaccine availability and coverage are, perhaps, as alarming as HIV as a risk to the global populace [5–8]. That HIV disease, unknown until 1981, should have joined respiratory and diarrheal diseases, tuberculosis, malaria, and vaccine-preventable diseases like measles as the most devastating of global infectious threats reminds us of the need for vigilance in recognition and response to emerging infectious diseases [9].

S.H. Vermund, M.D., Ph.D. (✉)
Vanderbilt Institute of Global Health, Vanderbilt University
School of Medicine, Nashville, TN, USA
e-mail: sten.vermund@Vanderbilt.edu

I.W. Fong (ed.), *Challenges in Infectious Diseases*, Emerging Infectious Diseases of the 21st Century 502, DOI 10.1007/978-1-4614-4496-1_1,

In countries most affected in southern Africa, HIV prevalence rates *in the general adult population* routinely exceed 1 in 10 adults and rise to as high as 1 in 2 in certain age/sex groups [10]. The self-perpetuating transmission cycles are facilitated by human sexual behaviors as well as the decade-long average incubation period of the virus. Rather than infecting and killing many persons quickly, like plague or influenza, HIV is transmitted more gradually and kills people well after they may have infected others [11, 12].

Advanced clinical or immunological disease has been termed the acquired immunodeficiency syndrome (AIDS), a concept still useful for surveillance but imprecise for use in clinical medicine; there are many more gradations and variations of HIV disease than the binary "AIDS" or "no AIDS" designation. Persons with AIDS-defining opportunistic infections (OI) or malignancies (OM) in the pretreatment era (before 1987) were typically severely immunologically suppressed; CD4+ T-lymphocyte counts under 200 cells/μL were ultimately included in the AIDS case definition as revised by the US Centers for Disease Control and Prevention (CDC) in 1993 [13]. But in the combination antiretroviral therapy (cART) era after 1996, persons with AIDS could achieve levels of immunological reconstitution sufficient to permit decades of disease-free life. Hence, in the era of cART, reaching a surveillance case definition of AIDS no longer suggests that an individual has current severe HIV disease if they have received cART. This chapter will refer to HIV disease in all its levels of severity, referring to AIDS only when discussing surveillance data that use AIDS as a surrogate for advanced HIV disease.

1.1.1 Global HIV Trends

As of the end of 2011, an estimated 34 million persons globally were living with HIV infection, 95–97% of whom were in low- and middle-income countries (LMIC) [14–16]. In 2012, the joint United Nations Programme on HIV/AIDS (UNAIDS) and the World Health Organization (WHO) estimate that the pandemic will pass the 30 million cumulative HIV mortality mark; in dozens of nations, HIV is the first ranking cause of death for young adults ages 20–44 years [14–16]. While continuing to expand in some nations (like Pakistan) and in some subpopulations (like Black men who have sex with men [MSM] in the United States), the prevalence has peaked and declined by varying degrees in a number of afflicted nations and/or population subgroups. In Thailand and Uganda, the success of control efforts predated the advent of cART and was attributed to behavioral and structural changes [17–21]. In southern sub-Saharan Africa where HIV rates are the highest, there is evidence of declining prevalence and incidence, as has been well documented in Zimbabwe [22–33]. Deaths may have contributed to declining prevalence [34], though in the face of expanded cART availability, declining prevalence and incidence may well be related [35].

In some parts of the world, incidence is stable and even rising, especially in selected vulnerable subgroups such as MSM in Asia, Black MSM in the USA, or injection drug users (IDU) in eastern Europe and central Asia [36–44]. Given that rates remain high in the general population, as in sub-Saharan Africa, and are persistent or rising in most at-risk populations throughout the world, no serious observer predicts the spontaneous demise of the pandemic [45–48].

Children are affected in many ways by the epidemic. They may be infected through mother-to-child transmission (MTCT) in utero, during delivery, or postpartum via breast milk [49–51]. HIV-exposed, but uninfected infants can suffer due to the loss of one or more parents due to HIV or due to their illness itself with its economic and social burden on the family [52]. Adolescents (or sexually abused children) can be infected sexually and may be challenging to engage in successful and sustained primary care [53]. Prevention of MTCT is challenged by programmatic obstacles that are amenable to quality improvement research and intervention [54–61]. Prevention programs are judged to be highly cost-effective and are the focus for intensive pregnancy screening and ART intervention [62]. Early infant diagnosis leading to earlier cART therapy is essential to improve outcomes for HIV-infected infants [63–65].

An alarming trend is one familiar to the field of STIs, namely, the replenishing of the at-risk population with sexually vulnerable youth; about half of the global population is under age 25, and this corresponds to the proportion of new infections globally attributable to this age group [66]. However, since the average age of sexual debut is in the teens, this suggests the intensity of risk for adolescents and youth once they become sexually active [67–71].

HIV morbidity and mortality have had a huge impact on economies of LMIC [72–74]. Given the link of HIV with vulnerable populations and/or poverty, such challenges as community development, orphans, household income, and gender-power issues have been exacerbated by the HIV pandemic [75–79]. Disease progression and transmission of other infectious diseases, notably tuberculosis, are accelerated by HIV coinfection [80–86]. Cancers such as Kaposi's sarcoma (human herpesvirus type 8 [HHV-8] coinfection) and cervical cancer (human papillomavirus [HPV] coinfection) loom large as major risks [87, 88]. In addition, the progression of HIV and its infectiousness is exacerbated by other coinfections [89–91]. Food insecurity may limit cART adherence when appetites surge with immune reconstitution and increased energy and metabolic demands [92–96]. Hence, the global community is increasingly embracing a more holistic response to the HIV pandemic, including community development, task shifting for health care workers, and horizontal health system reform, while acknowledging the need for sustained emergency responses [97–100]. HIV may be among the most important health care challenges in endemic nations, but it is hardly the only one.

1.1.2 HIV by Continent/Region

1.1.2.1 Sub-Saharan Africa

Over a third of the infected persons globally live in ten nations of southern Africa, by far the worst afflicted region. South Africa, for example, was the 25th most populous nation with 49 million persons in mid-2009 (http://www.census.gov/

population/international/data/idb/rank.php, accessed January 6, 2012). Yet it ranked first for the number of persons living with HIV/AIDS with an estimated 5.6 million persons (range 5.4–5.9 million) in 2009 (http://www.unaids.org/en/regionscountries/countries/southafrica/, accessed January 6, 2012). South African adults ages 15–49 years had an estimated 2009 prevalence rate of 17.8% (range 17.2–18.3%); nearly two million children had been orphaned by 2009. Averages mask extremes; some subpopulations in their mid-20s were over 50% HIV infected [10, 101].

The sub-Saharan African epidemic is driven by heterosexual contact [102, 103]. Injection drug use and male-to-male sexual contact may be increasing and represent future risk [104–110]. Iatrogenic spread has also been reported through reuse of contaminated needles and use of contaminated blood products in health care settings [111, 112]. However, the overwhelming burden of transmission is and remains of heterosexual origin. MTCT is still common in sub-Saharan Africa due to failures to achieve high coverage of HIV testing in pregnancy and proper mother-infant coverage with ART [54, 60, 61, 113–119].

1.1.2.2 East and Southeast Asia

The epidemic in Southeast Asia, China, Japan, Philippines, Indonesia, and other parts of the region is a complex one. While less intense than in Africa, the Asian epidemic remains intractable with persistent transmission in vulnerable populations. Countries like Japan, Korea, and Mongolia primarily report imported HIV cases with low indigenous transmission rates; however, high-risk populations such as MSM in Japan and STI patients in Mongolia suggest concern [120, 121]. In the Philippines, vulnerable populations have had surprisingly low rates of infection, but some observers believe that, over time, autochthonous HIV transmission will increase [122]. In Southeast Asia and Indonesia, heterosexual, MSM, and IDU transmission are all prevalent [104, 123–126]. In countries like Thailand, successes are notable in reducing transmission among IDU and heterosexual transmission with needle exchange and universal condom advocacy, respectively [21, 127, 128]. China has had some progress in addressing its serious problem of HIV among IDUs, but the epidemic among MSM is rising; fortunately, heterosexual spread is not common in the world's most populous nation, even among sex workers [129–131]. An unusual outbreak of HIV in rural central China spread due to pooled red cell reinfusions to blood and plasma donors who were illegally and unethically recruited in the 1990s [132, 133].

1.1.2.3 South Asia

India has experienced a substantial heterosexual epidemic concentrated in its southern states, with IDU-related transmission in northeastern states; the northern states have much lower incidence and prevalence [134]. Despite prevalence rates far lower than in sub-Saharan Africa, India, the second most populous nation on the globe, ranks just behind South Africa and Nigeria for the highest number of HIV-infected persons (about 2.5 million in 2009) living in the nation [135]. MSM are at risk throughout south Asia, including *hijras*, who are men who dress as women and have a long-standing cultural niche in such nations as India, Pakistan, and Bangladesh [136–141]. An explosive growth in HIV prevalence seen in Pakistan in 2002 underscores the fact that where risk behavior persists, HIV is likely to spread eventually [142–144].

1.1.2.4 Eastern Europe and Central Asia

Although same sex and heterosexual transmissions occur in Eastern Europe and Central Asia, most HIV transmission has been from IDU [145]. A number of countries continue to have growth in their epidemics, even as prevalence rates stabilize or even decline elsewhere in the world [146]. While rates in Eastern Europe and Central Asia have not reached the levels elsewhere, exceedingly poor policies that have not nurtured risk reduction among IDUs have exacerbated the epidemic, most notably in Russia that continues to ban any form of opiate substitution therapy (i.e., methadone or buprenorphine) [147–151]. Where aggressive risk reduction has been promulgated using clean needle and syringe exchange, results have been very promising [152]. All of this is sadly reminiscent of the policy blind spots in the United States that banned Federal support of clean needle exchange until congress lifted the ban in 2009; current US policies and plans are based more on prevention evidence rather than political concerns [153, 154].

1.1.2.5 Middle East and North Africa

Sexual transmission of HIV is reported in the Middle East and North Africa, particularly among MSM [155]. Migrant workers in the Gulf States are deported, if infected, and can serve to introduce HIV in their home countries [156]. Commercial sex workers have not had high rates, perhaps due to cultural and biological influences of near-universal male circumcision and lower partner exchange rates in the general population [157, 158]. IDU has been the largest driver of transmission in this low-prevalence region [159, 160]. Given its suppressive human rights policies, it is a paradox that Iran has been at the regional forefront of an assertive response to use of opiate substitution therapy to reduce drug craving and HIV risk, including services in prisons [161–163].

1.1.2.6 North America and Western Europe

The HIV epidemic in North America and Western Europe has been driven by MSM, IDU, and, to a lesser extent, heterosexual transmission [3]. Sexual vulnerability is higher in persons practicing unprotected anal intercourse and using alcohol and/or illicit drugs proximate to sexual activity [164–166]. Party drugs (e.g., nitrates, amphetamines, and cocaine) have been associated with higher risk sexual activity, an observation dating from before we even knew that HIV caused AIDS [167–169]. Persons addicted to crack cocaine and methamphetamine may practice high-risk sex, and both women and men may sell sex for drugs or money to support drug habits [170–173, 179]. Adolescents are vulnerable to peer pressures to have sex and use drugs [174, 175]. Affected subgroups have changed over time in the USA, for example, increasing numbers of Black and minority ethnic MSM and women together contribute over half the incident cases [40, 154, 176]. Molecular phylogenetic approaches have established historical links between HIV strains from central Africa to those in the USA and thence to Europe [3]. As in other high-income nations, HIV screening has virtually eliminated blood/blood product-related transmissions. Since the 1980s, breastfeeding was discouraged among HIV-infected mothers and since the 1990s, peripartum ART prophylaxis in the HIV-infected pregnant women and the exposed newborn. These strategies have reduced mother-to-child transmission to a rare public health problem, though some perinatal cases are still seen [177, 178, 180, 181].

Given the value of HIV therapy in reducing infectiousness, as demonstrated by the HIV Prevention Trials Network 052 protocol (HPTN 052, discussed later in this chapter), it is disappointing that only 19–28% (range of 2010 estimates) of Americans infected with HIV were on cART with successful suppression of HIV viral load [182–185]. High-access cities like Vancouver and San Francisco do much better and may be seeing prevention benefits from high HIV testing and cART coverage [35, 186, 187]. Aggressive testing and cART use within the context of excellent primary care may also contribute to lower-than-expected HIV rates in Western European countries, though other cultural elements and aggressive prevention interventions make this hard to disentangle. Declining incidence due to wider coverage with cART has been suggested in other high-income nations as well, for example, Taiwan [188].

1.1.2.7 Central and South America

There is diversity in the south and central American epidemic, but the dominant mode of transmission seems to be anal sex among MSM [189–193]. IDU contributes substantially in some regions such as urban Brazil but is a less common risk factor than in North America, Europe, or Asia [194–199]. Alcohol and noninjection drug use fuel unsafe sexual behaviors [200–205]. Heterosexual transmission occurs and bisexual men are thought to be an important bridge population [206, 207]. Perinatal transmission is less common with most antenatal programs in endemic areas offering HIV testing and ART, albeit imperfectly [208, 209].

1.1.2.8 Caribbean

The second highest prevalence rates in the world, after sub-Saharan Africa, occur in the Caribbean region [210–214]. The epidemic is diverse with the worst affected nation, Haiti, experiencing a heterosexual-dominant pattern [215–217]. Dominican Republic and Guyana also have substantial heterosexual transmission [218–221]. MSM are more common in most of the other islands [190, 222–225]. Puerto Rico is a territory of the USA with close ties to major US cities like New York and Miami (connected by so-called "air bridges" of low cost, passport-free travel); Puerto Rico has experienced substantial IDU-related transmission [226–233]. Cuba is well known for its mass HIV screening and quarantine approach to HIV, segregating HIV-infected persons into their own communities; this has alternatively been criticized for human rights restrictions and been praised for limiting the epidemic's spread [234–238]. Adolescents, as in the rest of world, are of special concern for sexual risk behaviors [239–243].

Selected mainland countries like Guyana (in South America) and Belize (in Central America) are often grouped with Caribbean countries due to proximity and sociopolitical synergies, even though they are not islands. Both Guyana and Belize are in the Caribbean Community and Common Market (CARICOM) and have formal public health ties with the English-speaking islands through the Caribbean Epidemiology Centre (CAREC) in Trinidad.

1.1.2.9 Australia and Oceania

Australia has had a persistent and aggressive risk reduction program from early days of their epidemic [244–247]. Their widespread and "user-friendly" approaches to clean needle exchange and availability of opiate substitutions therapy through primary care practitioners are credited for keeping HIV rates exceedingly low in IDUs [246, 248–251]. MSM are a principal challenge in parts of the region, though Oceania confronts pockets of heterosexual transmission [252–255].

In summary, each global region has its specific challenges to confront in HIV control. Even at the microgeographic level, there can be differences of just miles or even city blocks where IDU drives a micro-transmission dynamic vs. sexual activity driving a local epidemic. Infection control efforts must be based in an epidemiologic knowledge of the transmission drivers and sociocultural contexts of risk behaviors in a given region, or even a given neighborhood, "Know your epidemic" has become the adage that reminds us that a given prevention approach will not work in all settings. At the same time, there are great truths in the global pandemic: behavior change is a vital component of any part of the effort to control transmission; high cART coverage may reduce community-level transmission; risk reduction strategies can work to reduce HIV transmissions even if the underlying challenges (e.g., IDU, sex work) are not altered markedly; risk behaviors are steeped in cultural context and traditions that are not easily changed; and human rights underlie the global community's response, successful or unsuccessful, as respect for vulnerable persons is the first step toward engagement and assistance. Regional and national data are updated yearly by UNAIDS (http://www.unaids.org/en/).

1.2 Biological Mechanisms

1.2.1 Unique HIV Characteristics

It is unhelpful to consider HIV merely as an infectious disease, but also to consider it a chronic disease. Only with this merger of the infectious disease-chronic disease "dichotomy" can one understand the challenges ahead for HIV control. The lifespan of the infected individual can vary from years to decades; this is not a classic infection paradigm followed by either immunological control/recovery or death, as applies to so many other viruses. Examples of the classic infectious disease paradigm are vaccine-preventable diseases of childhood like measles and arboviruses like yellow fever.

In contrast, lentiviruses (i.e., slow viruses; Table 1.1) are characterized by years and even decades of gradual pathogenic impact. The HIV-infected individual will have transient, incomplete immunological control that is overwhelmed over time by viral escape mutations and immunological collapse [256]. This is why access to cART is so vital, in order to permit the body to restore partial immunological function by suppressing viral replication and stopping the mass destruction of CD4+ T-lymphocytes.

Retroviruses have ribonucleic acid (RNA) as their genetic material, requiring the virus to use a reverse transcriptase enzyme to convert RNA into deoxyribonucleic acid (DNA). The DNA can then integrate into the host cell genome with the genetic instructions hijacking the cell's protein manufacturing machinery to replicate HIV. While perhaps half of HIV-infected persons with the infection have nonspecific "flu" symptoms, others may not be aware that they are ill at all [257]. Whether or not someone has experienced symptoms of acute HIV infection, in following years, HIV-infected persons do not feel ill and may transmit HIV for many years until diagnosed and treated or until illness and death.

Given that most HIV diseases are asymptomatic, routine HIV testing must be promoted to identify asymptomatic disease. Screening of at-risk persons is a mainstay of diagnosis, and prevention is analogous to the disease control strategy for STIs and tuberculosis [258]. Within the pool of HIV-infected persons, additional screening is essential, as for cervical precancerous lesions, Kaposi's sarcoma lesions, tuberculosis, and other conditions far more prevalent in the HIV-infected individual.

Table 1.1 Lentiviruses (Lentivirus = genus; Retroviruses = family)

Bovine/equine lentiviruses	Feline/ovine/caprine	Primate, including human
Bovine immunodeficiency virus	Feline immunodeficiency virus	Human immunodeficiency virus type 1
Jembrana disease virus	Puma lentivirus	Human immunodeficiency virus type 2
Equine infectious anemia virus	Caprine arthritis encephalitis virus Visna-Maedi virus	Simian immunodeficiency virus

1.2.2 *Viral Entry and Replication*

HIV uses a particular protein, CD4, to recognize cells, serve as a receptor for fusion, entry, and infection. CD4 is short for "cluster of differentiation 4," a terminology used in cell cytometry and immunology, representing a surface glycoprotein on key cells that provide immunological surveillance, namely, T helper lymphocytes, macrophages, monocytes, and dendritic cells. In humans, this protein is encoded by a CD4 gene that, if mutated, may reduce susceptibility to infection. The HIV-1 uses its protruding viral envelope protein known as gp120 to bind to CD4; gp stand for glycoprotein and 120 represents the molecular weight of this particular protein. HIV must bind to a CD4 receptor, creating a conformational shift in the gp120 that enables the virus to bind to chemokine co-receptors expressed on the host cell. Two types of co-receptors are used by HIV. One is termed CCR5 or C-C chemokine receptor type 5 that is coded by the human CCR5 gene. The other is known as CXCR-4 or C-X-C chemokine receptor type 4 (also known as fusin), a protein encoded by the CXCR4 gene. Once gp120-CD4 engagement has permitted viral docking with one of these two beta chemokine receptors, a structural change then occurs in viral protein gp41 (together, gp120 and gp41 make up gp160), enabling HIV to insert its fusion peptide into the CD4+ cell. HIV then fuses with the host cell membrane. CD4's primary function is a vital one, namely, serving to assist T cell receptors (TCR) on antigen-presenting cells [259]. That HIV lives in and takes over the machinery of the CD4+ T cell is much like the legend of the Greek soldiers within the Trojan horse, destroying the very cell that is designed to help defend against outside invaders.

1.2.3 *Viral Variation and Evolution*

HIV-1 has many variants, referred to as subtypes or clades, due to recombinant viruses generated through co-circulation of different viruses. High recombination and mutation rates result in the generation of circulating recombinant forms, or "CRFs" [3, 4]. Over decades of viral expansion, the genetic complexity of HIV has increased globally such that over 40 CRFs have been recognized as of 2011 [260, 261]. HIV-1 genetic diversity is greatest in west-central Africa where hunters of chimpanzees may have been infected with an HIV precursor in the early twentieth century when they captured, killed, and skinned their primate "bushmeat." It is thought that chimpanzee HIV antecedents entered human populations in central Africa in the 1930s, with only indolent human-to-human transmission [262, 263]. Later, conditions of migration, urbanization, loss of sexual taboos, injection-related contaminations, and global travel facilitated entry of HIV into higher risk communities. In central Africa, most major clades have been isolated (represented by alphabet letters A through K, minus "B" and "E" clades that occur elsewhere) [264, 265]. Many observers suggest that there are few major biological differences among HIV clades, though there is evidence that C clade may be more pathogenic [266, 267]. Viral diversity continues to emerge and may be due to stochastic variations from founder infections with subsequent transmission within vulnerable populations [268, 269]. Dating of divergence events can be estimated using "molecular clocks" [270–272]. It appears that a divergence of major clades occurred in central Africa in the mid-twentieth century [273]. Now that phylodynamic approaches permit estimations of sequence evolution rates, we can also use these estimates as parameters for epidemic modeling of sexual and other transmission networks [3]. Given that the world now confronts tremendous HIV genetic diversity, also driven by antiretroviral drug pressures, viral diversity is a principal challenge for future vaccine and antiretroviral drug development [264, 274–278].

1.3 Current Therapy and Prognosis

1.3.1 Development of Antiretroviral Drugs

The scientific achievement represented by the discovery and development of antiretroviral drugs is among the great stories of applied scholarship in the late twentieth century [279–281]. The first discovered antiretroviral drug was zidovudine (ZDV) (also called azidothymidine [AZT]), a thymine analog in the drug family of nucleoside reverse transcriptase inhibitors (NRTI) [282]. When zidovudine is present, its thymine mimicry results in reverse transcriptase mistakenly adding it to the DNA strand; reverse transcription is then terminated since the zidovudine moiety does not accept the next nucleotide being added to the DNA [283].

Once ZDV was made available for clinical trials and then for commercial sale, there were early indications of clinical benefits in both clinical trials and also in larger population "real world use" conditions [284–287]. However, viral mutation rates are high and drug resistant strains emerged quickly, severely limiting the duration of drug benefit [288–295]. When new NRTI drugs were developed, dual therapy proved superior to monotherapy, but the revolutionary change occurred with the advent of new classes of antiretroviral drugs that attacked the virus at different stages of its life cycle. Using combination antiretroviral therapy (cART), many patients who were adherent to their cART regimens could suppress HIV replication indefinitely. Current guidelines are permissive of a variety of alternative cART regimens [296]. In settings with adequate resources, nearly everyone with a detectable HIV viral load is recommended to be treated, regardless of CD4+ cell counts (Table 1.2). Unfortunately for patients and for their uninfected sexual partners, low- and middle-income countries are typically limited to starting therapy at the World Health Organization (WHO) threshold of WHO clinical status 3 or 4 and/or CD4+ cell counts <350 μL^{-1}, or may even start at a lower threshold like <250 cells/μL, due to resource constraints.

1.3.2 Licensed Antiretroviral Therapy

There are six licensed classes of antiretroviral drugs (Table 1.3). Among the NRTI drugs, zidovudine, emtricitabine (FTC), lamivudine (3TC), abacavir (ABC), tenofovir disoproxil fumarate (TDF), didanosine (ddI or dideoxyinosine), and stavudine (d4T) are all in use. Stavudine has an unfavorable profile of side effects, but is still used widely in low-income countries due to its low generic cost. Non-nucleoside reverse transcriptase inhibitors (NNRTI) include efavirenz (EFV), both immediate and extended release forms of nevirapine (NVP), delavirdine (DLV), and newer drugs rilpivirine and etravirine.

Protease inhibitors (PIs) are often boosted with another protease inhibitor, ritonavir, to inhibit a cytochrome P450-3A4 (CYP3A4), a liver enzyme that metabolizes protease inhibitors. Ritonovir boosting both increases efficacy and reduces side effects of other PIs. PIs include amprenavir (APV), tipranavir (TPV), indinavir (IDV), saquinavir mesylate (SQV), lopinavir (LPV), ritonavir (RTV), fosamprenavir calcium (FOS-APV), darunavir (DRV), atazanavir sulfate (ATV), and nelfinavir mesylate (NFV).

Three newer classes have single licensed drugs in each class, as of 2011, though more will be licensed in the future (Table 1.3). Raltegravir works to inhibit integrase and is called an integrase strand transfer inhibitor. Maraviroc is a CCR5 blocker and inhibits viral entry, though it does not work against CXCR4 receptor strains of HIV. The single fusion inhibitor is enfuvirtide, (T-20), given subcutaneously twice daily.

Some drugs are specifically formulated for pediatric use (see http://www.fda.gov/ForConsumers/ByAudience/ForPatientAdvocates/HIVandAIDSActivities/ucm118951.htm, accessed January 22, 2012). Availability of pediatric formulations often lags, by years sometimes, the licensure of drugs suitable for adult consumption, a serious problem for the care of children with HIV infection [297]. Antiretroviral chemotherapy principles are similar for adults and children, but the availability of pediatric formulations sometimes skews therapeutic decision making.

Many drugs are licensed generics in the USA (see http://www.fda.gov/ForConsumers/ByAudience/ForPatientAdvocates/HIVandAIDSActivities/ucm118944.htm, accessed January 22, 2012). The generic market is expanding, and not all of the products have been through the FDA licensure process. The US FDA has approved a number of drugs for use in the President's Emergency Plan for AIDS Relief (PEPFAR) focused in Africa, Asia, and the Caribbean (see http://www.fda.gov/InternationalPrograms/FDABeyondOurBordersForeignOffices/AsiaandAfrica/ucm119231.htm, accessed January 22, 2012). The use of generics in PEPFAR has reduced costs and increased efficiency of programs but took a long time to negotiate given reluctance of Western pharmaceutical manufacturers to forego perceived patent rights [298, 299]. There are still daunting fiscal, regulatory, and operational challenges in obtaining the newest antiretroviral drugs for the global market [300].

Table 1.2 Initial antiretroviral therapy (ART) and consideration in patients with specific conditions[a]

Condition	Regimen components: Possible backbone drugs	Regimen components: Third agent	Considerations
High atherosclerotic cardiovascular risk	Emtricitabine, lamivudine, tenofovir	Efavirenz, nevirapine, atazanavir/r, raltegravir	Initiation of ART, regardless of CD4 cell count, is recommended [34] If possible avoid abacavir, fosamprenavir/r indinavir/r, lopinavir/r because of an associated increased risk of cardiovascular events [63, 97]
Chronic kidney disease	Abacavir,[b] emtricitabine, lamivudine: avoid tenofovir (glomerular and tubular toxicity), atazanavir, and indinavir (nephrolithiasis)	Efavirenz, raltegravir, nevirapine, maraviroc, PI/r	Initiate ART regardless of CD4 cell count (Blla) Avoid potentially nephrotoxic drugs (Alla) [53] When potentially nephrotoxic drugs must be used, monitor renal function closely For patients with reduced estimated glomerular filtration rate, dose adjustment for drugs with renal metabolism (emtricitabine, lamivudine, temofovir, maraviroc) should be considered
Chronic HBV infection	Emtricitabine, lamivudine, tenofovir. Use 2 HBV-active drugs. Do not use abacavir or abacavir/lamivudine alone for treatment of HBV in coinfected patients	Efavirenz, raltegravir, PI/r should be monitored for hepatotoxicity Avoid nevirapine except for women with CD4 <250 μL^{-1} and men with <400 μL^{-1} Maraviroc should be used with caution in patients with liver disease	ART that includes tenofovir/emtricitabine should be used irrespective of CD4 cell count [20] (Blla) Monitor alanine aminotransferase after ART initiation and after withdrawal of suppressive therapy [22–24] In patients with moderate to severe liver impairment, dose adjustment for drugs metabolized by the liver should be considered Alcohol should be avoided

Chronic HCV infection requiring therapy	Emtricitabine, lamivudine, tenofovir	Efavirenz, raltegavir, Pl/r should be monitored for hepatotoxicity	ART should generally be initiated first in all patients with HCV coinfection regardless of CD4 cell count to slow liver disease progression (Blla), except possibly in patients with HCV genotype 2 or 3 infection and a high CD4 cell count, for whom current HCV therapy has a higher probability of a sustained virologic response [26, 28] (Blll)
		Avoid nevirapine except for women with CD4 <250 μL^{-1} and men with <400 μL^{-1}	Avoid zidovudine, didanosine, zalcitabine, and stavudine, as well as abacavir [25, 27]
		Maraviroc should be used with caution in patients with liverdisease	Alcohol should be avoided by all coinfected patients
Pregnant women	Complete recommendations for the use of antiviral therapy in pregnant women are available at http://www.aidsinfo.nih.gov/ContentFiles/PerinatalGL.pdf, and http://www.europeanaidsclinicalsociety.org/guidelins.asp [17, 18]		ART is recommended to prevent the transmission of the virus to the fetus or infant (Ala) Efavirenz should generally be avoided, especially in the first trimester of pregnancy (teratogenic effect)

(continued)

Table 1.2 (continued)

Condition	Regimen components: Possible backbone drugs	Regimen components: Third agent	Considerations
Opportunistic infections, including tuberculosis	Any, according to the "What to Start" section	Choice of agent will be influenced by drug interactions, especially with rifampin and rifabutin	ART should be initiated as soon as possible in patients with opportunistic infections, including tuberculosis, with attention to drug interactions and the potential for immune reconstitution inflammatory syndromes (Ala) [36, 37]. Drug interactions likely to require dose adjustments; consult drug interaction dosing references (http://www.hiv-druginteractions.org, and http://hivinsite.ucsf.edu/insite?page=ar-00-02) [38, 39]

From [296]. Adapted with the permission of the publisher

Abbreviations: *ART* antiretroviral therapy, *HBV* hepatitis B virus, *HCV* hepatitis C virus, *PI* protease inhibitor, */r* ritonavir boosted

[a] Details, cautions, considerations, and supporting data are described in the text. Levels of evidence are described in the eBox (available at http://www.jama.com)

[b] In HLA B*5701-negative patients; has been associated with increased risk of myocardial infarction. Lower efficacy in patients with >100,000 copies/mL of HIV RNA at baseline (see text)

Table 1.3 Antiretroviral drugs used in 2011 in the treatment of HIV infection, with licensure date at the Food and Drug Administration

Multi-class combination products			
Brand name™	Generic name	Manufacturer name	Approval date
Atripla	Efavirenz, emtricitabine, and tenofovir disoproxil fumarate	Bristol-Myers Squibb & Gilead Sciences	July 2006
Complera	Emtricitabine, rilpivirine, and tenofovir disoproxil fumarate	Gilead Sciences	August 2011
Nucleoside reverse transcriptase inhibitors (NRTIs)			
Combivir	Lamivudine and zidovudine	GlaxoSmithKline	September 1997
Emtriva	Emtricitabine, FTC	Gilead Sciences	July 2003
Epivir	Lamivudine, 3TC	GlaxoSmithKline	November 1995
Epzicom	Abacavir and lamivudine	GlaxoSmithKline	August 2004
Retrovir	Zidovudine, azidothymidine, AZT, ZDV	GlaxoSmithKline	March 1987
Trizivir	Abacavir, zidovudine, and lamivudine	GlaxoSmithKline	November 2000
Truvada	Tenofovir disoproxil fumarate and emtricitabine	Gilead Sciences	August 2004
Videx EC	Enteric coated didanosine, ddI EC	Bristol-Myers Squibb	October 2000
Videx	Didanosine, dideoxyinosine, ddI	Bristol-Myers Squibb	October 1991
Viread	Tenofovir disoproxil fumarate, TDF	Gilead	October 2001
Zerit	Stavudine, d4T	Bristol-Myers Squibb	June 1994
Ziagen	Abacavir sulfate, ABC	GlaxoSmithKline	December 1998
Non-nucleoside reverse transcriptase inhibitors (NNRTIs)			
Edurant	Rilpivirine	Tibotec Therapeutics	May 2011
Intelence	Etravirine	Tibotec Therapeutics	January 2008
Rescriptor	Delavirdine, DLV	Pfizer	April 1997
Sustiva	Efavirenz, EFV	Bristol-Myers Squibb	September 1998
Viramune(Immediate Release)	Nevirapine, NVP	Boehringer Ingelheim	June 1996
Viramune XR (extended release)	Nevirapine, NVP	Boehringer Ingelheim	March 2011

(continued)

Table 1.3 (continued)

Multi-class combination products			
Brand name™	Generic name	Manufacturer name	Approval date
Protease inhibitors (PIs)			
Agenerase	Amprenavir, APV	GlaxoSmithKline	April 1999
Aptivus	Tipranavir, TPV	Boehringer Ingelheim	June 2005
Crixivan	Indinavir, IDV,	Merck	March 1996
Invirase	Saquinavir mesylate, SQV	Hoffmann-La Roche	December 1995
Kaletra	Lopinavir and ritonavir, LPV/RTV	Abbott Laboratories	September 2000
Lexiva	Fosamprenavir calcium, FOS-APV	GlaxoSmithKline	October 2003
Norvir	Ritonavir, RTV	Abbott Laboratories	March 1996
Prezista	Darunavir	Tibotec Therapeutics	June 2006
Reyataz	Atazanavir sulfate, ATV	Bristol-Myers Squibb	June 2003
Viracept	Nelfinavir mesylate, NFV	Agouron Pharmaceuticals	March 1997
Fusion inhibitor			
Fuzeon	Enfuvirtide, T-20	Hoffmann-La Roche & Trimeris	March 2003
Entry inhibitor – CCR5 co-receptor antagonist			
Selzentry	Maraviroc, MVC	Pfizer	August 2007
HIV integrase strand transfer inhibitor			
Isentress	Raltegravir, RAL	Merck & Co.	October 2007

Adapted from FDA web site, accessed January 22, 2012: http://www.fda.gov/ForConsumers/byAudience/ForPatientAdvocates/HIVandAIDSActivities/ucm118915.htm

1.3.3 Current Recommended Regimens

As of 2010–2011, recommended components of initial antiretroviral regimens include [296] the following:

- Tenofovir (TDF) and emtricitabine (FTC), two NRTIs that are available as fixed-dose combination alone and also available with efavirenz, an NNRTI that is suitable for cART. Advantages of TDF/FTC are once daily dosing and a high genetic barrier to resistance (TDF, not FTC). Side effects are not prominent, but include renal dysfunction and decreased bone mineral density associated with TDF.
  - An alternative is the combination of abacavir/lamivudine that is also once daily in a fixed-dose combination of two NRTI drugs. However, this combination has weaker antiviral efficacy in treatment-naive patients with baseline HIV-1 RNA >100,000 copies/mL than TDF/FTC. Abacavir has cardiovascular side effects, and screening for HLA-B*5701 is advisable to reduce risk of abacavir hypersensitivity.
- To complete the cART regimen, either TDF/FTC or abacavir/lamivudine should be complemented with the NNRTI, efavirenz. HIV can mutate easily to evade NNRTI drugs so efavirenz resistance occurs very rapidly outside the context of cART. Alternatives to efavirenz are indicated for patients with major psychiatric illness, in their first trimester of pregnancy, or for women with an intention to become pregnant.
- Atazanavir boosted with ritonavir (both protease inhibitors) is a once daily alternative as the backbone of a cART regimen. It leaves open options for future regimens as it can be used with NRTIs, preserving the use of NNRTIs for a later date when they might be needed. There is less lipidogenic potential than when lopinavir boosted with ritonavir is used. Use can be complicated by hyperbilirubinemia, need for acid-reducing agents, and risk of nephrolithiasis.
- Darunavir boosted with ritonavir (both protease inhibitors) is another once daily alternative as the backbone of a cART regimen in treatment-naïve patients. It is superior to lopinavir boosted with ritonavir.
- Raltegravir is an integrase inhibitor given twice daily. It has low potential to interact with other drugs, which is an advantage in its use. HIV can mutate quickly to evade this drug.
- Lopinavir boosted with ritonavir is a co-formulated pair of protease inhibitors that is heat stable and can be given once daily. Side effects include hyperlipidemia and gastrointestinal symptoms.
- Fosamprenavir boosted with ritonavir represent two protease inhibitors with a profile similar to lopinavir/ritonavir, useful when other preferred drugs are not tolerated.
- Maraviroc is a CCR5 antagonist that targets the host protein CCR5 viral co-receptor. Since one needs to ensure that CXCR4 virus is not present, one needs to perform a costly viral tropism assay before use. With limited clinical experience in treatment-naïve patients, there are theoretical reasons to avoid its use in other than multiple drug failure patients who do not have CXCR4 receptor HIV strains circulating [301].

- Enfuvirtide is an HIV fusion inhibitor used in combination therapy for "salvage" therapy in patients with multi-drug-resistant HIV. The peptide is biomimetic, that is, designed to mimic components of the HIV-1 fusion machinery, and the drug displaces normal fusion components to prevent successful virus-cell fusion. Enfuvirtide therapy is extremely costly, and its inconvenient dosing (subcutaneously twice daily) regimen further limits its global relevance.

1.3.4 Challenges in Patient Care

Patient management issues are complex for HIV disease (Table 1.2). Rather than the death sentence for so many in the pretreatment era, HIV disease is now a chronic, manageable disease. It requires HIV testing, linkage to care, cART availability, national guidelines permitting cART administration, and adherence to lifelong therapeutic regimens. In the United States, only a quarter of persons infected with HIV are on suppressive cART, showing how inadequate current systems are to meet the full need [183–185]. In low- and middle-income countries, it is likely that fewer than 10% of persons infected with HIV are on cART with successful viral suppression. Special challenges exist with comorbidities that may inhibit proper health care access and/or adherence to cART regimens. These include mental health problems such as depression and substance use including opiates, stimulants, and alcohol [302–321]. In addition, stigmatized persons who do not feel comfortable "coming out" into the mainstream of clinical care may not reach care or be retained in care; this is thought to be an important driver of the epidemic in Black men who have sex with men (MSM) in the United States, for example [38, 40, 41, 176, 322–329]. Adolescents present special challenges in care, and adherence rates have been suboptimal in this population [53, 330–337]. Children in care depend on the capabilities of their parents or guardians; many children have been orphaned and some do not know that they are HIV infected, making it difficult for them to participate in their ongoing care [338–344].

ART itself has an array of complications that require recognition and management [296]. PIs are associated with lipid abnormalities and cardiovascular list. Efavirenz is contraindicated in pregnancy. NRTIs can have serious, albeit rare, lactic acidosis. Stavudine can cause severe peripheral neuropathies. Beyond the scope of this chapter, these side effects require preventive and therapeutic management from a clinician experienced in HIV drug regimens and their alternatives.

The tremendous impact on morbidity and mortality of cART in high-income countries has been well documented [322, 345–347]. Similar benefits are seen in low- and middle-income countries, but they depend on the programmatic efficiencies; resources available from PEPFAR; the Global Fund to Fight AIDS, Tuberculosis and Malaria; local ministries of health; and the ability of programs to find, recruit, and retain HIV-infected persons in cART-based care (Table 1.4) [348–352]. Scaling

Table 1.4 Essential elements to nurture successful and complete transition of HIV care and treatment programs to national governments and local organizations

Essential elements	Goals
Health workforce development	Increase the numbers of health care providers, with special attention to coverage of rural care, including task shifting to nurses, clinical officers, laboratory and pharmacy technicians, care partners, and/or community health workers
Integration of services	Enable HIV/AIDS care and treatment to be handled by sustainable primary care programs, with key linkages to sexually transmitted infection and tuberculosis control, and family planning, for example
Physical infrastructures	Empower communities to access basic electricity, water, medical waste disposal, and clinic space for physical examinations, patient education/waiting, laboratory, and surgery
Pharmacy logistics systems	Ensure that inventory management, shipping, and storage systems avoid stock-outs of supplies (e.g., test kits, blood draw equipment) and antiretroviral, antibiotic, and other drugs
Laboratory development	Decentralize laboratory work, as much as possible and affordable, with point-of-care diagnostic tests
Quality of care and iterative evaluation	Build sustainable quality improvement research and systems improvement efforts into HIV care programs
Hub-and-spoke models of care	Bring primary and HIV/AIDS care closer to people who are remote from major clinical services
Data management systems	Build sustainable, affordable electronic medical record systems to harmonize systems created for the emergency HIV response
Community engagement to support programs	Implement innovative models of outreach, retention, and adherence support at the community level, tapping into the inherent strengths of patient-to-patient and family-to-patient support schemes as a form of task shifting
Cultural changes in the health sector	Train staff and reform procedures to protect patient confidentiality and privacy; provide more respectful, client-friendly services; and ensure that all communications are in languages spoken by patients
Management and administration	Train and capacitate health systems to use modern business practices for financial and logistical management

Adapted from Vermund et al. [353]. With permission of the publisher

up of programs has been both challenging and inspiring; new models for the management of chronic diseases in resource-limited settings are now extant, offering promise for a wide variety of diseases requiring ongoing care for their management [48, 59, 64, 354–371].

1.4 Combination Prevention

1.4.1 Know Your Local Epidemic

The epidemiology of the HIV epidemic in high-income countries is distinct in some ways from the situation in many low- and middle-income nations, so we present these in two separate sections [36]. In all settings, HIV is a complex disease based on human behavior and affected by stigma and prejudice as well as fear and family stress [316, 372]. HIV/AIDS is transmitted similarly to patterns for other sexual and blood-borne agents. When persons have multiple sexual partners (i.e., high mixing rate phenomena) and do not use condoms, HIV transmission is more probable [102]. Reuse of syringes and needles, receipt of contaminated blood or blood products, or occupational needle sticks in a health care setting can result in parenteral transmission of HIV. Mother-to-child transmission in utero (pre-partum), during delivery (intra-partum), or from breastfeeding (postpartum) is an additional major transmission route, though this is now rare in high-income countries due to screening and cART use among pregnant women [49, 373–376].

HIV is an STI and is spread similarly to Hepatitis B virus (HBV) [377, 378]. That HIV infection is not curable means that persons can transmit the infection for many years. STIs can be spread through blood-borne routes, as with herpes simplex type 2 (HSV-2), syphilis, gonorrhea, and Chlamydia, but sexual routes are the dominant mode of transmission. Hepatitis C virus (HCV) is transmitted overwhelmingly through blood-borne routes, in contrast, with sexual and perinatal cases occurring rarely. Another human lentivirus, human T-lymphotropic virus type 1 (HTLV-1) is transmitted most often via breast milk; HTLV-2 transmission is well documented via needle exchange. While HIV is similar to other STIs in its route of transmission, its CD4+ T-lymphocyte tropism makes it unique.

1.4.2 Sociopolitical Obstacles

While we have many tools to prevent HIV, it has been rare that policymakers and health care leaders have mobilized effectively to deploy them [379]. A failure to protect the blood supply in the early 1980s resulted in the infection of blood and blood product recipients such as persons with hemophilia. Sexual risk reduction remains a taboo topic in political, religious, and social circles, despite the fact that delaying adolescent coital debut and reducing numbers of sexual partners are widely supported goals. Condoms are opposed for two reasons: that they may lead to higher risk behaviors and that they violate certain religious views; evidence is lacking for the former and the latter may be changing. For example, Pope Benedict XVI stated in his recent book that "there may be a basis in the case of some individuals, as perhaps when a male prostitute uses a condom, where this can be a first step in the direction of a moralization, a first assumption of responsibility"(the Pope later indicated that he also was referring to female prostitutes) [380]. Failure to provide clean needles and syringes for injection drug users (IDU) in the USA from 1987 to 1995 led to 4,394–9,666 infections, about a third of incident IDU cases (33% of the incidence in IDUs) with an attendant cost of US$244 to 538 million [153]. Public health professionals advocate evidence-based prevention, rather than using HIV/AIDS as a political tool [145].

1.4.3 Behavior

Behavior change is a vital component of any prevention intervention since even biomedical intervention must be adhered to. However, behavior change as a primary mode of risk reduction has been disappointing. For example, Project EXPLORE was designed to reduce HIV incidence in homosexual men in 6 US cities using a 10-visit educational intervention with periodic reinforcements [381–383]. The 18.2% reduction (95% CI −4.7 to 36.0) in HIV incidence in the intervention group compared to a control group receiving a short intervention did not suggest that the intervention was robust [383]. The benefits were lower in substance users and persons with mental health problems [384–386]. Current prevention efforts in higher income Western nations are employing many approaches: cART to reduce infectiousness and result in prevention, preexposure prophylaxis (PrEP) using cART in seronegative persons to prevent infection, and increased testing and linkage to cART, so-called serosorting (HIV-infected persons having sex only with other infected persons, with negatives seeking negatives), substance abuse treatment (including needle exchange and alcohol treatment), contingency cash transfers (rewards for lower risk behaviors), and "ABC" approaches of *A*bstinence/*B*e faithful/*C*ondom advocacy [171, 184, 387–395]. CDC has promulgated evidence-based interventions for risk reduction in the USA [396–400]. Abstinence-only education does not work to reduce risk and actually was associated with higher pregnancy rates than more comprehensive educational approaches that highlighted STI prevention with condom use [401–403]. While "ABC" principals to guide public health interventions are deemed important, they are not adequate to stem the global pandemic [41, 184, 404, 405]. Structural interventions to reduce drug use, like improved schools and after-school opportunities for youth, must be considered. Risk reduction approaches on a large scale that offer universal testing, strong linkages to care, and assertive and liberal use of cART-based care, combined with community partnerships to reduce stigma, are more modern approaches.

1.4.4 Elements of Combination Prevention

Combination prevention seems to be the best strategy to reduce transmission. Single "magic bullets" are unlikely to work well enough to alter an epidemic profile in the absence of other strategic efforts. For example, even a future vaccine for HIV would require multiple visits for full immunization and would require a large-scale population mobilization and program expansion unprecedented for adolescents and adults.

Combination packages will differ by target at-risk population and epidemiologic context [406]. For example, IDUs will need needle exchange and addiction treatment as centerpieces of their approach, while sex workers will need support to use barriers, seek alternative employment, or perhaps use preexposure prophylaxis (PrEP) and STI screening and treatment. Those interventions with the strongest evidence of efficacy to reduce HIV transmission (infectiousness) or acquisition (susceptibility) include voluntary medical male circumcision (VMMC) [101, 407–409]. ART for prevention was begun as a concept with the definitive demonstration of prevention of mother-to-child transmission (PMTCT) with ART dating from 1994 [410]. Observational data from 2000 to 2001 suggested that ART would reduce sexual transmission [411, 412]. Yet not until 2011 was the HPTN 052 trial definitive in demonstrating cART as a major tool to reduce infectiousness and sexual transmission [182].

Other strategies have been less consistently beneficial in clinical trials. Treatment of curable sexually transmitted infections (STIs) worked in one Tanzanian epidemic context to reduce HIV transmission, but has failed in other epidemic contexts [413]. Tenofovir-containing PrEP(cART among HIV-seronegative at-risk persons) has been successful in CAPRISA 004 (topical microbicide for women), oral use in iPrEx (MSM), and Partners PrEP and TDF-2 studies (heterosexual men and women) but not in the large VOICE trial or the FemPrEP studies (heterosexual women) [414–417]. The Thai vaccine prime-boost strategy published in 2009 was partially effective, but the vaccine companies are not seeking licensure for marketing of either the prime or boost products, given their modest effect [418, 419].

Clinical trial data are not available for some interventions, but observational data suggest that they will be effective nonetheless. Effectiveness in HIV prevention has been demonstrated or strongly suggested using male and, possibly, female condoms, opioid substitution therapy for IDUs, contraception for HIV-infected women to reduce unintended pregnancies, needle exchange for drug users, and a variety of behavioral and structural interventions [405].

1.4.5 Testing and Linkage to Care

Knowledge of one's HIV serostatus is the gateway to a host of HIV prevention or care services. Persons testing HIV seropositive typically reduce their sexual transmission risk behaviors [420–422]. In sub-Saharan Africa, only a fraction (<20%) of

African adults have been tested for HIV, yet the HPTN 043 NIMH Project ACCESS study demonstrates how community mobilization can increase testing rates up to tenfold [423, 424]. Persons who do not know the serostatus of themselves and their partners are 50–66% less likely to use condoms [18, 425]. HIV testing access includes provider-initiated, routine, or opt-out testing and voluntary home-based HIV counseling and testing (HBCT) [413, 421]. HBCT may be cost-effective for population-level scale-up in generalized epidemics despite its higher programmatic costs [426].

The HPTN 052 trial has been called a "game-changer" by the director of UNAIDS. If enough persons can be tested and linked to care, ART that reduces viral replication could limit the HIV transmission by 96%, as per the clinical trial results. In nine countries, HPTN 052 investigators enrolled 1,763 couples in which one partner was HIV-1-positive and the other was HIV-1-negative; 54% of the subjects were from Africa, and 50% of infected partners were men. HIV-1-infected subjects with 350–550 CD4+ cells/μL were assigned randomly to receive ART either immediately (early therapy) or after a decline in the CD4 count to 250 cells/μL (or 350 when national guidelines were changed) or the onset of HIV-1-related symptoms (delayed therapy). Of the 28 linked transmissions, only one occurred in the early-therapy group (hazard ratio = 0.04; 95%CI: 0.01, 0.27). Subjects receiving early therapy were healthier. The key to making HPTN 052 clinical trial results a reality is coverage: maximum testing, effective linkage to care, and high coverage and adherence to cART. Given that WHO has estimated a 23% yearly ART attrition rate in Africa, this latter issue alone will be a huge challenge [427].

Behavioral risk reduction remains a cornerstone of HIV control. All biomedical approaches will depend on testing, accessing the service, and willingness to adhere to the prevention modality (e.g., VMMC, future HIV vaccine or microbicide, cART regimen, consistent and correct condom use). Prevention for positives to reduce risky behaviors looks promising with counseling focused on building motivation and developing skills [428]. Evidence suggests that successful interventions are based on sound behavioral theory, such as the health belief model, that addresses mental health and substance-use issues and focuses on adherence [304]. Despite the fact that no clinical trials have been done, it is clear from high-caliber observational studies that correct and consistent condom use is a vital tool for HIV/STI risk reduction [18, 19, 429].

1.5 Future Directions

A new construct for viewing the global HIV pandemic has been proposed by Beyrer et al. [44]. Based on a systematic review of published and unpublished literature from 2000 to 2009, the authors selected 133 HIV prevalence studies from 50 countries to apply an algorithmic approach for categorization. Four scenarios for LMICs were suggested: (1) settings where MSM are the predominant contributor to HIV transmission, (2) settings where HIV transmission among MSM occurs in the context of epidemics driven by IDUs, (3) settings where HIV transmission among MSM occurs in the context of well-established HIV transmission among heterosexuals, and (4) settings where both sexual and parenteral modes contribute significantly to HIV transmission. Perhaps this new paradigm can help guide prevention strategies by reminding policymakers and HIV control workers as to what populations are the largest drivers of local transmission dynamics.

Among the major achievements in confronting the HIV pandemic have been the development and deployment of cART that can turn a previously fatal disease into a chronic, manageable one. However, lower income nations have huge health service challenges that must be addressed for PEPFAR achievements to be expanded and sustained (Table 1.4). Even in the USA and Western Europe, there is a sense of HIV fatigue such that economic downturns from 2008 onward seem to invite cuts in HIV programs to satisfy fiscal exigencies. However, we know from the experiences of the past that failure to prevent HIV or to treat it early once infection has occurred will simply cost society more in the long run, given the high direct costs of illness and indirect costs of disability or death [46, 345, 430–432]. Prevention, including testing and early cART treatment, is a good societal and economic investment.

Acknowledgment I am very grateful to Megan E. Johnson, M.S. who was invaluable in assembling and finalizing the references.

References

1. McEvedy C (1988) The bubonic plague. Sci Am 258:118–123
2. Haensch S, Bianucci R, Signoli M et al (2010) Distinct clones of *Yersinia pestis* caused the black death. PLoS Pathog 6:e1001134
3. Vermund SH, Leigh-Brown AJ (2012) The HIV epidemic: high-income countries. In: Bushman FD, Nabel GJ, Swanstrom R (eds) HIV: from biology to prevention and treatment, 1st edn. Cold Spring Harbor Laboratory Press, New York, pp 385–408
4. Shao Y, Williamson C (2012) The HIV-1 epidemic: low-to middle-income countries. In: Bushman FD, Nabel GJ, Swanstrom R (eds) HIV: from biology to prevention and treatment, 1st edn. Cold Spring Harbor Laboratory Press, New York, pp 367–383
5. Stephenson I (2005) Are we ready for pandemic influenza H5N1? Expert Rev Vac 4:151–155
6. Monto AS (2009) The risk of seasonal and pandemic influenza: prospects for control. Clin Infect Dis 48(Suppl 1):S20–S25
7. Fedson DS (2009) Meeting the challenge of influenza pandemic preparedness in developing countries. Emerg Infect Dis 15:365–371
8. Fedson DS (2006) Vaccine development for an imminent pandemic: why we should worry, what we must do. Hum Vac 2:38–42
9. Chavers LS, Vermund SH (2007) An introduction to emerging and reemerging infectious diseases. In: Lashley FR, Durham JD (eds) Emerging infectious diseases: trends and issues, 2nd edn. Springer Publishing Company, New York, pp 3–24
10. Karim QA, Kharsany AB, Frohlich JA et al (2011) Stabilizing HIV prevalence masks high HIV incidence rates amongst rural and urban women in KwaZulu-Natal, South Africa. Int J Epidemiol 40:922–930
11. Baggaley RF, Fraser C (2010) Modelling sexual transmission of HIV: testing the assumptions, validating the predictions. Curr Opin HIV AIDS 5:269–276

12. Blower S, Schwartz EJ, Mills J (2003) Forecasting the future of HIV epidemics: the impact of antiretroviral therapies & imperfect vaccines. AIDS Rev 5:113–125
13. Center for Disease Control and Prevention, 1993 revised classification system for HIV infection and expanded surveillance case definition for AIDS among adolescents and adults. MMWR: Morb Mort Wkly Rep Recomm Rep/RR-17 41:1–5
14. (UNAIDS) JUNPoHA (2011) UNAIDS: World AIDS day report, 2011. Report No.: 978-92-9173-904-2. Joint United Nations Programme on HIV/AIDS (UNAIDS), Geneva, Switzerland
15. (UNAIDS) JUNPoHA (2010) Global report: UNAIDS report on global AIDS epidemic 2010. Joint United Nations Programme on HIV/AIDS (UNAIDS), Geneva, Switzerland
16. Ki-moon B, Zuma J, Piot P et al (2011) AIDS at 30: Nations at the crossroads: Joint United Nations Programme on HIV/AIDS (UNAIDS)
17. Kipp W, Chapman E, Jhangri GS et al (2009) Fourteen years of surveillance of HIV-1 prevalence among pregnant women attending antenatal care clinics in western Uganda. Int J STD AIDS 20:499–502
18. Stoneburner RL, Low-Beer D (2004) Population-level HIV declines and behavioral risk avoidance in Uganda. Science 304:714–718
19. Hanenberg RS, Rojanapithayakorn W, Kunasol P, Sokal DC (1994) Impact of Thailand's HIV-control programme as indicated by the decline of sexually transmitted diseases. Lancet 344:243–245
20. Nelson KE, Celentano DD, Eiumtrakol S et al (1996) Changes in sexual behavior and a decline in HIV infection among young men in Thailand. N Engl J Med 335:297–303
21. Celentano DD, Nelson KE, Lyles CM et al (1998) Decreasing incidence of HIV and sexually transmitted diseases in young Thai men: evidence for success of the HIV/AIDS control and prevention program. AIDS 12:F29–F36
22. Hargrove JW, Humphrey JH, Mahomva A et al (2011) Declining HIV prevalence and incidence in perinatal women in Harare, Zimbabwe. Epidemics 3:88–94
23. Marsh KA, Nyamukapa CA, Donnelly CA et al (2011) Monitoring trends in HIV prevalence among young people, aged 15 to 24 years, in Manicaland, Zimbabwe. J Intern AIDS Soc 14:27
24. Halperin DT, Mugurungi O, Hallett TB et al (2011) A surprising prevention success: why did the HIV epidemic decline in Zimbabwe? PLoS Med 8:e1000414
25. Gregson S, Nyamukapa C, Schumacher C et al (2011) Did national HIV prevention programs contribute to HIV decline in Eastern Zimbabwe? Evidence from a prospective community survey. Sex Transm Dis 38:475–482
26. International Group on Analysis of Trends in HIVP, Behaviours in Young People in Countries most Affected by HIV (2010) Trends in HIV prevalence and sexual behaviour among young people aged 15-24 years in countries most affected by HIV. Sex Transm Infect 86 (Suppl 2):ii72–ii83
27. Gregson S, Gonese E, Hallett TB et al (2010) HIV decline in Zimbabwe due to reductions in risky sex? Evidence from a comprehensive epidemiological review. Int J Epidemiol 39:1311–1323
28. Gouws E, Stanecki KA, Lyerla R, Ghys PD (2008) The epidemiology of HIV infection among young people aged 15-24 years in southern Africa. AIDS 22(Suppl 4):S5–S16
29. Lopman B, Gregson S (2008) When did HIV incidence peak in Harare, Zimbabwe? Back-calculation from mortality statistics. PLoS One 3:e1711
30. Dube S, Boily MC, Mugurungi O, Mahomva A, Chikhata F, Gregson S (2008) Estimating vertically acquired HIV infections and the impact of the prevention of mother-to-child transmission program in Zimbabwe: insights from decision analysis models. J Acquir Immune Defic Syndr 48:72–81
31. Lopman B, Nyamukapa C, Mushati P et al (2008) HIV incidence in 3 years of follow-up of a Zimbabwe cohort–1998–2000 to 2001–03: contributions of proximate and underlying determinants to transmission. Int J Epidemiol 37:88–105
32. Mahomva A, Greby S, Dube S et al (2006) HIV prevalence and trends from data in Zimbabwe, 1997-2004. Sex Transm Infect 82(Suppl 1):i42–i47

33. Gregson S, Garnett GP, Nyamukapa CA et al (2006) HIV decline associated with behavior change in eastern Zimbabwe. Science 311:664–666
34. Wawer MJ, Serwadda D, Gray RH et al (1997) Trends in HIV-1 prevalence may not reflect trends in incidence in mature epidemics: data from the Rakai population-based cohort, Uganda. AIDS 11:1023–1030
35. Das M, Chu PL, Santos GM et al (2010) Decreases in community viral load are accompanied by reductions in new HIV infections in San Francisco. PLoS One 5:e11068
36. Kilmarx PH (2009) Global epidemiology of HIV. Curr Opin HIV AIDS 4:240–246
37. Baral S, Sifakis F, Cleghorn F, Beyrer C (2007) Elevated risk for HIV infection among men who have sex with men in low- and middle-income countries 2000-2006: a systematic review. PLoS Med 4:e339
38. Oster AM, Wiegand RE, Sionean C et al (2011) Understanding disparities in HIV infection between black and white MSM in the United States. AIDS 25:1103–1112
39. Lieb S, Prejean J, Thompson DR et al (2011) HIV prevalence rates among men who have sex with men in the southern United States: population-based estimates by race/ethnicity. AIDS Behav 15:596–606
40. El-Sadr WM, Mayer KH, Hodder SL (2010) AIDS in America–forgotten but not gone. N Engl J Med 362:967–970
41. Vermund SH, Hodder SL, Justman JE et al (2010) Addressing research priorities for prevention of HIV infection in the United States. Clin Infect Dis 50(Suppl 3):S149–S155
42. Hamers FF, Downs AM (2003) HIV in central and eastern Europe. Lancet 361:1035–1044
43. Aceijas C, Stimson GV, Hickman M et al (2004) Global overview of injecting drug use and HIV infection among injecting drug users. AIDS 18:2295–2303
44. Beyrer C, Wirtz AL, Walker D, Johns B, Sifakis F, Baral SD (2011) The global HIV epidemics among men who have sex with men. World Bank, Washington, DC
45. Larson HJ, Bertozzi S, Piot P (2011) Redesigning the AIDS response for long-term impact. WHO Bull 89:846–852
46. Schwartlander B, Stover J, Hallett T et al (2011) Towards an improved investment approach for an effective response to HIV/AIDS. Lancet 377:2031–2041
47. Hogan DR, Salomon JA (2005) Prevention and treatment of human immunodeficiency virus/acquired immunodeficiency syndrome in resource-limited settings. WHO Bull 83:135–143
48. Vergara AE, Assan A, Vermund SH (2009) Principles and experiences in national antiretroviral therapy roll-out. In: Marlink RG, Teitelman SJ (eds) From the ground up: building comprehensive HIV/AIDS care programs in resource-limited settings. Elizabeth Glaser Pediatric AIDS Foundation, Washington, DC, pp 1–14
49. Fowler MG, Gable AR, Lampe MA, Etima M, Owor M (2010) Perinatal HIV and its prevention: progress toward an HIV-free generation. Clin Perinatol 37:699–719
50. Mofenson LM (2010) Prevention in neglected subpopulations: prevention of mother-to-child transmission of HIV infection. Clin Infect Dis 50(Suppl 3):S130–S148
51. Goldenberg RL, Stringer JS, Sinkala M, Vermund SH (2002) Perinatal HIV transmission: developing country considerations. J Matern Fetal Neonatal Med 12:149–158
52. Newell ML, Brahmbhatt H, Ghys PD (2004) Child mortality and HIV infection in Africa: a review. AIDS 18(Suppl 2):S27–S34
53. Ding H, Wilson CM, Modjarrad K, McGwin G Jr, Tang J, Vermund SH (2009) Predictors of suboptimal virologic response to highly active antiretroviral therapy among human immunodeficiency virus-infected adolescents: analyses of the reaching for excellence in adolescent care and health (REACH) project. Arch Pediatr Adolesc Med 163:1100–1105
54. Stringer EM, Ekouevi DK, Coetzee D et al (2010) Coverage of nevirapine-based services to prevent mother-to-child HIV transmission in 4 African countries. JAMA 304:293–302
55. Megazzini KM, Sinkala M, Vermund SH et al (2010) A cluster-randomized trial of enhanced labor ward-based PMTCT services to increase nevirapine coverage in Lusaka, Zambia. AIDS 24:447–455
56. Stringer EM, Chi BH, Chintu N et al (2008) Monitoring effectiveness of programmes to prevent mother-to-child HIV transmission in lower-income countries. WHO Bull 86:57–62

57. Reithinger R, Megazzini K, Durako SJ, Harris DR, Vermund SH (2007) Monitoring and evaluation of programmes to prevent mother to child transmission of HIV in Africa. BMJ 334:1143–1146
58. Potter D, Goldenberg RL, Chao A et al (2008) Do targeted HIV programs improve overall care for pregnant women? Antenatal syphilis management in Zambia before and after implementation of prevention of mother-to-child HIV transmission programs. J Acquir Immune Defic Syndr 47:79–85
59. Bolton-Moore C, Mubiana-Mbewe M, Cantrell RA et al (2007) Clinical outcomes and CD4 cell response in children receiving antiretroviral therapy at primary health care facilities in Zambia. JAMA 298:1888–1899
60. Stringer JS, Sinkala M, Maclean CC et al (2005) Effectiveness of a city-wide program to prevent mother-to-child HIV transmission in Lusaka, Zambia. AIDS 19:1309–1315
61. Stringer EM, Sinkala M, Stringer JS et al (2003) Prevention of mother-to-child transmission of HIV in Africa: successes and challenges in scaling-up a nevirapine-based program in Lusaka, Zambia. AIDS 17:1377–1382
62. Galarraga O, Wirtz VJ, Figueroa-Lara A et al (2011) Unit costs for delivery of antiretroviral treatment and prevention of mother-to-child transmission of HIV: a systematic review for low- and middle-income countries. Pharmacoeconomics 29:579–599
63. Ciaranello AL, Park JE, Ramirez-Avila L, Freedberg KA, Walensky RP, Leroy V (2011) Early infant HIV-1 diagnosis programs in resource-limited settings: opportunities for improved outcomes and more cost-effective interventions. BMC Med 9:59
64. Ciampa PJ, Burlison JR, Blevins M et al (2011) Improving retention in the early infant diagnosis of HIV program in rural Mozambique by better service integration. J Acquir Immune Defic Syndr 58:115–119
65. Violari A, Cotton MF, Gibb DM et al (2008) Early antiretroviral therapy and mortality among HIV-infected infants. N Engl J Med 359:2233–2244
66. UNAIDS: World AIDS Day Report 2011: core epidemiology slides. Joint United Nations Programme on HIV/AIDS (UNAIDS), 2011. http://www.slideshare.net/UNAIDS/unaids-world-aids-day-report-2011-core-slides-10250153. Accessed 22 Jan 2012
67. Kourtis AP, Kraft JM, Gavin L, Kissin D, McMichen-Wright P, Jamieson DJ (2006) Prevention of sexually transmitted human immunodeficiency virus (HIV) infection in adolescents. Curr HIV Res 4:209–219
68. Underhill K, Operario D, Montgomery P (2007) Systematic review of abstinence-plus HIV prevention programs in high-income countries. PLoS Med 4:e275
69. Gavin L, MacKay AP, Brown K et al (2009) Sexual and reproductive health of persons aged 10-24 years – United States, 2002-2007. MMWR Surveill Summ 58:1–58
70. DiClemente RJ, Crittenden CP, Rose E et al (2008) Psychosocial predictors of HIV-associated sexual behaviors and the efficacy of prevention interventions in adolescents at-risk for HIV infection: what works and what doesn't work? Psychosom Med 70:598–605
71. Spiegel HM, Futterman DC (2009) Adolescents and HIV: prevention and clinical care. Curr HIV/AIDS Rep 6:100–107
72. Boutayeb A (2009) The impact of HIV/AIDS on human development in African countries. BMC Public Health 9(Suppl 1):S3
73. Ferreira PC, Pessoa S, Santos MR (2011) The impact of AIDS on income and human capital. Econ Inq 49:1104–1116
74. Galarraga O, Colchero MA, Wamai RG, Bertozzi SM (2009) HIV prevention cost-effectiveness: a systematic review. BMC Public Health 9(Suppl 1):S5
75. Thurlow J, Gow J, George G (2009) HIV/AIDS, growth and poverty in KwaZulu-Natal and South Africa: an integrated survey, demographic and economy-wide analysis. J Int AIDS Soc 12:18
76. Hunter SS, Bulirwa E, Kisseka E (1993) AIDS and agricultural production. Report of a land utilization survey, Masaka and Rakai districts of Uganda. Land Use Policy 10:241–258
77. Nabyonga-Orem J, Bazeyo W, Okema A, Karamagi H, Walker O (2008) Effect of HIV/AIDS on household welfare in Uganda rural communities: a review. East Afr Med J 85:187–196

78. Hosegood V, Preston-Whyte E, Busza J, Moitse S, Timaeus IM (2007) Revealing the full extent of households' experiences of HIV and AIDS in rural South Africa. Soc Sci Med 65:1249–1259
79. Andrews G, Skinner D, Zuma K (2006) Epidemiology of health and vulnerability among children orphaned and made vulnerable by HIV/AIDS in sub-Saharan Africa. AIDS Care 18:269–276
80. Lawn SD, Wood R (2011) Tuberculosis in antiretroviral treatment services in resource-limited settings: addressing the challenges of screening and diagnosis. J Infect Dis 204 (Suppl 4):S1159–S1167
81. Venkatesh KK, Swaminathan S, Andrews JR, Mayer KH (2011) Tuberculosis and HIV co-infection: screening and treatment strategies. Drugs 71:1133–1152
82. Wood R, Lawn SD, Johnstone-Robertson S, Bekker LG (2011) Tuberculosis control has failed in South Africa–time to reappraise strategy. South Afr Med J 101:111–114
83. Martinson NA, Hoffmann CJ, Chaisson RE (2011) Epidemiology of tuberculosis and HIV: recent advances in understanding and responses. Proc Am Thorac Soc 8:288–293
84. Kwan CK, Ernst JD (2011) HIV and tuberculosis: a deadly human syndemic. Clin Microbiol Rev 24:351–376
85. Lawn SD, Zumla AI (2011) Tuberculosis. Lancet 378:57–72
86. Nachega JB, Rosenkranz B, Simon G, Chaisson RE, Diacon A, Taljaard J (2011) Management of adult active tuberculosis disease in era of HIV pandemic, current practices and future perspectives. Infect Disord Drug Targets 11:134–143
87. Sahasrabuddhe VV, Parham GP, Mwanahamuntu MH, Vermund SH (2012) Cervical cancer prevention in low- and middle-income countries: feasible, affordable, essential. Cancer Prev Res 5:11–17
88. Casper C (2011) The increasing burden of HIV-associated malignancies in resource-limited regions. Annu Rev Med 62:157–170
89. Barnabas RV, Webb EL, Weiss HA, Wasserheit JN (2011) The role of coinfections in HIV epidemic trajectory and positive prevention: a systematic review and meta-analysis. AIDS 25:1559–1573
90. Modjarrad K, Vermund SH (2010) Effect of treating co-infections on HIV-1 viral load: a systematic review. Lancet Infect Dis 10:455–463
91. Modjarrad K, Vermund SH (2011) An addition to the effect of treating co-infections on HIV-1 viral load. Lancet Infect Dis 11:81
92. Koethe JR, Heimburger DC (2010) Nutritional aspects of HIV-associated wasting in sub-Saharan Africa. Am J Clin Nutr 91:1138S–1142S
93. Koethe JR, Chi BH, Megazzini KM, Heimburger DC, Stringer JS (2009) Macronutrient supplementation for malnourished HIV-infected adults: a review of the evidence in resource-adequate and resource-constrained settings. Clin Infect Dis 49:787–798
94. van Oosterhout JJ, Ndekha M, Moore E, Kumwenda JJ, Zijlstra EE, Manary M (2010) The benefit of supplementary feeding for wasted Malawian adults initiating ART. AIDS Care 22:737–742
95. Ahoua L, Umutoni C, Huerga H et al (2011) Nutrition outcomes of HIV-infected malnourished adults treated with ready-to-use therapeutic food in sub-Saharan Africa: a longitudinal study. J Int AIDS Soc 14:2
96. Manary M, Ndekhat M, van Oosterhout JJ (2010) Supplementary feeding in the care of the wasted HIV infected patient. Malawi Med J 22:46–48
97. Peterse I, Swartz L (2002) Primary health care in the era of HIV/AIDS. some implications for health systems reform. Soc Sci Med 55:1005–1013
98. Benatar SR (2004) Health care reform and the crisis of HIV and AIDS in South Africa. N Engl J Med 351:81–92
99. Dohrn J, Nzama B, Murrman M (2009) The impact of HIV scale-up on the role of nurses in South Africa: time for a new approach. J Acquir Immune Defic Syndr 52(Suppl 1):S27–S29
100. Chopra M, Lawn JE, Sanders D et al (2009) Achieving the health Millennium Development Goals for South Africa: challenges and priorities. Lancet 374:1023–1031

101. Auvert B, Ballard R, Campbell C et al (2001) HIV infection among youth in a South African mining town is associated with herpes simplex virus-2 seropositivity and sexual behaviour. AIDS 15:885–898
102. Vermund SH, Allen KL, Karim QA (2009) HIV-prevention science at a crossroads: advances in reducing sexual risk. Curr Opin HIV AIDS 4:266–273
103. Eyawo O, de Walque D, Ford N, Gakii G, Lester RT, Mills EJ (2010) HIV status in discordant couples in sub-Saharan Africa: a systematic review and meta-analysis. Lancet Infect Dis 10:770–777
104. Vlahov D, Robertson AM, Strathdee SA (2010) Prevention of HIV infection among injection drug users in resource-limited settings. Clin Infect Dis 50(Suppl 3):S114–S121
105. McCurdy SA, Ross MW, Williams ML, Kilonzo GP, Leshabari MT (2010) Flashblood: blood sharing among female injecting drug users in Tanzania. Addiction 105:1062–1070
106. Smith AD, Tapsoba P, Peshu N, Sanders EJ, Jaffe HW (2009) Men who have sex with men and HIV/AIDS in sub-Saharan Africa. Lancet 374:416–422
107. Baral S, Adams D, Lebona J et al (2011) A cross-sectional assessment of population demographics, HIV risks and human rights contexts among men who have sex with men in Lesotho. J Int AIDS Soc 14:36
108. Rispel LC, Metcalf CA, Cloete A, Reddy V, Lombard C (2011) HIV prevalence and risk practices among men who have sex with men in two South African cities. J Acquir Immune Defic Syndr 57:69–76
109. Merrigan M, Azeez A, Afolabi B et al (2011) HIV prevalence and risk behaviours among men having sex with men in Nigeria. Sex Transm Infect 87:65–70
110. Johnston LG, Holman A, Dahoma M et al (2010) HIV risk and the overlap of injecting drug use and high-risk sexual behaviours among men who have sex with men in Zanzibar (Unguja), Tanzania. Int J Drug Policy 21:485–492
111. Simonsen L, Kane A, Lloyd J, Zaffran M, Kane M (1999) Unsafe injections in the developing world and transmission of bloodborne pathogens: a review. WHO Bull 77:789–800
112. Centers for Disease Control & Prevention (2011) Progress toward strengthening national blood transfusion services–14 countries, 2008–2010. MMWR Morb Mortal Wkly Rep 60:1577–1582
113. Hussain A, Moodley D, Naidoo S, Esterhuizen TM (2011) Pregnant women's access to PMTCT and ART services in South Africa and implications for universal antiretroviral treatment. PLoS One 6:e27907
114. Stinson K, Boulle A, Coetzee D, Abrams EJ, Myer L (2010) Initiation of highly active antiretroviral therapy among pregnant women in Cape Town, South Africa. Trop Med Int Health 15:825–832
115. Ekouevi DK, Coffie PA, Becquet R et al (2008) Antiretroviral therapy in pregnant women with advanced HIV disease and pregnancy outcomes in Abidjan, Cote d'Ivoire. AIDS 22:1815–1820
116. Kumwenda J, Matchere F, Mataya R et al (2011) Coverage of highly active antiretroviral therapy among postpartum women in Malawi. Int J STD AIDS 22:368–372
117. Chen JY, Ogwu AC, Svab P et al (2010) Antiretroviral treatment initiation among HIV-infected pregnant women with low CD4(+) cell counts in Gaborone, Botswana. J Acquir Immune Defic Syndr 54:102–106
118. Bancheno WM, Mwanyumba F, Mareverwa J (2010) Outcomes and challenges of scaling up comprehensive PMTCT services in rural Swaziland, Southern Africa. AIDS Care 22: 1130–1135
119. Horwood C, Haskins L, Vermaak K, Phakathi S, Subbaye R, Doherty T (2010) Prevention of mother to child transmission of HIV (PMTCT) programme in KwaZulu-Natal, South Africa: an evaluation of PMTCT implementation and integration into routine maternal, child and women's health services. Trop Med Int Health 15:992–999
120. Davaalkham J, Unenchimeg P, Baigalmaa C et al (2009) High-risk status of HIV-1 infection in the very low epidemic country, Mongolia, 2007. Int J STD AIDS 20:391–394

121. Nemoto T (2004) HIV/AIDS surveillance and prevention studies in Japan: summary and recommendations. AIDS Educ Prev 16:27–42
122. Farr AC, Wilson DP (2010) An HIV epidemic is ready to emerge in the Philippines. J Int AIDS Soc 13:16
123. van Griensven F, de Lind van Wijngaarden JW (2010) A review of the epidemiology of HIV infection and prevention responses among MSM in Asia. AIDS 24(Suppl 3):S30–S40
124. Sharma M, Oppenheimer E, Saidel T, Loo V, Garg R (2009) A situation update on HIV epidemics among people who inject drugs and national responses in South-East Asia Region. AIDS 23:1405–1413
125. Ruxrungtham K, Brown T, Phanuphak P (2004) HIV/AIDS in Asia. Lancet 364:69–82
126. Couture MC, Sansothy N, Sapphon V et al (2011) Young women engaged in sex work in Phnom Penh, Cambodia, have high incidence of HIV and sexually transmitted infections, and amphetamine-type stimulant use: new challenges to HIV prevention and risk. Sex Transm Dis 38:33–39
127. Park LS, Siraprapasiri T, Peerapatanapokin W, Manne J, Niccolai L, Kunanusont C (2010) HIV transmission rates in Thailand: evidence of HIV prevention and transmission decline. J Acquir Immune Defic Syndr 54:430–436
128. Ainsworth M, Beyrer C, Soucat A (2003) AIDS and public policy: the lessons and challenges of “success” in Thailand. Health Policy 64:13–37
129. Wu Z, Sullivan SG, Wang Y, Rotheram-Borus MJ, Detels R (2007) Evolution of China’s response to HIV/AIDS. Lancet 369:679–690
130. Xiao Y, Kristensen S, Sun J, Lu L, Vermund SH (2007) Expansion of HIV/AIDS in China: lessons from Yunnan Province. Soc Sci Med 64:665–675
131. Tucker JD, Cohen MS (2011) China’s syphilis epidemic: epidemiology, proximate determinants of spread, and control responses. Curr Opin Infect Dis 24:50–55
132. Qian HZ, Vermund SH, Wang N (2005) Risk of HIV/AIDS in China: subpopulations of special importance. Sex Transm Infect 81:442–447
133. Qian HZ, Vermund SH, Kaslow RA et al (2006) Co-infection with HIV and hepatitis C virus in former plasma/blood donors: challenge for patient care in rural China. AIDS 20: 1429–1435
134. Chandrasekaran P, Dallabetta G, Loo V, Rao S, Gayle H, Alexander A (2006) Containing HIV/AIDS in India: the unfinished agenda. Lancet Infect Dis 6:508–521
135. Dandona L, Lakshmi V, Kumar GA, Dandona R (2006) Is the HIV burden in India being overestimated? BMC Public Health 6:308
136. Siddiqui AU, Qian HZ, Altaf A, Cassell H, Shah SA, Vermund SH (2011) Condom use during commercial sex among clients of Hijra sex workers in Karachi, Pakistan (cross-sectional study). BMJ Open 1:e000154
137. Sahastrabuddhe S, Gupta A, Stuart E et al (2012) Sexually transmitted infections and risk behaviors among transgender persons (Hijras) of Pune, India. J Acquir Immune Defic Syndr 59:72–78
138. Shaw SY, Emmanuel F, Adrien A et al (2011) The descriptive epidemiology of male sex workers in Pakistan: a biological and behavioural examination. Sex Transm Infect 87:73–80
139. Phillips AE, Lowndes CM, Boily MC et al (2010) Men who have sex with men and women in Bangalore, South India, and potential impact on the HIV epidemic. Sex Transm Infect 86:187–192
140. Solomon SS, Srikrishnan AK, Sifakis F et al (2010) The emerging HIV epidemic among men who have sex with men in Tamil Nadu, India: geographic diffusion and bisexual concurrency. AIDS Behav 14:1001–1010
141. Verma R, Shekhar A, Khobragade S et al (2010) Scale-up and coverage of Avahan: a large-scale HIV-prevention programme among female sex workers and men who have sex with men in four Indian states. Sex Transm Infect 86(Suppl 1):i76–i82
142. Altaf A, Saleem N, Abbas S, Muzaffar R (2009) High prevalence of HIV infection among injection drug users (IDUs) in Hyderabad and Sukkur, Pakistan. J Pak Med Assoc 59: 136–140

143. Vermund SH, White H, Shah SA et al (2006) HIV/AIDS in Pakistan: has the explosion begun? J Pak Med Assoc 56:S1–S2
144. Kazi AM, Shah SA, Jenkins CA, Shepherd BE, Vermund SH (2010) Risk factors and prevalence of tuberculosis, human immunodeficiency virus, syphilis, hepatitis B virus, and hepatitis C virus among prisoners in Pakistan. Int J Infect Dis 14(Suppl 3):e60–e66
145. Mathers BM, Degenhardt L, Ali H et al (2010) HIV prevention, treatment, and care services for people who inject drugs: a systematic review of global, regional, and national coverage. Lancet 375:1014–1028
146. Kelly JA, Amirkhanian YA (2003) The newest epidemic: a review of HIV/AIDS in Central and Eastern Europe. Int J STD AIDS 14:361–371
147. Bridge J, Lazarus JV, Atun R (2010) HIV epidemics and prevention responses in Asia and Eastern Europe: lessons to be learned? AIDS 24(Suppl 3):S86–S94
148. Rechel B (2010) HIV/AIDS in the countries of the former Soviet Union: societal and attitudinal challenges. Cent Eur J Public Health 18:110–115
149. Elovich R, Drucker E (2008) On drug treatment and social control: Russian narcology's great leap backwards. Harm Reduct J 5:23
150. Tkatchenko-Schmidt E, Renton A, Gevorgyan R, Davydenko L, Atun R (2008) Prevention of HIV/AIDS among injecting drug users in Russia: opportunities and barriers to scaling-up of harm reduction programmes. Health Policy 85:162–171
151. Kalichman SC, Kelly JA, Sikkema KJ, Koslov AP, Shaboltas A, Granskaya J (2000) The emerging AIDS crisis in Russia: review of enabling factors and prevention needs. Int J STD AIDS 11:71–75
152. Platt L, Rhodes T, Hickman M et al (2008) Changes in HIV prevalence and risk among new injecting drug users in a Russian city of high HIV prevalence. J Acquir Immune Defic Syndr 47:623–631
153. Lurie P, Drucker E (1997) An opportunity lost: HIV infections associated with lack of a national needle-exchange programme in the USA. Lancet 349:604–608
154. Millett GA, Crowley JS, Koh H et al (2010) A way forward: the National HIV/AIDS Strategy and reducing HIV incidence in the United States. J Acquir Immune Defic Syndr 55(Suppl 2):S144–S147
155. Mumtaz G, Hilmi N, McFarland W et al (2010) Are HIV epidemics among men who have sex with men emerging in the Middle East and North Africa?: a systematic review and data synthesis. PLoS Med 8:e1000444
156. Shah SA, Khan OA, Kristensen S, Vermund SH (1999) HIV-infected workers deported from the Gulf States: impact on Southern Pakistan. Int J STD AIDS 10:812–814
157. Mumtaz G, Hilmi N, Akala FA et al (2011) HIV-1 molecular epidemiology evidence and transmission patterns in the Middle East and North Africa. Sex Transm Infect 87:101–106
158. Abu-Raddad LJ, Hilmi N, Mumtaz G et al (2010) Epidemiology of HIV infection in the Middle East and North Africa. AIDS 24(Suppl 2):S5–S23
159. Sawires S, Birnbaum N, Abu-Raddad L, Szekeres G, Gayle J (2009) Twenty-five years of HIV: lessons for low prevalence scenarios. J Acquir Immune Defic Syndr 51(Suppl 3): S75–S82
160. Todd CS, Nassiramanesh B, Stanekzai MR, Kamarulzaman A (2007) Emerging HIV epidemics in Muslim countries: assessment of different cultural responses to harm reduction and implications for HIV control. Curr HIV/AIDS Rep 4:151–157
161. Farnia M, Ebrahimi B, Shams A, Zamani S (2010) Scaling up methadone maintenance treatment for opioid-dependent prisoners in Iran. Int J Drug Policy 21:422–424
162. Zamani S, Farnia M, Torknejad A et al (2010) Patterns of drug use and HIV-related risk behaviors among incarcerated people in a prison in Iran. J Urban Health 87:603–616
163. Zamani S, Farnia M, Tavakoli S et al (2010) A qualitative inquiry into methadone maintenance treatment for opioid-dependent prisoners in Tehran, Iran. Int J Drug Policy 21: 167–172
164. Shoptaw S, Reback CJ (2007) Methamphetamine use and infectious disease-related behaviors in men who have sex with men: implications for interventions. Addiction 102(Suppl 1):130–135

165. Colfax G, Shoptaw S (2005) The methamphetamine epidemic: implications for HIV prevention and treatment. Curr HIV/AIDS Rep 2:194–199
166. Miller M (2003) The dynamics of substance use and sex networks in HIV transmission. J Urban Health 80:iii88–iii96
167. Goedert JJ (1984) Recreational drugs: relationship to AIDS. Ann N Y Acad Sci 437: 192–199
168. Drumright LN, Patterson TL, Strathdee SA (2006) Club drugs as causal risk factors for HIV acquisition among men who have sex with men: a review. Subst Use Misuse 41:1551–1601
169. Woolf SE, Maisto SA (2009) Alcohol use and risk of HIV infection among men who have sex with men. AIDS Behav 13:757–782
170. Wilson T, DeHovitz JA (1997) STDs, HIV, and crack cocaine: a review. AIDS Patient Care STDS 11:62–66
171. Corsi KF, Booth RE (2008) HIV sex risk behaviors among heterosexual methamphetamine users: literature review from 2000 to present. Curr Drug Abuse Rev 1:292–296
172. Zierler S, Krieger N (1997) Reframing women's risk: social inequalities and HIV infection. Annu Rev Public Health 18:401–436
173. Norris J, Masters NT, Zawacki T (2004) Cognitive mediation of women's sexual decision making: the influence of alcohol, contextual factors, and background variables. Annu Rev Sex Res 15:258–296
174. Senf JH, Price CQ (1994) Young adults, alcohol and condom use: what is the connection? J Adolesc Health 15:238–244
175. Fortenberry JD (1998) Alcohol, drugs, and STD/HIV risk among adolescents. AIDS Patient Care STDS 12:783–786
176. Millett GA, Peterson JL, Wolitski RJ, Stall R (2006) Greater risk for HIV infection of black men who have sex with men: a critical literature review. Am J Public Health 96:1007–1019
177. Lindegren ML, Byers RH Jr, Thomas P et al (1999) Trends in perinatal transmission of HIV/AIDS in the United States. JAMA 282:531–538
178. Wortley PM, Lindegren ML, Fleming PL (2001) Successful implementation of perinatal HIV prevention guidelines. A multistate surveillance evaluation. MMWR Morb Mort Wkly Rep Recomm Rep/CDC 50:17–28
179. Freeman P, Walker BC, Harris DR et al (2011) Methamphetamine use and risk for HIV among young men who have sex with men in 8 US cities. Arch Pediatr Adolesc Med 165: 736–740
180. Whitmore SK, Taylor AW, Espinoza L, Shouse RL, Lampe MA, Nesheim S (2012) Correlates of mother-to-child transmission of HIV in the United States and Puerto Rico. Pediatrics 129:e74–e81
181. European Collaborative Study in E, Bailey H, Townsend C, Cortina-Borja M, Thorne C (2011) Insufficient antiretroviral therapy in pregnancy: missed opportunities for prevention of mother-to-child transmission of HIV in Europe. Antivir Ther16:895–903
182. Cohen MS, Chen YQ, McCauley M et al (2011) Prevention of HIV-1 infection with early antiretroviral therapy. N Engl J Med 365:493–505
183. Centers for Disease Control & Prevention (2011) Vital signs: HIV prevention through care and treatment–United States. MMWR Morb Mortal Wkly Rep 60:1618–1623
184. Burns DN, Dieffenbach CW, Vermund SH (2010) Rethinking prevention of HIV type 1 infection. Clin Infect Dis 51:725–731
185. Gardner EM, McLees MP, Steiner JF, Del Rio C, Burman WJ (2011) The spectrum of engagement in HIV care and its relevance to test-and-treat strategies for prevention of HIV infection. Clin Infect Dis 52:793–800
186. Montaner JS, Lima VD, Barrios R et al (2010) Association of highly active antiretroviral therapy coverage, population viral load, and yearly new HIV diagnoses in British Columbia, Canada: a population-based study. Lancet 376:532–539
187. Caceres CF, Stall R (2003) Commentary: The human immunodeficiency virus/AIDS epidemic among men who have sex with men in Latin America and the Caribbean: it is time to bridge the gap. Int J Epidemiol 32:740–743

188. Fang CT, Hsu HM, Twu SJ et al (2004) Decreased HIV transmission after a policy of providing free access to highly active antiretroviral therapy in Taiwan. J Infect Dis 190:879–885
189. McGowan CC, Cahn P, Gotuzzo E et al (2007) Cohort Profile: Caribbean, Central and South America Network for HIV research (CCASAnet) collaboration within the International Epidemiologic Databases to Evaluate AIDS (IeDEA) programme. Int J Epidemiol 36:969–976
190. Caceres CF (2002) HIV among gay and other men who have sex with men in Latin America and the Caribbean: a hidden epidemic? AIDS 16(Suppl 3):S23–S33
191. Coplan PM, Gortmaker S, Hernandez-Avila M, Spiegelman D, Uribe-Zuniga P, Mueller NE (1996) Human immunodeficiency virus infection in Mexico City. Rectal bleeding and anal warts as risk factors among men reporting sex with men. Am J Epidemiol 144:817–827
192. McCarthy MC, Wignall FS, Sanchez J et al (1996) The epidemiology of HIV-1 infection in Peru, 1986-1990. AIDS 10:1141–1145
193. Bastos FI, Caceres C, Galvao J, Veras MA, Castilho EA (2008) AIDS in Latin America: assessing the current status of the epidemic and the ongoing response. Int J Epidemiol 37:729–737
194. Lima ES, Friedman SR, Bastos FI et al (1994) Risk factors for HIV-1 seroprevalence among drug injectors in the cocaine-using environment of Rio de Janeiro. Addiction 89:689–698
195. Hacker MA, Malta M, Enriquez M, Bastos FI (2005) Human immunodeficiency virus, AIDS, and drug consumption in South America and the Caribbean: epidemiological evidence and initiatives to curb the epidemic. Pan Am J Public Health 18:303–313
196. Rodriguez CM, Marques LF, Touze G (2002) HIV and injection drug use in Latin America. AIDS 16(Suppl 3):S34–S41
197. Caiaffa WT, Proietti FA, Carneiro-Proietti AB et al (2003) The dynamics of the human immunodeficiency virus epidemics in the south of Brazil: increasing role of injection drug users. Clin Infect Dis 37(Suppl 5):S376–S381
198. Khalsa JH, Francis H, Mazin R (2003) Bloodborne and sexually transmitted infections in drug abusers in the United States, Latin America, the Caribbean, and Spain. Clin Infect Dis 37(Suppl 5):S331–S337
199. Mesquita F, Doneda D, Gandolfi D et al (2003) Brazilian response to the human immunodeficiency virus/acquired immunodeficiency syndrome epidemic among injection drug users. Clin Infect Dis 37(Suppl 5):S382–S385
200. Bastos FI, Caiaffa W, Rossi D, Vila M, Malta M (2007) The children of mama coca: coca, cocaine and the fate of harm reduction in South America. Int J Drug Policy 18:99–106
201. Damacena GN, Szwarcwald CL, de SouzaJunior PR, Dourado I (2011) Risk factors associated with HIV prevalence among female sex workers in 10 Brazilian cities. J Acquir Immune Defic Syndr 57(Suppl 3):S144–S152
202. Cortez FC, Boer DP, Baltieri DA (2011) Psychosocial pathways to inconsistent condom use among male sex workers: personality, drug misuse and criminality. Sex Health 8:390–398
203. Anastario M, Manzanero R, Blanco R et al (2011) HIV infection, sexual risk behaviour and condom use in the Belize defense force. Int J STD AIDS 22:73–9
204. Bassols AM, Boni R, Pechansky F (2010) Alcohol, drugs, and risky sexual behavior are related to HIV infection in female adolescents. Rev Bras Psiquiatr 32:361–368
205. von Diemen L, De Boni R, Kessler F, Benzano D, Pechansky F (2010) Risk behaviors for HCV- and HIV-seroprevalence among female crack users in Porto Alegre, Brazil. Arch Women's Ment Health 13:185–191
206. Ramirez J, Suarez E, de la Rosa G, Castro MA, Zimmerman MA (1994) AIDS knowledge and sexual behavior among Mexican gay and bisexual men. AIDS Educ Prev 6:163–174
207. Konda KA, Celentano DD, Kegeles S, Coates TJ, Caceres CF, Group NCHSPT (2011) Latent class analysis of sexual risk patterns among esquineros (street corner men) a group of heterosexually identified, socially marginalized men in urban coastal Peru. AIDS Behav 15:862–868
208. D'Ippolito M, Read JS, Korelitz J et al (2007) Missed opportunities for prevention of mother-to-child transmission of human immunodeficiency virus type 1 in Latin America and the Caribbean: the NISDI perinatal study. Pediatr Infect Dis J 26:649–653

209. Read JS, Cahn P, Losso M et al (2007) Management of human immunodeficiency virus-infected pregnant women at Latin American and Caribbean sites. Obstet Gynecol 109:1358–1367
210. Figueroa JP (2003) HIV/AIDS in the Caribbean. The need for a more effective public health response. West Indian Med J 52:156–158
211. Figueroa JP (2008) The HIV epidemic in the Caribbean: meeting the challenges of achieving universal access to prevention, treatment and care. West Indian Med J 57:195–203
212. Figueroa JP (2004) An overview of HIV/AIDS in Jamaica: strengthening the response. West Indian Med J 53:277–282
213. Calleja JM, Walker N, Cuchi P, Lazzari S, Ghys PD, Zacarias F (2002) Status of the HIV/AIDS epidemic and methods to monitor it in the Latin America and Caribbean region. AIDS 16(Suppl 3):S3–S12
214. Inciardi JA, Syvertsen JL, Surratt HL (2005) HIV/AIDS in the Caribbean Basin. AIDS Care 17(Suppl 1):S9–S25
215. Castro A, Farmer P (2005) Understanding and addressing AIDS-related stigma: from anthropological theory to clinical practice in Haiti. Am J Public Health 95:53–59
216. Pape J, Johnson WD Jr (1993) AIDS in Haiti: 1982-1992. Clin Infect Dis 17(Suppl 2):S341–S345
217. Dorjgochoo T, Noel F, Deschamps MM et al (2009) Risk factors for HIV infection among Haitian adolescents and young adults seeking counseling and testing in Port-au-Prince. J Acquir Immune Defic Syndr 52:498–508
218. Seguy N, Denniston M, Hladik W et al (2008) HIV and syphilis infection among gold and diamond miners–Guyana, 2004. West Indian Med J 57:444–449
219. Schumacher S, Norin J, Bolu O, DuBois A, Wolford J, Shaffer N (2009) HIV testing and counselling for prevention of mother-to-child transmission at labour and delivery in Guyana. West Indian Med J 58:112–113
220. Allen CF, Edwards M, Williamson LM et al (2006) Sexually transmitted infection service use and risk factors for HIV infection among female sex workers in Georgetown, Guyana. J Acquir Immune Defic Syndr 43:96–101
221. Palmer CJ, Validum L, Loeffke B et al (2002) HIV prevalence in a gold mining camp in the Amazon region, Guyana. Emerg Infect Dis 8:330–331
222. van Griensven F, de Lindvan Wijngaarden JW, Baral S, Grulich A (2009) The global epidemic of HIV infection among men who have sex with men. Curr Opin HIV AIDS 4:300–307
223. Padilla M, Castellanos D, Guilamo-Ramos V, Reyes AM, Sanchez Marte LE, Soriano MA (2008) Stigma, social inequality, and HIV risk disclosure among Dominican male sex workers. Soc Sci Med 67:380–388
224. Finlinson HA, Colon HM, Robles RR, Soto M (2006) Sexual identity formation and AIDS prevention: an exploratory study of non-gay-identified Puerto Rican MSM from working class neighborhoods. AIDS Behav 10:531–539
225. Tabet SR, de Moya EA, Holmes KK et al (1996) Sexual behaviors and risk factors for HIV infection among men who have sex with men in the Dominican Republic. AIDS 10: 201–206
226. Gelpi-Acosta C, Hagan H, Jenness SM, Wendel T, Neaigus A (2011) Sexual and injection-related risks in Puerto Rican-born injection drug users living in New York City: A mixed-methods analysis. Harm Reduct J 8:28
227. Clatts MC, Rodriguez-Diaz CE, Garcia H, Vargas-Molina RL, Jovet-Toledo GG, Goldsamt LA (2011) Preliminary evidence of significant gaps in continuity of HIV care among excarcerated populations in Puerto Rico. J Int Assoc Phys AIDS Care 10:339–341
228. Colon-Lopez V, Rodriguez-Diaz CE, Ortiz AP, Soto-Salgado M, Suarez E, Perez CM (2011) HIV-related risk behaviors among a sample of men who have sex with men in Puerto Rico: an overview of substance use and sexual practices. Puerto Rico Health Sci J 30:65–68
229. Norman LR, Devieux JG, Rosenberg R, Malow RM (2011) HIV-testing practices and a history of substance use among women living in public housing in Puerto Rico. J Int Assoc Phys AIDS Care 10:260–265

230. Rodriguez-Diaz CE, Reece M, Rivera-Alonso B, Laureano-Landron I, Dodge B, Malow RM (2011) Behind the bars of paradise: HIV and substance use among incarcerated populations in Puerto Rico. J Int Assoc Phys AIDS Care 10:266–272
231. Mino M, Deren S, Colon HM (2011) HIV and drug use in Puerto Rico: findings from the ARIBBA study. J Int Assoc Phys AIDS Care 10:248–259
232. Zerden Lde S, Marilis Lopez L, Lundgren LM (2010) Needle sharing among Puerto Rican injection drug users in Puerto Rico and Massachusetts: place of birth and residence matter. Subst Use Misuse 45:1605–1622
233. Perez CM, Marrero E, Melendez M et al (2010) Seroepidemiology of viral hepatitis, HIV and herpes simplex type 2 in the household population aged 21–64 years in Puerto Rico. BMC Infect Dis 10:76
234. Machado LY, Blanco M, Dubed M, Díaz HM, Ruiz NM, Váldes N, Romay D, Lobaina LI. (2011) HIV Type 1 Genetic Diversity in Newly Diagnosed Cuban Patients. AIDS Res Hum Retroviruses. 2011 Dec 19. [Epub ahead of print] PubMed PMID: 22059433
235. Gorry C (2011) Cuba's national HIV/AIDS program. MEDICC Rev 13:5–8
236. Hsieh YH, Wang YS, de Arazoza H, Lounes R (2010) Modeling secondary level of HIV contact tracing: its impact on HIV intervention in Cuba. BMC Infect Dis 10:194
237. Anderson T (2009) HIV/AIDS in Cuba: lessons and challenges. Rev Panam Salud Publica = Pan Am J Public Health 26:78–86
238. Gorry C (2008) Cuba's HIV/AIDS program: controversy, care and cultural shift. MEDICC Rev 10:10–14
239. Rojas P, Malow R, Ruffin B, Rothe EM, Rosenberg R (2011) The HIV/AIDS epidemic in the Dominican Republic: Key contributing factors. J Int Assoc Phys AIDS Care 10:306–315
240. Halperin DT, de Moya EA, Perez-Then E, Pappas G, Garcia Calleja JM (2009) Understanding the HIV epidemic in the Dominican Republic: a prevention success story in the Caribbean? J Acquir Immune Defic Syndr 51(Suppl 1):S52–S59
241. Garris I, Rodriguez EM, De Moya EA et al (1991) AIDS heterosexual predominance in the Dominican Republic. J Acquir Immune Defic Syndr 4:1173–1178
242. Andrews BE (2011) Prevalence and correlates of HIV testing among Caribbean youth. Int J STD AIDS 22:722–726
243. O'Toole BJ, McConkey R, Casson K, Goetz-Goldberg D, Yazdani A (2007) Knowledge and attitudes of young people in Guyana to HIV/AIDS. Int J STD AIDS 18:193–197
244. Mao L, Kippax SC, Holt M, Prestage GP, Zablotska IB, de Wit JB (2011) Rates of condom and non-condom-based anal intercourse practices among homosexually active men in Australia: deliberate HIV risk reduction? Sex Transm Infect 87:489–493
245. Kang M, Skinner R, Usherwood T (2010) Interventions for young people in Australia to reduce HIV and sexually transmissible infections: a systematic review. Sex Health 7:107–128
246. Jones L, Pickering L, Sumnall H, McVeigh J, Bellis MA (2010) Optimal provision of needle and syringe programmes for injecting drug users: A systematic review. Int J Drug Policy 21:335–342
247. Minichiello V, Marino R, Browne J (2001) Knowledge, risk perceptions and condom usage in male sex workers from three Australian cities. AIDS Care 13:387–402
248. Miller ER, Hellard ME, Bowden S, Bharadwaj M, Aitken CK (2009) Markers and risk factors for HCV, HBV and HIV in a network of injecting drug users in Melbourne, Australia. J Infect 58:375–382
249. Falster K, Kaldor JM, Maher L (2009) collaboration of Australian Needle and Syringe Programs. Hepatitis C virus acquisition among injecting drug users: a cohort analysis of a national repeated cross-sectional survey of needle and syringe program attendees in Australia, 1995–2004. J Urban Health. 2009 Jan;86(1):106–118. PubMed PMID: 18979201; PubMed Central PMCID: PMC2629525
250. Maher L, Li J, Jalaludin B et al (2007) Impact of a reduction in heroin availability on patterns of drug use, risk behaviour and incidence of hepatitis C virus infection in injecting drug users in New South Wales, Australia. Drug Acohol Depend 89:244–250

251. Dolan K, Rutter S, Wodak AD (2003) Prison-based syringe exchange programmes: a review of international research and development. Addiction 98:153–158
252. Vallely A, Page A, Dias S et al (2010) The prevalence of sexually transmitted infections in Papua New Guinea: a systematic review and meta-analysis. PLoS One 5:e15586
253. Washington CH, Singer LM, McCaig T et al (2008) The prevalence of HIV infection in women attending antenatal clinics in Fiji. P N G Med J 51:56–59
254. Vanualailai J, Deo A, Sharma B, Chandra S (2003) Nonlinear dynamics of the observed HIV-positive population size in Fiji. Pac Health Dialog 10:45–52
255. Corner H, Rissel C, Smith B et al (2005) Sexual health behaviours among Pacific Island youth in Vanuatu, Tonga and the Federated States of Micronesia. Health Promot J Aus 16:144–150
256. Bushman FD, Nabel GJ, Swanstrom R (2011) HIV: from biology to prevention and treatment, 1st edn. Cold Spring Harbor Laboratory Press, New York
257. Cohen MS, Shaw GM, McMichael AJ, Haynes BF (2011) Acute HIV-1 Infection. N Engl J Med 364:1943–1954
258. Reid SE, Reid CA, Vermund SH (2004) Antiretroviral therapy in sub-Saharan Africa: adherence lessons from tuberculosis and leprosy. Int J STD AIDS 15:713–716
259. Wilen CB, Tilton JC, Doms RW (2012) HIV: cell binding and entry. In: Bushman FD, Nabel GJ, Swanstrom R (eds) HIV: from biology to prevention and treatment, 1st edn. Cold Spring Harbor Laboratory Press, New York, pp 23–32
260. Robertson DL, Anderson JP, Bradac JA et al (2000) HIV-1 nomenclature proposal. Science 288:55–56
261. Kuiken C, Foley B, Leitner T et al (eds) HIV sequence compendium 2010. Theoretical Biology and Biophysics Group, Los Alamos National Laboratory, NM, LA-UR 10-03684, New Mexico
262. Sharp PM, Hahn BH (2010) The evolution of HIV-1 and the origin of AIDS. Biol Sci 365:2487–2494
263. Gao F, Bailes E, Robertson DL et al (1999) Origin of HIV-1 in the chimpanzee Pan troglodytes troglodytes. Nature 397:436–441
264. Kalish ML, Robbins KE, Pieniazek D et al (2004) Recombinant viruses and early global HIV-1 epidemic. Emerg Infect Dis 10:1227–1234
265. Rambaut A, Robertson DL, Pybus OG, Peeters M, Holmes EC (2001) Human immunodeficiency virus. Phylogeny and the origin of HIV-1. Nature 410:1047–1048
266. Novitsky V, Ndung'u T, Wang R et al (2011) Extended high viremics: a substantial fraction of individuals maintain high plasma viral RNA levels after acute HIV-1 subtype C infection. AIDS 25:1515–1522
267. Novitsky V, Wang R, Lagakos S, Essex M (2010) HIV-1 subtype C phylodynamics in the global epidemic. Viruses 2:33–54
268. Hemelaar J, Gouws E, Ghys PD, Osmanov S (2011) WHO-UNAIDS Network for HIV Isolation and Characterisation. Global trends in molecular epidemiology of HIV-1 during 2000–2007. AIDS. 2011 Mar 13;25(5):679–689. PubMed PMID: 21297424
269. Rambaut A, Posada D, Crandall KA, Holmes EC (2004) The causes and consequences of HIV evolution. Nat Rev Genet 5:52–61
270. Veras NM, Gray RR, Brigido LF, Rodrigues R, Salemi M (2011) High-resolution phylogenetics and phylogeography of human immunodeficiency virus type 1 subtype C epidemic in South America. J Gen Virol 92:1698–1709
271. Lewis F, Hughes GJ, Rambaut A, Pozniak A, Leigh Brown AJ (2008) Episodic sexual transmission of HIV revealed by molecular phylodynamics. PLoS Med 5:e50
272. Suchard MA, Weiss RE, Sinsheimer JS (2001) Bayesian selection of continuous-time Markov chain evolutionary models. Mol Biol Evol 18:1001–1013
273. Korber B, Muldoon M, Theiler J et al (2000) Timing the ancestor of the HIV-1 pandemic strains. Science 288:1789–1796
274. Gifford RJ, de Oliveira T, Rambaut A et al (2007) Phylogenetic surveillance of viral genetic diversity and the evolving molecular epidemiology of human immunodeficiency virus type 1. J Virol 81:13050–13056

275. Takebe Y, Liao H, Hase S et al (2010) Reconstructing the epidemic history of HIV-1 circulating recombinant forms CRF07_BC and CRF08_BC in East Asia: the relevance of genetic diversity and phylodynamics for vaccine strategies. Vaccine 28(Suppl 2):B39–B44
276. Hughes GJ, Fearnhill E, Dunn D et al (2009) Molecular phylodynamics of the heterosexual HIV epidemic in the United Kingdom. PLoS Pathog 5:e1000590
277. Deng X, Liu H, Shao Y, Rayner S, Yang R (2008) The epidemic origin and molecular properties of B′: a founder strain of the HIV-1 transmission in Asia. AIDS 22:1851–1858
278. Shafer RW, Rhee SY, Bennett DE (2008) Consensus drug resistance mutations for epidemiological surveillance: basic principles and potential controversies. Antivir Ther 13(Suppl 2):59–68
279. Mitsuya H, Broder S (1987) Strategies for antiviral therapy in AIDS. Nature 325:773–778
280. Broder S (2010) Twenty-five years of translational medicine in antiretroviral therapy: promises to keep. Sci Transl Med 2:39ps3
281. Broder S (2010) The development of antiretroviral therapy and its impact on the HIV-1/AIDS pandemic. Antiviral Res 85:1–18
282. Mitsuya H, Yarchoan R, Kageyama S, Broder S (1991) Targeted therapy of human immunodeficiency virus-related disease. FASEB J 5:2369–2381
283. Maeda K, Mitsuya H (2007) Development of therapeutics for AIDS: structure-based molecular targeting. Tuberculosis 87(Suppl 1):S31–S34
284. Volberding PA, Lagakos SW, Koch MA et al (1990) Zidovudine in asymptomatic human immunodeficiency virus infection. A controlled trial in persons with fewer than 500 CD4-positive cells per cubic millimeter. The AIDS Clinical Trials Group of the National Institute of Allergy and Infectious Diseases. N Engl J Med 322:941–949
285. Fischl MA, Richman DD, Hansen N et al (1990) The safety and efficacy of zidovudine (AZT) in the treatment of subjects with mildly symptomatic human immunodeficiency virus type 1 (HIV) infection. A double-blind, placebo-controlled trial. The AIDS Clinical Trials Group. Ann Intern Med 112:727–737
286. Graham NM, Zeger SL, Park LP et al (1992) The effects on survival of early treatment of human immunodeficiency virus infection. N Engl J Med 326:1037–1042
287. Graham NM, Zeger SL, Park LP et al (1991) Effect of zidovudine and Pneumocystis carinii pneumonia prophylaxis on progression of HIV-1 infection to AIDS. The Multicenter AIDS Cohort Study. Lancet 338:265–269
288. Concorde Coordinating Committee (1994) Concorde: MRC/ANRS randomised double-blind controlled trial of immediate and deferred zidovudine in symptom-free HIV infection. Lancet 343:871–881
289. Volberding PA, Lagakos SW, Grimes JM et al (1994) The duration of zidovudine benefit in persons with asymptomatic HIV infection. Prolonged evaluation of protocol 019 of the AIDS Clinical Trials Group. JAMA 272:437–442
290. Vella S, Giuliano M, Dally LG et al (1994) Long-term follow-up of zidovudine therapy in asymptomatic HIV infection: results of a multicenter cohort study. The Italian Zidovudine Evaluation Group. J Acquir Immune Defic Syndr 7:31–38
291. Gardner LI, Harrison SH, Hendrix CW et al (1998) Size and duration of zidovudine benefit in 1003 HIV-infected patients: U.S. Army, Navy, and Air Force natural history data. Military Medical Consortium for Applied Retroviral Research. J Acquir Immune Defic Syndr 17:345–353
292. Simberkoff MS, Hartigan PM, Hamilton JD et al (1996) Long-term follow-up of symptomatic HIV-infected patients originally randomized to early versus later zidovudine treatment; report of a Veterans Affairs Cooperative Study. VA Cooperative Study Group on AIDS Treatment. J Acquir Immune Defic Syndr 11:142–150
293. Ioannidis JP, Cappelleri JC, Lau J et al (1995) Early or deferred zidovudine therapy in HIV-infected patients without an AIDS-defining illness. Ann Intern Med 122:856–866
294. Volberding PA, Lagakos SW, Grimes JM et al (1995) A comparison of immediate with deferred zidovudine therapy for asymptomatic HIV-infected adults with CD4 cell counts of 500 or more per cubic millimeter. AIDS Clinical Trials Group. N Engl J Med 333:401–407

295. Cooper DA, Gatell JM, Kroon S et al (1993) Zidovudine in persons with asymptomatic HIV infection and CD4+ cell counts greater than 400 per cubic millimeter. The European-Australian Collaborative Group. N Engl J Med 329:297–303
296. Thompson MA, Aberg JA, Cahn P et al (2010) Antiretroviral treatment of adult HIV infection: 2010 recommendations of the International AIDS Society-USA panel. JAMA 304:321–333
297. Dionisio D, Gass R, McDermott P et al (2007) What strategies to boost production of affordable fixed-dose anti-retroviral drug combinations for children in the developing world? Curr HIV Res 5:155–187
298. Holmes CB, Coggin W, Jamieson D et al (2010) Use of generic antiretroviral agents and cost savings in PEPFAR treatment programs. JAMA 304:313–320
299. Marques UR, Guimaraes VS, Sternberg C (2005) Brazil's AIDS controversy: antiretroviral drugs, breaking patents, and compulsory licensing. Food Drug Law J 60:471–477
300. Waning B, Kyle M, Diedrichsen E et al (2010) Intervening in global markets to improve access to HIV/AIDS treatment: an analysis of international policies and the dynamics of global antiretroviral medicines markets. Global Health 6:9
301. Parra J, Portilla J, Pulido F et al (2011) Clinical utility of maraviroc. Clin Drug Invest 31:527–542
302. Nel A, Kagee A (2011) Common mental health problems and antiretroviral therapy adherence. AIDS Care 23:1360–1365
303. Gonzalez A, Barinas J, O'Cleirigh C (2011) Substance use: impact on adherence and HIV medical treatment. Curr HIV/AIDS Rep 8:223–234
304. Blashill AJ, Perry N, Safren SA (2011) Mental health: a focus on stress, coping, and mental illness as it relates to treatment retention, adherence, and other health outcomes. Curr HIV/AIDS Rep 8:215–222
305. Meyer JP, Springer SA, Altice FL (2011) Substance abuse, violence, and HIV in women: a literature review of the syndemic. J Women's Health 20:991–1006
306. Altice FL, Kamarulzaman A, Soriano VV, Schechter M, Friedland GH (2010) Treatment of medical, psychiatric, and substance-use comorbidities in people infected with HIV who use drugs. Lancet 376:367–387
307. Bravo P, Edwards A, Rollnick S, Elwyn G (2010) Tough decisions faced by people living with HIV: a literature review of psychosocial problems. AIDS Rev 12:76–88
308. Shuper PA, Neuman M, Kanteres F, Baliunas D, Joharchi N, Rehm J (2010) Causal considerations on alcohol and HIV/AIDS–a systematic review. Alcohol Alcohol 45:159–166
309. Kresina TF, Bruce RD, McCance-Katz EF (2009) Medication assisted treatment in the treatment of drug abuse and dependence in HIV/AIDS infected drug users. Curr HIV Res 7:354–364
310. Fuller BE, Loftis JM, Rodriguez VL, McQuesten MJ, Hauser P (2009) Psychiatric and substance use disorders comorbidities in veterans with hepatitis C virus and HIV coinfection. Curr Opin Psychiatry 22:401–408
311. Pence BW (2009) The impact of mental health and traumatic life experiences on antiretroviral treatment outcomes for people living with HIV/AIDS. J Antimicrob Chemother 63:636–640
312. Stirratt MJ, Gordon CM (2008) Adherence to biomedical HIV prevention methods: considerations drawn from HIV treatment adherence research. Curr HIV/AIDS Rep 5:186–192
313. Whetten K, Reif S, Whetten R, Murphy-McMillan LK (2008) Trauma, mental health, distrust, and stigma among HIV-positive persons: implications for effective care. Psychosom Med 70:531–538
314. Hartzell JD, Janke IE, Weintrob AC (2008) Impact of depression on HIV outcomes in the HAART era. J Antimicrob Chemother 62:246–255
315. Ingersoll KS, Cohen J (2008) The impact of medication regimen factors on adherence to chronic treatment: a review of literature. J Behav Med 31:213–224
316. Remien RH, Mellins CA (2007) Long-term psychosocial challenges for people living with HIV: let's not forget the individual in our global response to the pandemic. AIDS 21 (Suppl 5):S55–S63

317. Patel V, Araya R, Chatterjee S et al (2007) Treatment and prevention of mental disorders in low-income and middle-income countries. Lancet 370:991–1005
318. Conway B (2007) The role of adherence to antiretroviral therapy in the management of HIV infection. J Acquir Immune Defic Syndr 45(Suppl 1):S14–S18
319. Olatunji BO, Mimiaga MJ, O'Cleirigh C, Safren SA (2006) Review of treatment studies of depression in HIV. Top HIV Med 14:112–124
320. Springer SA, Altice FL (2005) Managing HIV/AIDS in correctional settings. Curr HIV/AIDS Rep 2:165–170
321. Chander G, Himelhoch S, Moore RD (2006) Substance abuse and psychiatric disorders in HIV-positive patients: epidemiology and impact on antiretroviral therapy. Drugs 66:769–789
322. Lauby JL, Marks G, Bingham T et al (2012) Having supportive social relationships is associated with reduced risk of unrecognized HIV infection among black and Latino men who have sex with men. AIDS Behav 16:508–515
323. Millett GA, Ding H, Marks G et al (2011) Mistaken assumptions and missed opportunities: correlates of undiagnosed HIV infection among black and Latino men who have sex with men. J Acquir Immune Defic Syndr 58:64–71
324. Reisner SL, Mimiaga MJ, Bland S et al (2010) Problematic alcohol use and HIV risk among Black men who have sex with men in Massachusetts. AIDS Care 22:577–587
325. Mimiaga MJ, Reisner SL, Fontaine YM et al (2010) Walking the line: stimulant use during sex and HIV risk behavior among Black urban MSM. Drug Alcohol Depend 110:30–37
326. Mimiaga MJ, Reisner SL, Bland S et al (2009) Health system and personal barriers resulting in decreased utilization of HIV and STD testing services among at-risk black men who have sex with men in Massachusetts. AIDS Patient Care STDS 23:825–835
327. Reisner SL, Mimiaga MJ, Skeer M et al (2009) Clinically significant depressive symptoms as a risk factor for HIV infection among black MSM in Massachusetts. AIDS Behav 13: 798–810
328. Bond L, Wheeler DP, Millett GA, LaPollo AB, Carson LF, Liau A (2009) Black men who have sex with men and the association of down-low identity with HIV risk behavior. Am J Public Health 99(Suppl 1):S92–S95
329. Lauby JL, Millett GA, LaPollo AB, Bond L, Murrill CS, Marks G (2008) Sexual risk behaviors of HIV-positive, HIV-negative, and serostatus-unknown Black men who have sex with men and women. Arch Sex Behav 37:708–719
330. DeLaMora P, Aledort N, Stavola J (2006) Caring for adolescents with HIV. Curr HIV/AIDS Rep 3:74–78
331. Reisner SL, Mimiaga MJ, Skeer M, Perkovich B, Johnson CV, Safren SA (2009) A review of HIV antiretroviral adherence and intervention studies among HIV-infected youth. Top HIV Med 17:14–25
332. Dowshen N, D'Angelo L (2011) Health care transition for youth living with HIV/AIDS. Pediatrics 128:762–771
333. Koenig LJ, Nesheim S, Abramowitz S (2011) Adolescents with perinatally acquired HIV: emerging behavioral and health needs for long-term survivors. Curr Opin Obstet Gynecol 23:321–327
334. Murphy DA, Moscicki AB, Vermund SH, Muenz LR (2000) Psychological distress among HIV(+) adolescents in the REACH study: effects of life stress, social support, and coping. The Adolescent Medicine HIV/AIDS Research Network. J Adolesc Health 27: 391–398
335. Murphy DA, Durako SJ, Moscicki AB et al (2001) No change in health risk behaviors over time among HIV infected adolescents in care: role of psychological distress. J Adolesc Health 29:57–63
336. Vermund SH, Wilson CM, Rogers AS, Partlow C, Moscicki AB (2001) Sexually transmitted infections among HIV infected and HIV uninfected high-risk youth in the REACH study. Reaching for Excellence in Adolescent Care and Health. J Adolesc Health 29: 49–56

337. Murphy DA, Mitchell R, Vermund SH, Futterman D, Adolescent Medicine HIVARN (2002) Factors associated with HIV testing among HIV-positive and HIV-negative high-risk adolescents: the REACH Study. Reaching for Excellence in Adolescent Care and Health. Pediatrics 110:e36
338. Yanagisawa S, Poudel KC, Jimba M (2010) Sibling caregiving among children orphaned by AIDS: synthesis of recent studies for policy implications. Health Policy 98:121–130
339. Zhao G, Li X, Fang X, Zhao J, Yang H, Stanton B (2007) Care arrangements, grief and psychological problems among children orphaned by AIDS in China. AIDS Care 19:1075–1082
340. Bhargava A, Bigombe B (2003) Public policies and the orphans of AIDS in Africa. BMJ 326:1387–1389
341. Vaz LM, Maman S, Eng E, Barbarin OA, Tshikandu T, Behets F (2011) Patterns of Disclosure of HIV Status to Infected Children in a Sub-Saharan African Setting. J Dev Behav Pediatr. 2011 Feb 11. [Epub ahead of print] PubMed PMID: 21317803; PubMed Central PMCID: PMC3128187
342. Vaz LM, Eng E, Maman S, Tshikandu T, Behets F (2010) Telling children they have HIV: lessons learned from findings of a qualitative study in sub-Saharan Africa. AIDS Patient Care STDS 24:247–256
343. Corneli A, Vaz L, Dulyx J, Omba S, Rennie S, Behets F (2009) The role of disclosure in relation to assent to participate in HIV-related research among HIV-infected youth: a formative study. J Int AIDS Soc 12:17
344. Vaz L, Corneli A, Dulyx J et al (2008) The process of HIV status disclosure to HIV-positive youth in Kinshasa, Democratic Republic of the Congo. AIDS Care 20:842–852
345. Walensky RP, Paltiel AD, Losina E et al (2006) The survival benefits of AIDS treatment in the United States. J Infect Dis 194:11–19
346. Vermund SH (2006) Millions of life-years saved with potent antiretroviral drugs in the United States: a celebration, with challenges. J Infect Dis 194:1–5
347. Lundgren JD, Mocroft A (2006) The impact of antiretroviral therapy on AIDS and survival. J HIV Ther 11:36–38
348. McCoy D, Chopra M, Loewenson R et al (2005) Expanding access to antiretroviral therapy in sub-saharan Africa: avoiding the pitfalls and dangers, capitalizing on the opportunities. Am J Public Health 95:18–22
349. Schwartlander B, Grubb I, Perriens J (2006) The 10-year struggle to provide antiretroviral treatment to people with HIV in the developing world. Lancet 368:541–546
350. Ojikutu B (2007) Introduction: the realities of antiretroviral therapy rollout: overcoming challenges to successful programmatic implementation. J Infect Dis 196(Suppl 3): S445–S448
351. Rosen S, Sanne I, Collier A, Simon JL (2005) Rationing antiretroviral therapy for HIV/AIDS in Africa: choices and consequences. PLoS Med 2:e303
352. Lamptey P, Wilson D (2005) Scaling up AIDS treatment: what is the potential impact and what are the risks? PLoS Med 2:e39
353. Vermund SH, Sidat M, Weil LF et al (2012) Transitioning HIV care and treatment programs in southern Africa to full local management. AIDS 26(10):1303–1310
354. Moon TD, Burlison JR, Sidat M et al (2010) Lessons Learned while Implementing an HIV/AIDs care and treatment program in rural Mozambique. Retrovir Res Treat 3:1–14
355. Menzies NA, Berruti AA, Berzon R et al (2011) The cost of providing comprehensive HIV treatment in PEPFAR-supported programs. AIDS 25:1753–1760
356. Filler SJ, Berruti AA, Menzies N et al (2011) Characteristics of HIV care and treatment in PEPFAR-supported sites. J Acquir Immune Defic Syndr 57:e1–e6
357. Stringer JS, Zulu I, Levy J et al (2006) Rapid scale-up of antiretroviral therapy at primary care sites in Zambia: feasibility and early outcomes. JAMA 296:782–793
358. Banda Y, Chapman V, Goldenberg RL et al (2007) Use of traditional medicine among pregnant women in Lusaka, Zambia. J Altern Complement Med 13:123–127
359. Klausner JD, Serenata C, O'Bra H et al (2011) Scale-up and continuation of antiretroviral therapy in South African treatment programs, 2005-2009. J Acquir Immune Defic Syndr 56:292–295

360. Biesma RG, Brugha R, Harmer A, Walsh A, Spicer N, Walt G (2009) The effects of global health initiatives on country health systems: a review of the evidence from HIV/AIDS control. Health Policy Plan 24:239–252
361. Abimiku AG, Institute of Human Virology UoMSoMPP (2009) Building laboratory infrastructure to support scale-up of HIV/AIDS treatment, care, and prevention: in-country experience. Am J Clin Pathol 131:875–886
362. Yiannoutsos CT, An MW, Frangakis CE et al (2008) Sampling-based approaches to improve estimation of mortality among patient dropouts: experience from a large PEPFAR-funded program in Western Kenya. PLoS One 3:e3843
363. Schoni-Affolter F, Keiser O, Mwango A et al (2011) Estimating loss to follow-up in HIV-infected patients on antiretroviral therapy: the effect of the competing risk of death in Zambia and Swaziland. PLoS One 6:e27919
364. Moon TD, Burlison JR, Blevins M et al (2011) Enrolment and programmatic trends and predictors of antiretroviral therapy initiation from president's emergency plan for AIDS Relief (PEPFAR)-supported public HIV care and treatment sites in rural Mozambique. Int J STD AIDS 22:621–627
365. Groh K, Audet CM, Baptista A et al (2011) Barriers to antiretroviral therapy adherence in rural Mozambique. BMC Public Health 11:650
366. Cook RE, Ciampa PJ, Sidat M et al (2011) Predictors of successful early infant diagnosis of HIV in a rural district hospital in Zambezia, Mozambique. J Acquir Immune Defic Syndr 56:e104–e109
367. Koethe JR, Limbada MI, Giganti MJ et al (2010) Early immunologic response and subsequent survival among malnourished adults receiving antiretroviral therapy in Urban Zambia. AIDS 24:2117–2121
368. Giganti MJ, Levy JW, Banda Y et al (2010) Methods and baseline results of a repeated cross-sectional survey to assess the public health impact of antiretroviral therapy in Lusaka, Zambia. Am J Trop Med Hyg 82:971–977
369. Chi BH, Cantrell RA, Mwango A et al (2010) An empirical approach to defining loss to follow-up among patients enrolled in antiretroviral treatment programs. Am J Epidemiol 171:924–931
370. Morris MB, Chapula BT, Chi BH et al (2009) Use of task-shifting to rapidly scale-up HIV treatment services: experiences from Lusaka, Zambia. BMC Health Serv Res 9:5
371. Krebs DW, Chi BH, Mulenga Y et al (2008) Community-based follow-up for late patients enrolled in a district-wide programme for antiretroviral therapy in Lusaka, Zambia. AIDS Care 20:311–317
372. Mahajan AP, Sayles JN, Patel VA et al (2008) Stigma in the HIV/AIDS epidemic: a review of the literature and recommendations for the way forward. AIDS 22(Suppl 2):S67–S79
373. Whitmore SK, Zhang X, Taylor AW, Blair JM (2011) Estimated number of infants born to HIV-infected women in the United States and five dependent areas, 2006. J Acquir Immune Defic Syndr 57(3):218–222
374. Whitmore SK, Patel-Larson A, Espinoza L, Ruffo NM, Rao S (2010) Missed opportunities to prevent perinatal human immunodeficiency virus transmission in 15 jurisdictions in the United States during 2005-2008. Women Health 50:414–425
375. Birkhead GS, Pulver WP, Warren BL, Hackel S, Rodriguez D, Smith L (2010) Acquiring human immunodeficiency virus during pregnancy and mother-to-child transmission in New York: 2002-2006. Obstet Gynecol 115:1247–1255
376. Centers for Disease Control and Prevention (CDC) (2010) Racial/ethnic disparities among children with diagnoses of perinatal HIV infection – 34 states, 2004–2007. MMWR Morb Mortal Wkly Rep 59:97–101. Erratum in: MMWR Morb Mortal Wkly Rep. 2010 Feb 12;59(5):136. PubMed PMID: 20134398
377. Dwyre DM, Fernando LP, Holland PV (2011) Hepatitis B, hepatitis C and HIV transfusion-transmitted infections in the 21st century. Vox Sang 100:92–98
378. Barth RE, Huijgen Q, Taljaard J, Hoepelman AI (2010) Hepatitis B/C and HIV in sub-Saharan Africa: an association between highly prevalent infectious diseases. A systematic review and meta-analysis. Int J Infect Dis 14:e1024–e1031

379. Mahy M, Warner-Smith M, Stanecki KA, Ghys PD (2009) Measuring the impact of the global response to the AIDS epidemic: challenges and future directions. J Acquir Immune Defic Syndr 52(Suppl 2):S152–S159
380. Xvi PB, Seewald P (2010) Light of the world: the Pope, the Church, and the Signs of the Times, 1st edn. Ignatius Press, San Francisco
381. Koblin BA, Chesney MA, Husnik MJ et al (2003) High-risk behaviors among men who have sex with men in 6 US cities: baseline data from the EXPLORE Study. Am J Public Health 93:926–932
382. Chesney MA, Koblin BA, Barresi PJ et al (2003) An individually tailored intervention for HIV prevention: baseline data from the EXPLORE Study. Am J Public Health 93:933–938
383. Koblin B, Chesney M, Coates T (2004) Effects of a behavioural intervention to reduce acquisition of HIV infection among men who have sex with men: the EXPLORE randomised controlled study. Lancet 364:41–50
384. Colfax G, Vittinghoff E, Husnik MJ et al (2004) Substance use and sexual risk: a participant- and episode-level analysis among a cohort of men who have sex with men. Am J Epidemiol 159:1002–1012
385. Colfax G, Coates TJ, Husnik MJ et al (2005) Longitudinal patterns of methamphetamine, popper (amyl nitrite), and cocaine use and high-risk sexual behavior among a cohort of San Francisco men who have sex with men. J Urban Health 82:i62–i70
386. Salomon EA, Mimiaga MJ, Husnik MJ et al (2009) Depressive symptoms, utilization of mental health care, substance use and sexual risk among young men who have sex with men in EXPLORE: implications for age-specific interventions. AIDS Behav 13:811–821
387. El-Bassel N, Gilbert L, Witte S, Wu E, Hunt T, Remien RH (2010) Couple-based HIV prevention in the United States: advantages, gaps, and future directions. J Acquir Immune Defic Syndr 55(Suppl 2):S98–S101
388. Crawford ND, Vlahov D (2010) Progress in HIV reduction and prevention among injection and noninjection drug users. J Acquir Immune Defic Syndr 55(Suppl 2):S84–S87
389. Read JS (2010) Prevention of mother-to-child transmission of HIV: antiretroviral strategies. Clin Perinatol 37:765–776
390. Cohen MS, Gay CL, Busch MP, Hecht FM (2010) The detection of acute HIV infection. J Infect Dis 202(Suppl 2):S270–S277
391. Reynolds SJ, Quinn TC (2010) Setting the stage: current state of affairs and major challenges. Clin Infect Dis 50(Suppl 3):S71–S76
392. DeGruttola V, Smith DM, Little SJ, Miller V (2010) Developing and evaluating comprehensive HIV infection control strategies: issues and challenges. Clin Infect Dis 50(Suppl 3):S102–S107
393. Buchbinder S (2009) The epidemiology of new HIV infections and interventions to limit HIV transmission. Top HIV Med 17:37–43
394. Rotheram-Borus MJ, Swendeman D, Chovnick G (2009) The past, present, and future of HIV prevention: integrating behavioral, biomedical, and structural intervention strategies for the next generation of HIV prevention. Annu Rev Clin Psychol 5:143–167
395. Barrow RY, Berkel C, Brooks LC, Groseclose SL, Johnson DB, Valentine JA (2008) Traditional sexually transmitted disease prevention and control strategies: tailoring for African American communities. Sex Transm Dis 35:S30–S39
396. Margaret Dolcini M, Gandelman AA, Vogan SA et al (2010) Translating HIV interventions into practice: community-based organizations' experiences with the diffusion of effective behavioral interventions (DEBIs). Soc Sci Med 71:1839–1846
397. Harshbarger C, Simmons G, Coelho H, Sloop K, Collins C (2006) An empirical assessment of implementation, adaptation, and tailoring: the evaluation of CDC's national diffusion of VOICES/VOCES. AIDS Educ Prev 18:184–197
398. Wingood GM, DiClemente RJ (2006) Enhancing adoption of evidence-based HIV interventions: promotion of a suite of HIV prevention interventions for African American women. AIDS Educ Prev 18:161–170

399. Collins C, Harshbarger C, Sawyer R, Hamdallah M (2006) The diffusion of effective behavioral interventions project: development, implementation, and lessons learned. AIDS Educ Prev 18:5–20
400. Lyles CM, Crepaz N, Herbst JH, Kay LS (2006) Evidence-based HIV behavioral prevention from the perspective of the CDC's HIV/AIDS Prevention Research Synthesis Team. AIDS Educ Prev 18:21–31
401. Ott MA, Santelli JS (2007) Abstinence and abstinence-only education. Curr Opin Obstet Gynecol 19:446–452
402. Kohler PK, Manhart LE, Lafferty WE (2008) Abstinence-only and comprehensive sex education and the initiation of sexual activity and teen pregnancy. J Adolesc Health 42:344–351
403. Trenholm C, Devaney B, Fortson K, Clark M, Bridgespan LQ, Wheeler J (2008) Impacts of abstinence education on teen sexual activity, risk of pregnancy, and risk of sexually transmitted diseases. J Policy Anal Manage 27:255–276
404. Dworkin SL, Ehrhardt AA (2007) Going beyond "ABC" to include "GEM": critical reflections on progress in the HIV/AIDS epidemic. Am J Public Health 97:13–18
405. Kurth AE, Celum C, Baeten JM, Vermund SH, Wasserheit JN (2011) Combination HIV prevention: significance, challenges, and opportunities. Curr HIV/AIDS Rep 8:62–72
406. Glasgow RE, Vogt TM, Boles SM (1999) Evaluating the public health impact of health promotion interventions: the RE-AIM framework. Am J Public Health 89:1322–1327
407. Auvert B, Taljaard D, Lagarde E, Sobngwi-Tambekou J, Sitta R, Puren A (2005) Randomized, controlled intervention trial of male circumcision for reduction of HIV infection risk: the ANRS 1265 trial. PLoS Med 2:e298
408. Bailey RC, Moses S, Parker CB et al (2007) Male circumcision for HIV prevention in young men in Kisumu, Kenya: a randomised controlled trial. Lancet 369:643–656
409. Gray RH, Kigozi G, Serwadda D et al (2007) Male circumcision for HIV prevention in men in Rakai, Uganda: a randomised trial. Lancet 369:657–666
410. Connor EM, Sperling RS, Gelber R et al (1994) Reduction of maternal-infant transmission of human immunodeficiency virus type 1 with zidovudine treatment. Pediatric AIDS Clinical Trials Group Protocol 076 Study Group. N Engl J Med 331:1173–1180
411. Fideli US, Allen SA, Musonda R et al (2001) Virologic and immunologic determinants of heterosexual transmission of human immunodeficiency virus type 1 in Africa. AIDS Res Hum Retroviruses 17:901–910
412. Quinn TC, Wawer MJ, Sewankambo N et al (2000) Viral load and heterosexual transmission of human immunodeficiency virus type 1 Rakai Project Study Group. N Engl J Med 342:921–929
413. Korenromp EL, White RG, Orroth KK et al (2005) Determinants of the impact of sexually transmitted infection treatment on prevention of HIV infection: a synthesis of evidence from the Mwanza, Rakai, and Masaka intervention trials. J Infect Dis 191(Suppl 1):S168–S178
414. Abdool Karim Q, Abdool Karim SS, Frohlich JA et al (2010) Effectiveness and safety of tenofovir gel, an antiretroviral microbicide, for the prevention of HIV infection in women. Science 329:1168–1174
415. Grant RM, Lama JR, Anderson PL et al (2010) Preexposure chemoprophylaxis for HIV prevention in men who have sex with men. N Engl J Med 363:2587–2599
416. Celum C, Baeten JM (2012) Tenofovir-based pre-exposure prophylaxis for HIV prevention: evolving evidence. Curr Opin Infect Dis 25:51–57
417. Krakower D, Mayer KH (2011) Promising prevention approaches: tenofovir gel and prophylactic use of antiretroviral medications. Curr HIV/AIDS Rep 8:241–248
418. Rerks-Ngarm S, Pitisuttithum P, Nitayaphan S et al (2009) Vaccination with ALVAC and AIDSVAX to prevent HIV-1 infection in Thailand. N Engl J Med 361:2209–2220
419. Johnston MI, Fauci AS (2011) HIV vaccine development–improving on natural immunity. N Engl J Med 365:873–875
420. Denison JA, O'Reilly KR, Schmid GP, Kennedy CE, Sweat MD (2008) HIV voluntary counseling and testing and behavioral risk reduction in developing countries: a meta-analysis, 1990–2005. AIDS Behav 12:363–373

421. Allen S, Tice J, Van de Perre P et al (1992) Effect of serotesting with counselling on condom use and seroconversion among HIV discordant couples in Africa. BMJ 304:1605–1609
422. Wilson D, Halperin DT (2008) "Know your epidemic, know your response": a useful approach, if we get it right. Lancet 372:423–426
423. Khumalo-Sakutukwa G, Morin SF, Fritz K et al (2008) Project Accept (HPTN 043): a community-based intervention to reduce HIV incidence in populations at risk for HIV in sub-Saharan Africa and Thailand. J Acquir Immune Defic Syndr 49:422–431
424. Sweat M, Morin S, Celentano D et al (2011) Community-based intervention to increase HIV testing and case detection in people aged 16-32 years in Tanzania, Zimbabwe, and Thailand (NIMH Project Accept, HPTN 043): a randomised study. Lancet Infect Dis 11:525–532
425. Stoneburner RL, Low-Beer D (2004) Sexual partner reductions explain human immunodeficiency virus declines in Uganda: comparative analyses of HIV and behavioural data in Uganda, Kenya, Malawi, and Zambia. Int J Epidemiol 33:624
426. Bunnell R, Cherutich P (2008) Universal HIV testing and counselling in Africa. Lancet 371:2148–2150
427. Renaud-Thery FDC, Ken S, Thierry S, Perriens J (2010) Adult antiretroviral therapy in resource limited settings: a systematic review of first-line treatment failure and attrition rates. In: 17th conference on retroviruses and opportunistic Infections, San Francisco, CA
428. Bunnell R, Ekwaru JP, Solberg P et al (2006) Changes in sexual behavior and risk of HIV transmission after antiretroviral therapy and prevention interventions in rural Uganda. AIDS 20:85–92
429. Vandenbruaene M (2007) Interview: King Kennard Holmes–chair of the Department of Global Health of the University of Washington. Lancet Infect Dis 7:516–520
430. Wagner B, Blower S (2010) Costs of eliminating HIV in South Africa have been underestimated. Lancet 376:953–954
431. Wilson DP, Blower SM (2005) Designing equitable antiretroviral allocation strategies in resource-constrained countries. PLoS Med 2:e50
432. Wagner BG, Kahn JS, Blower S (2010) Should we try to eliminate HIV epidemics by using a 'Test and Treat' strategy? AIDS 24:775–776

Chapter 2
Multidrug-Resistant Bacteria: The Emerging Crisis

Daniel Livorsi*, Edward Stenehjem*, and Robert Gaynes

2.1 Introduction

Over the past 50 years, significant advances in drug development, surgical techniques, medical therapy, and device manufacturing have propelled the field of medicine to new heights. Organ transplantation is more common and successful than ever; patients with HIV are able to maintain stable immune function with one pill a day; critical care monitoring has never been so advanced; and chronic medical conditions are treated effectively with a wide variety of medical options. Managing complex patients like these would be nearly impossible without the use of effective antimicrobial therapy to treat inevitable infections. These advancements, however, are actively being threatened by an increase in multidrug-resistant organisms (MDROs). Without urgent action and increased education, MDROs have the potential to reverse decades of medical innovation.

Although the term is used frequently, MDROs do not have a universal definition. A MDRO must be resistant to at least one class of antimicrobials but, more commonly, are resistant to most classes of antibiotics available. Among the gram-positive organisms, methicillin-resistant *Staphylococcus aureus* (MRSA) and vancomycin-resistant *Enterococcus faecium* (VRE) represent the greatest therapeutic challenges. The adaptive power of *S. aureus* became clear in the 1960s when the

---

*The authors Daniel Livorsi and Edward Stenehjem have equally contributed.

D. Livorsi, M.D. (✉) • E. Stenehjem, M.D. • R. Gaynes, M.D.
Division of Infectious Diseases, Department of Medicine,
Emory University School of Medicine, Atlanta, GA, USA

Atlanta VA Medical Center,
1670 Clairmont Ave, Atlanta, GA 30033, USA
e-mail: dlivorsi@alumni.rice.edu

I.W. Fong (ed.), *Challenges in Infectious Diseases*, Emerging Infectious Diseases of the 21st Century 502, DOI 10.1007/978-1-4614-4496-1_2,

first cases of MRSA were identified. Since 1960, *S. aureus* has developed resistance to β-lactam compounds, and now, more than 50% of the *S. aureus* isolates recovered in United States (US) hospitals are methicillin-resistant [1, 2]. Compared to MRSA, VRE is less virulent but poses significant therapeutic challenges. Many *E. faecium* isolates in US critical care units are now resistant to vancomycin, ampicillin, and/or aminoglycosides. The changing epidemiology and the high-level resistance in these organisms leave clinicians few options when treating life-threatening VRE infections.

Over the past 10 years, the medical community has seen the development of several antibiotics active against resistant gram-positive organisms, including linezolid, daptomycin, tigecycline, quinupristin-dalfopristin, telavancin, and ceftaroline. These agents have expanded treatment options but also have their limitations. Resistance to each one has been observed in individuals not previously exposed to antibiotics. Future study on the efficacy of these agents and careful monitoring of the molecular epidemiology of the resistance mechanisms is of high priority.

The state of multidrug-resistant gram-positive organisms is now being overshadowed by the emergence of resistant gram-negative pathogens. In contrast to gram-positive organisms, the pharmaceutical pipeline for antibiotics active against MDR gram-negative organisms is dry with no new medications in advanced stages of clinical development. Due to this emergence of highly resistant pathogens, clinicians have been forced to use antibiotics with known significant toxicities and poorly studied benefits.

Initially, clinicians were accustomed to seeing significant resistance in a few known gram-negative pathogens, specifically *Pseudomonas aeruginosa* and *Acinetobacter baumannii*. Now, high-level resistance has spread to members of the *Enterobacteriaceae* family and caused significant treatment challenges in both hospitalized and community patients. The production of extended-spectrum β-lactamases (ESBLs) is common in the *Enterobacteriaceae* family and has resulted in many clinicians using carbapenems as first-line therapy for these infections.

The medical community has become accustomed to carbapenems being active against most, if not all, gram-negative infections. This trend, however, is changing rapidly. Through multiple mechanisms, gram-negative organisms have become resistant to the carbapenems and have been responsible for multiple hospital outbreaks. Case reports of carbapenem-resistant *K. pneumoniae* (CRKP) were first identified in the USA in 1996 [3] and were followed shortly by an outbreak in New York City in 2003 [4]. Of growing concern is the discovery of a new mechanism of carbapenem resistance mediated by the New Delhi metallo-β-lactamase enzyme (NDM-1) [5]. First identified in India, isolates containing NDM-1 have also been identified in other countries, including the USA [6].

Although the majority of pathogens causing human disease remain sensitive to our standard antimicrobials, a group of pathogens have *escaped* our first-line therapies and account for the majority of resistance problems in the modern hospital. This group of organisms, referred to as the ESKAPE organisms, consists of *E. faecium, S. aureus, K. pneumoniae, A. baumannii, P. aeruginosa,* and *Enterobacter* species. The ESKAPE organisms cause the majority of multidrug-resistant infections, cause significant morbidity and mortality, and will be the focus of this review.

2.2 Clinical Significance of MDROs

Infections due to MDROs have a significant negative impact on morbidity, mortality, and hospital expenditures [7–10]. This negative impact is likely due to increased virulence of the pathogen, delay in appropriate antibiotic therapy, and predisposing host factors. Determining how these factors influence the outcome of infections is challenging and an area of active research.

2.2.1 MRSA

Resistance to methicillin is not the only difference between MRSA and methicillin-sensitive *S. aureus* (MSSA) isolates. Through unclear mechanisms, patients colonized with MRSA develop more subsequent infections with the colonizing strain than patients colonized with MSSA [11]. In addition, higher case fatality rates have been seen with MRSA bacteremia [12, 13], post-sternotomy mediastinitis [14], and surgical-site infections [15] when compared to equivalent infections with MSSA. Delays in the administration of appropriate antibiotics, less efficacious antibiotics, and intrinsic characteristics of certain MRSA strains (i.e., Panton-Valentine leukocidin production) may all contribute to worse clinical outcomes.

2.2.2 VRE

Vancomycin-resistant *Enterococcus* (VRE) is associated with worse outcomes than vancomycin-susceptible isolates. A 2005 meta-analysis compared VRE bloodstream infections to vancomycin-sensitive infections using strict inclusion criteria to control for severity of underlying illness. The odds of death in VRE patients was more than twice as high as patients with vancomycin-susceptible infections [16]. In neutropenic patients with VRE bacteremia, an increasing duration of bacteremia was associated with increased mortality [17]. This association suggests that time to appropriate antibiotics is likely a significant factor in determining outcome of bloodstream infections with VRE. In other studies, VRE infection has been associated with increased morbidity, length of stay, and hospital costs [18].

2.2.3 MDR Gram-Negative Bacilli

Gram-negative pathogens play a significant role in hospital-acquired infections and community-acquired urinary tract infections. In the US, gram-negative infections account for 25% of all nosocomial bloodstream infections, and the rate of antibiotic resistance is increasing [19]. Multidrug-resistant gram-negative organisms are also a common cause of ventilator-associated pneumonia [20]. Multiple studies have evaluated the clinical impact of resistance in gram-negative infections. Carbapenem resistance was associated with an increased risk of death in patients with *Acinetobacter* bacteremia [21]. In Israel, ESBL production and a delay in adequate therapy were significant predictors for mortality among patients with *Enterobacteriaceae* bacteremia [22]. Another study found multidrug-resistant *Enterobacter* infections to be associated with increased mortality, hospital stay, and hospital charges [23]. Failure rates and mortality rates were more than doubled in patients with ESBL-positive *K. pneumoniae* bloodstream infections as compared to non-ESBL producers [24].

With growing levels of resistance, clinicians now face difficult decisions when initiating antibiotic therapy for critically ill patients. Appropriate and timely antibiotic therapy has consistently been shown to be a major predictor of survival and outcome in patients with sepsis [25–27]. Knowing the epidemiology of resistance at one's own institution is of paramount importance.

2.3 Economics of Resistance

In many studies, antibiotic resistance is associated with increased morbidity, length of stay, and mortality. Estimates of additional costs of care due to resistant pathogens have ranged from US$7,212 to $98,575 per infection with an additional length of stay between 2 and 15.3 days [28]. This increased cost may, in part, be due to higher pharmaceutical costs, increased duration of hospitalization, increased severity of illness, and need for more invasive procedures and monitoring. In general, sensitive organisms are treated with easily obtainable and standard antimicrobials. Resistant infections, at times, require newer (daptomycin, linezolid) or more toxic antibiotics (quinupristin-dalfopristin, polymyxin B), which can be more expensive. One study suggests that MDR gram-negative infections are significantly more costly than MRSA infections due to increased need for ICU care and monitoring [29]. The economic impact of MDR infections is not the only problem. The overuse of antibiotics can lead to resistance, multiple drug-related complications, fungal superinfections, and development of *Clostridium difficile* colitis.

2.4 Origins of Antibiotic Resistance

The origin of antibiotic resistance has long puzzled scientists. There is now a growing literature describing the interconnectedness of the natural environment and clinical environment and the effect humans have on the microbial ecology.

Environmental bacteria produce a wide array of antibacterial antibiotics and biologically active substances. These antibiotic-producing bacteria have developed resistance mechanisms to avoid self-intoxication from the very antibiotic they produce.

Antibiotic-resistance genes most likely originated in these antibiotic-producing bacteria and have subsequently spread to both nonpathogenic and pathogenic environmental bacteria.

Antibiotic resistance is not limited to pathogenic bacteria [30]. Certain environmental microbes may demonstrate more drug resistance than the bacteria typically associated with disease. There are approximately 5×10^{30} bacteria on the planet; the vast majority are nonpathogenic [31]. These microbes interact with an array of chemicals in the environment produced by other bacteria, fungi, plants, animals, and humans. Living in this environment over centuries, microbes have evolved complex processes for sensing, responding to, and metabolizing small molecules in addition to acquiring the resistance mechanisms found in antibiotic-producing organisms [32].

Researchers have now begun to focus on the antibiotic resistome to serve as a framework to understand the ecology of resistance [33]. The antibiotic resistome consists of all antibiotic-resistance genes in microbes found in free-living environments or as commensals of other organisms. One of the first glimpses of the diversity in the antibiotic resistome came in 2006 with the evaluation of spore-forming bacteria in various soil types. The 480 isolated strains of bacteria were tested against 21 different antibiotics ranging in mechanisms of action and time in clinical use. The investigators found resistance to every antibiotic tested and found the majority of soil strains to be multidrug resistant [34]. Studies from samples obtained deep below the earth's surface have also confirmed multidrug-resistant microbes that have likely never been in contact with human sources of antibiotics [35]. A quantitative study of soil found that the level of antibiotic-resistance genes has increased remarkably from the 1940s to the present, especially among genes that conferred resistance to tetracyclines and β-lactam antibiotics [36]. With baseline measurements prior to the antibiotic era, we have a rare glimpse into how the antibiotic resistome has changed with the addition of antibiotics into the environment. The environment is a rich source of antibiotic-resistance genes. Human activity has likely contributed to the expansion of the environmental resistome with our use of antibiotics in agriculture and medicine [37]. The question remains on how efficiently and under what circumstances genes from the environment can be transferred and successfully incorporated into the resistome of clinically known pathogens. Insight into the connection of these two environments will be critical to the understanding and prediction of future antibiotic resistance.

2.5 Antibiotic Use and Resistance

As discussed above, antibiotic-resistance mechanisms existed prior to the human discovery and clinical use of antibiotics. However, the clinical use of antibiotics has put additional pressure on microorganisms to allow resistant pathogens to thrive and facilitated the spread of multidrug-resistant bacteria in the community and hospital. The causal link between antibiotic use and development of resistance is often difficult to prove because the antibiotic exposure may be far removed from the isolation of the resistant bacteria.

Primary care physicians are responsible for a considerable portion of all antimicrobial prescriptions for urinary tract infections and respiratory infections. A recent meta-analysis of 24 studies evaluated the relationship between the prescription of antibiotics in primary care and the subsequent development of antibiotic resistance. In both urinary tract infections and respiratory infections, antibiotic usage was consistently associated with subsequent antibiotic resistance with an odds ratio of approximately 2.5. Longer duration and multiple courses of antibiotics were associated with higher rates of resistance [38]. A retrospective study in Colorado demonstrated a rise in fluoroquinolone-resistant *E. coli* after an institutional switch from trimethoprim-sulfamethoxazole to levofloxacin for the treatment of acute cystitis. As levofloxacin prescriptions increased, so did resistance rates. In multivariate analysis, hospitalization and previous use of levofloxacin were associated with fluoroquinolone-resistant *E. coli* [39].

The association of broad-spectrum β-lactam use and the development of resistance in gram-negative bacteria has also been studied. The fluctuations in antibiotic prescribing practices in a large community hospital in Germany allowed for a longitudinal analysis of the development of antibiotic resistance among *P. aeruginosa* isolates. In this study, increasing use of imipenem was associated with a dramatic increase in imipenem resistance; implementation of a strategy to limit the use of imipenem resulted in a decline in resistance [40]. Interestingly, the use of piperacillin-tazobactam and ceftazidime showed no association with the development of resistance in *P. aeruginosa,* a result seen in other studies as well [41, 42].

Case-control and cohort studies have also been utilized to evaluate antibiotic use as a risk factor for resistant gram-negative organisms. A recent study found that the risk of infection with carbapenem-resistant *K. pneumoniae* rose with increasing duration of prior treatment with β-lactam/β-lactamase inhibitor combinations, fluoroquinolones, and carbapenems [43]. An international, multisite study found ESBL production in *K. pneumoniae* bacteremias to be associated with the previous administration of β-lactam antibiotics containing an oxyimino group (ceftriaxone, ceftazidime, aztreonam) with a risk ratio of 3.9 [44]. While the majority of trials have found a consistent association between antibiotic use and drug resistance, not all studies have shown a clear association [45–47].

2.6 Mechanisms of Resistance

2.6.1 The Role of Genetic Variability

Antibiotic resistance can develop through a variety of pathways that introduce novel genetic elements into a bacterium's DNA (Fig. 2.1). These genetic changes can stem from internal processes within the bacterium or from external factors.

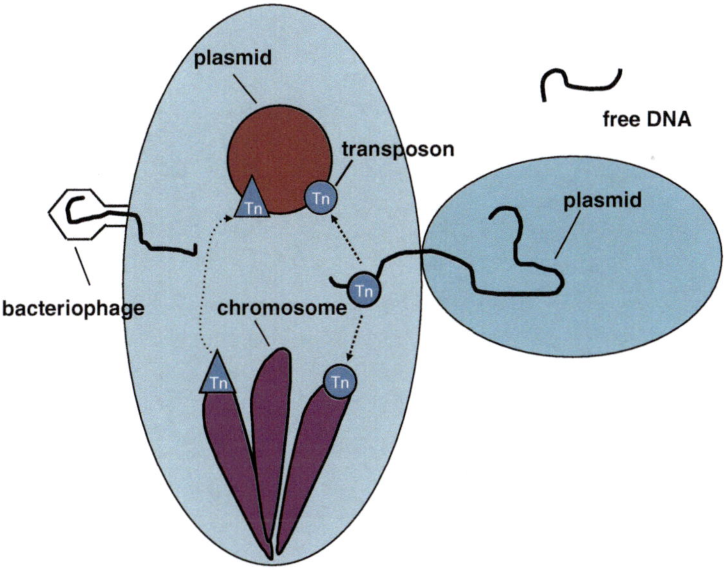

Fig. 2.1 Methods by which bacteria acquire new resistance genes (Used with permission from J. Steinberg)

Spontaneous point mutations in bacterial DNA can produce novel mechanisms of antibiotic resistance. In general, mutations occur at a rate of 10^{-5} to 10^{-9} per base pair per generation. Point mutations at key sequences of some older β-lactamase genes (TEM-1 and SHV-1) led to the emergence of extended-spectrum β-lactamases, or ESBLs [48].

Rearrangements of bacterial DNA can be also generated by mobile genetic elements. Integrons or transposons can move from one point to another within a bacterium's own chromosome or plasmid, thereby rearranging entire segments of the bacterial genome and potentially producing new resistance mechanisms. In addition, resistance genes can spread between different strains of bacteria through the uptake of naked DNA from the surrounding environment (transformation), the transfer of DNA via bacteriophages (transduction), or the exchange of mobile genetic elements, such as plasmids, through direct cell-to-cell contact (conjugation). The *vanA* gene for vancomycin resistance in *S. aureus* (VRSA), for example, was acquired through conjugation with VRE [49].

Bacterial subpopulations with effective resistance mechanisms will become prevalent under selective antibiotic pressure. In general, antibiotic resistance spreads through the dissemination of a successful clone. Strains of MRSA, termed USA 300 and EMRSA-16, are both examples of clones that have spread through vast geographic regions and are now major causes of human disease.

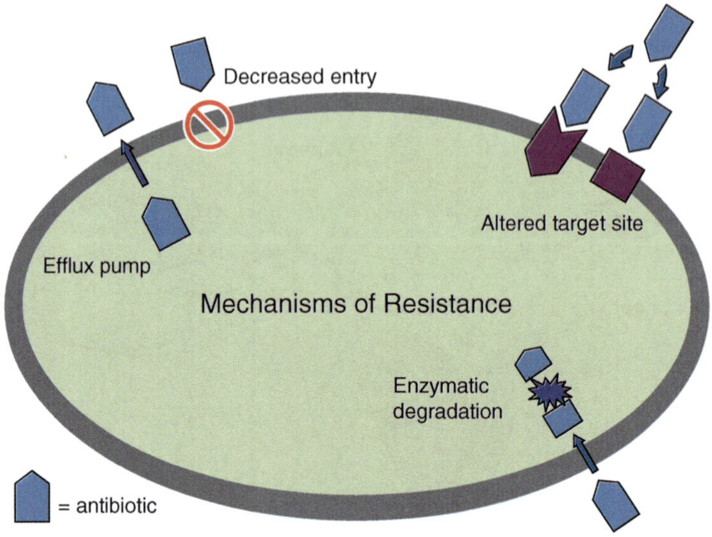

Fig. 2.2 Mechanisms of antibiotic resistance (Used with permission from J. Steinberg)

2.6.2 Mechanisms of Antibiotic Resistance in the ESKAPE Organisms

The ESKAPE organisms use four major resistance mechanisms to survive in the presence of antibiotics (Fig. 2.2). One common mechanism involves the production of an enzyme that inactivates the antibiotic. Aminoglycoside-modifying enzymes (AMEs) are a type of inactivating enzyme found in many bacteria, including *P. aeruginosa* and *A. baumannii*. AMEs phosphorylate, adenylate, or acetylate the aminoglycoside compound to eliminate its antibacterial effect. Like AMEs, β-lactamases also inactivate their substrate antibiotic. β-lactamases achieve this effect by splitting the amide bond of the β-lactam ring. These enzymes are the primary mechanism of resistance to β-lactam antibiotics. To date, hundreds of β-lactamases have been described [50], including the newest β-lactamases: ESBLs and carbapenem-hydrolyzing enzymes (e.g., KPCs, MBLs, and NDM-1). Using the amino acid structure of each enzyme, β-lactamases can be categorized into 4 molecular classes, A–D [51]. Based on their substrate spectrum and their responses to inhibitors, β-lactamases have also been classified into several functional groups [52].

A second mechanism of antibiotic resistance involves modification of the antibiotic's target site. *S. aureus* acquired methicillin resistance through modification of a penicillin-binding protein (PBP), the target site for β-lactam antibiotics. PBP2a, encoded by the *mecA* gene in MRSA, has low affinity for β-lactam antibiotics, which makes the bacteria resistant to nearly all β-lactam agents. Target site modification is an important cause of fluoroquinolone resistance in both gram-negative, for example, *P. aeruginosa*, and gram-positive bacteria, for example, *S. aureus*. Amino acid substitutions in the *gyrA* and *parC* genes modify the binding sites of DNA gyrase and topoisomerase IV, thereby producing fluoroquinolone resistance [53]. Finally, vancomycin resistance in *Enterococcus* also reflects modifications to the antibiotic target site. The *vanA* gene, carried by a plasmid, encodes an inducible protein that synthesizes peptidoglycan precursors with a modified terminus. Instead of the normal D-alanine-D-alanine sequence, *vanA* strains produce D-alanine-D-lactate. Vancomycin binds with less affinity, and high-level vancomycin resistance is produced.

To withstand the pressure of antibiotics, bacteria can prevent antibiotic entry into the bacterial cell, a third mechanism of resistance. The thickened cell wall in vancomycin-intermediate *S. aureus* (VISA) prevents the glycopeptide molecules from reaching their target near the cell membrane [54]. Changes to some bacteria's outer membrane proteins, or porins, result in diminished antibiotic transport into the periplasmic space and, in turn, diminished access to antibiotic target sites. In *P. aeruginosa*, the most common cause of imipenem resistance occurs via a mutational loss of a specific outer membrane protein, OprD [55]. Carbapenem resistance in *A. baumannii* has also been linked to the loss of porin channels [56].

Efflux of an antibiotic is the fourth mechanism of resistance. These efflux pumps, which are categorized into five superfamilies, use active transport to move the antibiotic molecule out of the bacterial cell. Multidrug efflux pumps, such as the MexAB-OprM system, are frequently expressed in multidrug-resistant *P. aeruginosa* [55]. The MexAB-OprM system produces resistance to a variety of antibiotics, including anti-pseudomonal penicillins, anti-pseudomonal cephalosporins, and fluoroquinolones. The plasmid-encoded Tet drug efflux pumps are the major mechanism of tetracycline resistance in enteric gram-negatives [57]. Antibiotic efflux, in addition to ribosomal methylation, is an important mechanism for resistance to macrolides and lincosamides [58].

Bacteria can display multiple mechanisms of resistance simultaneously. The wide array of antimicrobial-resistance mechanisms described in *A. baumannii* is impressive and demonstrates the organism's ability to adapt to changing environmental pressure. Its ability to upregulate or acquire resistance determinants has made it an emerging pathogen of great public health concern. As an example, a multidrug-resistant strain of *A. baumannii* was found to have a single resistance island containing 88 open reading frames, 82 of which were predicted to have originated from other gram-negative organisms and 45 different antimicrobial-resistance genes, which conferred resistance to seven classes of antibiotics [59]. This ability to harbor multiple genetic resistance mutations causes a highly variable and complex susceptibility profile. The most prevalent mechanism of β-lactam resistance is enzymatic degradation by β-lactamase enzymes. AmpC β-lactamases, ESBLs, and OXA and MBL carbapenemases are common in *A. baumannii* and confer resistance to most β-lactam antibiotics. Changes in outer membrane proteins, multidrug efflux pumps, and penicillin-binding proteins are also present and contribute to resistance. Aminoglycoside-modifying enzymes and efflux pumps commonly cause high-level aminoglycoside resistance, while mutations in the *gyrA* and *parC* confer resistance to fluoroquinolones [60].

Much like *A. baumannii, P. aeruginosa* demonstrates a complex array of resistance mechanisms. *P. aeruginosa* displays intrinsic resistance to macrolides and many β-lactams due to the relative impermeability of the outer membrane coupled with active drug efflux mechanisms. Fluoroquinolone resistance is common and often due to overexpressed efflux pumps and DNA gyrase mutations. Aminoglycoside resistance is often associated with the presence of modifying enzymes and active efflux pumps [61]. Resistance to anti-pseudomonal penicillins and anti-pseudomonal cephalosporins may occur because of overexpression of AmpC β-lactamases and/or acquisition of ESBLs. Many of these ESBLs are acquired through plasmid conjugation and have the potential for rapid spread of resistance to susceptible strains [62]. Carbapenems, typically resistant to hydrolysis by AmpC β-lactamases and ESBLs, are now becoming inactive in many *P. aeruginosa* infections due to increasing acquisition of carbapenemases [63].

2.7 Trends in Resistance

2.7.1 MRSA

Prior to the introduction of penicillin in the early 1940s, invasive *S. aureus* infection caused significant morbidity and mortality. The introduction of penicillin greatly reduced this burden of disease, but its effect was short lived [64]. Only 1 year after the introduction of penicillin, the first penicillin-resistant *S. aureus* was reported [65]. As use of penicillin increased in hospitals after World War II, penicillin-resistant *S. aureus* began to increase dramatically in response to increased antibiotic pressure [66]. Paralleling the current MRSA epidemic, resistance to penicillin was first identified in hospitalized patients and subsequently spread to the community. The production of a β-lactamase was responsible for the resistance of *S. aureus* to penicillin. This increase in resistance was the stimulus for the development of semisynthetic penicillins, which would remain active in the presence of inactivating enzymes. Methicillin was subsequently introduced in 1961 and was active against β-lactamase-producing *S. aureus.*

Within 1 year of methicillin's introduction, MRSA emerged as an important clinical pathogen in the United Kingdom [67]. MRSA is characterized by the expression of the *mecA* gene, which encodes a protein (PBP2a) with low affinity for β-lactam antibiotics. This *mecA* gene, carried by the staphylococcal cassette chromosome *mec* (SCC*mec*), was probably acquired from coagulase-negative *Staphylococcus* via horizontal transfer [68–70].

MRSA outbreaks in US hospitals were commonly described in the medical literature during the late 1960s and early 1970s [71, 72]. Over the next 20 years, MRSA infections became increasingly more common in hospitalized populations. The National Nosocomial Infections Surveillance (NNIS) system began collecting data on nosocomial infections in 1970. In the early 1980s, data from the NNIS system demonstrated a slow increase in MRSA nosocomial infections to a rate of 5–10% of all *S. aureus* isolates collected. Rates among small community hospitals remained low (<5%) at that time. The epidemiology of nosocomial MRSA infections dramatically changed in the late 1980s and early 1990s. By the early 1990s, the proportion of *S. aureus* isolates due to MRSA had increased to 20% among small community hospitals and was 40% in large urban medical centers [73, 74]. In 2003, MRSA accounted for 64% of all nosocomial *S. aureus* infections [1].

As nosocomial MRSA infections became more common in the late 1990s, sporadic cases of MRSA infections began to appear in the general community without identifiable MRSA risk factors [75]. Mimicking the trends seen with penicillin-resistant *S. aureus*, rates of community-acquired MRSA rose dramatically and now account for the majority of *S. aureus* skin and soft tissue infections. Although community-acquired strains and hospital-acquired strains share a common resistance to methicillin, the genetic lineage of the strains and resistance profiles were distinct. Hospital-acquired MRSA (HA-MRSA) strains were traditionally due to USA 100 and USA 200 based on PFGE typing and carried the SCCmec types I–III, while community-associated MRSA (CA-MRSA) were due to USA 300 and 400 and carried the SCCmec type IV. This clear distinction between HA and CA strains has now become blurred as strains commonly associated with CA-MRSA are now causing nosocomial infections [76, 77].

Over the past 20 years, *S. aureus* with intermediate susceptibility to vancomycin (VISA) and isolates resistant to vancomycin (VRSA) have been described in the medical literature. VISA strains arise from chromosomal mutations that result in a thickened cell wall. Based on current Clinical and Laboratory Standard Institute breakpoints, isolates with vancomycin minimum inhibitory concentrations (MICs) between 4 and 8 μg/ml are considered VISA. VISA isolates have been found in many countries worldwide, but accurate epidemiologic data is difficult to obtain due to varying methodologies in detection and lack of standardized diagnostic criteria.

More commonly found than VISA is heteroresistant VISA (hVISA): strains of vancomycin-susceptible *S. aureus* containing small subpopulations that are able to grow at a vancomycin concentration ≥4 μg/ml. The hVISA phenotype has been described in the USA, Japan, South Africa, and many other countries. A review of 13 epidemiologic studies from around the world found the prevalence of hVISA to be 2.16% of all MRSA isolates [78]. However, the clinical significance of hVISA infections remains unclear [79, 80].

S. aureus isolates with true high-level resistance to vancomycin (VRSA) were first described in the USA in 2002 [81]. The first case of VRSA was the result of conjugation between a strain of MRSA and a strain of VRE. A diabetic patient with a foot ulcer grew both VRE and VRSA from his wound site. The *vanA* gene was found in both isolates, and molecular analysis confirmed that the Tn1546 genetic element encoding *vanA* was responsible for the transfer of resistance [49].

VRSA has been identified in 11 cases worldwide, 9 of which have occurred in the USA [82]. Like the index case, most of these isolates have been recovered from patients with a prior history of VRE colonization/infection and extensive exposure to vancomycin. Transfer of the *vanA* cluster from enterococcus to MRSA has been identified as the genetic basis of resistance [83]. Fortunately, these isolates have appeared sporadically and do not appear to be spreading, but the threat of emergence clearly demonstrates how *S. aureus* continues to evolve in the face of increasing antibiotic pressure.

2.7.2 VRE

Initially viewed as a non-virulent inhabitant of the gastrointestinal flora, *Enterococcus* has now become a major clinical threat and is the third most common cause of nosocomial bloodstream infections in the USA [19].

Treatment of serious enterococcal infections has frustrated clinicians for over 50 years. In 1951, the addition of an aminoglycoside to penicillin was shown to act synergistically and increase cure rates of enterococcal bacteremia significantly [84]. For years, this combination of penicillin or ampicillin (or vancomycin in patients with a penicillin allergy) and an aminoglycoside remained standard of care for enterococcal bacteremia and endocarditis. In the 1970s and 1980s, however, high-level resistance to aminoglycosides was identified, and 50% of isolates were resistant [85, 86]. The loss of aminoglycosides as effective synergistic agents left clinicians without any bactericidal regimens for serious infections. At that time, *E. faecium* had also developed high-level ampicillin resistance in many strains, leaving vancomycin as the most effective antimicrobial.

VRE was first described in France and England in the late 1980s [87, 88]. Not long after, the NNIS system began monitoring levels of enterococcal isolates resistant to vancomycin in US hospitals. From 1991 to 2004, rates of vancomycin resistance in enterococcal isolates recovered from ICUs steadily increased to 28.5% [89]; this trend has continued through 2006 [90]. In 2003, the majority of vancomycin-resistant enterococcal infections were due to *E. faecium,* representing 91% of the VRE isolates.

Not only is the epidemiology of resistance changing, but the epidemiology of enterococcal infections is also changing. In previous years, *Enterococcus faecalis* accounted for the majority of enterococcal infections by at least a 9:1 ratio with very minimal vancomycin resistance reported. Now, *E. faecium* accounts for 20–36% of enterococcal infections in the USA [91] and is found to be vancomycin resistant in 60% of cases (compared to 2% of *E. faecalis* cases) [19].

Antibiotic selection pressure has also been identified as a factor that has contributed to the increase in VRE colonization and infection. Oral administration of glycopeptides in Belgium was associated with increased rates of VRE in feces [92], while the impact of parenteral vancomycin is more controversial [93, 94]. Anti-anaerobic drugs, cephalosporins, and extended-spectrum penicillins all may contribute to the risk of colonization and subsequent infection with VRE [95].

2.7.3 *Klebsiella Species*

K. pneumoniae is a common cause of nosocomial pneumonia, bloodstream infections, and urinary tract infections [96]. *K. pneumoniae* was one of the first organisms known to harbor ESBLs, a β-lactamase that generates resistance to third-generation cephalosporins and monobactams [97]. Hundreds of ESBL variants have been described, including SHV, TEV, and CTX-M types. ESBL-producing *K. pneumoniae* strains have easily spread within hospitals and healthcare communities [98].

During the past decade, there has been an emergence of organisms that express carbapenem-hydrolyzing β-lactamases. These β-lactamases include the metallo-β-lactamases (MBL), oxacillinases (OXA), and clavulanic acid-inhibited β-lactamases (class A). The genetic material encoding the carbapenem-hydrolyzing enzymes can be located chromosomally or, more commonly, on mobile plasmids or transposons.

The *K. pneumoniae* carbapenemase (KPC) was originally described in *K. pneumoniae*. Like ESBLs, KPCs are generally carried on plasmids and are typically associated with other genes that confer resistance. Currently, KPC-producing *K. pneumoniae* are the most common species of carbapenem-resistant *Enterobacteriaceae* in the USA and produce a class A carbapenemase, bla_{kpc}. Although the bla_{kpc} enzymes are most commonly identified in *K. pneumoniae,* they have now been reported in *E. coli, Salmonella cubana, Enterobacter cloacae, Proteus mirabilis,* and *Klebsiella oxytoca* [99].

A KPC-producing strain of *K. pneumoniae* was first detected in North Carolina, USA, in 1996 [3] and has since spread to over 24 US states. In 2007, the CDC reported that 8% of all *Klebsiella* healthcare-associated infection isolates in the USA were carbapenem resistant, compared to 1% in 2000 [100]. In this survey, the predominant cause of carbapenem resistance was bla_{kpc}. KPC-producing bacteria have also become endemic in Greece and Israel with sporadic reports in several other countries [99].

In 2010, reports of a novel carbapenemase garnered the attention of the media and medical community [5]. This new carbapenemase was first isolated from a *K. pneumoniae* urinary tract infection in a woman returning to Sweden from New Delhi, India [101]. The new carbapenemase, named bla_{NDM1} (New Delhi metallo-β-lactamase), was found on a transmissible genetic element and conferred a similar resistance profile as KPC-producing organisms. Although initially identified in *K. pneumoniae,* the genetic material responsible for the resistance has subsequently been transferred to other members of the *Enterobacteriaceae* family, including *E. coli.* Organisms harboring the NDM-1 mutations have been found widely throughout India, Pakistan, the United Kingdom, and Bangladesh and are now turning up in many countries across the world, including the USA [102]. In most cases, infections with NDM-1 can be linked to the Indian subcontinent; however, the rapid global spread of this organism ensures that secondary cases will soon be identified [6]. To halt the dissemination of NDM-1 producers, early identification of cases and prevention of their spread with screening, hand hygiene, and infection control will need to be strictly enforced [100].

2.7.4 *Acinetobacter baumannii*

A. baumannii is a non-fermenting, gram-negative bacterium that was considered a relatively minor pathogen only 15 years ago. The clinical significance of *A. baumannii* has grown due to its emerging resistance to available antimicrobials and its increased involvement in ICU outbreaks. *A. baumannii*, like other nosocomial pathogens, has a remarkable ability to colonize the hospital environment and target the most vulnerable patient populations. A common cause of ventilator-associated pneumonia, *A. baumannii* is endemic in many hospital intensive care units and causes significant morbidity and mortality [103]. The frequency of isolation in nosocomial pneumonia of *A. baumannii*, as reported by the NNIS system, showed a clear increasing trend from 1986 to 2003, while other nosocomial acquired gram-negative infections remained stable. Geographic differences in resistance patterns in the USA are also common; 68% of *A. baumannii* isolates in the northeast show 3-class resistance compared to 33% in the west [104].

An outbreak with *A. baumannii* in New York City in 2001 found variable antibiotic susceptibility patterns and frequently an interplay between several different mechanisms. In this outbreak, only 32% of isolates were susceptible to meropenem, and 14% were susceptible to levofloxacin. Almost all isolates (94%) remained sensitive to polymyxin [105]. Resistant *Acinetobacter* infections have emerged as a significant pathogen in military personnel returning from Iraq, Kuwait, and Afghanistan [106]. *A. baumannii* strains resistant to all commonly used antibiotics are now common in many ICUs and require the use of second-line agents, such as colistin and tigecycline.

2.7.5 *Pseudomonas aeruginosa*

Antimicrobial resistance is not a novel concept in *P. aeruginosa*. Resistant *P. aeruginosa* is a well-known cause of diverse nosocomial infections and cystic fibrosis exacerbations. In the US, *P. aeruginosa* is consistently the second most common cause of nosocomial pneumonia, behind *S. aureus,* and the leading cause among gram-negative pathogens [96]. In addition, it is the third most common cause of nosocomial urinary tract infections (16.3%) and the eighth most frequent cause of nosocomial bloodstream infections (3.4%). Data from the CDC's NNIS program from 1986 to 2003 demonstrated the consistency of *P. aeruginosa* infections in the ICU. Over the course of 16 years, *P. aeruginosa* caused 20% of all gram-negative nosocomial pneumonia cases without significant variation [96]. Although infection rates have been consistent over the course of many years, *P. aeruginosa* has shown significant increases in developing resistance to antimicrobials. When comparing the 2003 resistance rates to baseline levels from 1998 to 2002, resistance rates in nosocomial ICU infections to imipenem, fluoroquinolones, and third-generation cephalosporins increased 15, 9, and 20%, respectively [89]. Similarly, using a national surveillance program monitoring *P. aeruginosa* resistance, ciprofloxacin resistance was found to increase from 15% in 1993 to 32% in 2002. Similar trends were seen for imipenem and tobramycin. Notably, isolates with resistance to 2 or 3 antimicrobials increased significantly over the 10-year period, while single drug resistance stayed constant [107]. A more recent report from the CDC shows the level of multidrug-resistant *P. aeruginosa* (defined by resistance of one or more antimicrobials in at least 3 classes) may be stabilizing. Data from the NNIS and NHSN show the rates of multidrug resistance peaked in 2007 at 22% and have subsequently come down to 17% in 2008 [103].

2.7.6 *Enterobacter Species*

Enterobacter species are a common cause of nosocomial infection in the US [96] and cause significant morbidity and mortality [108]. As with other members of the *Enterobacteriaceae* family, resistance due to the production of ESBLs and inducible cephalosporinases is a common occurrence [109]. New reports of carbapenemase production via KPC and NDM-1 enzymes are of increasing concern [110, 111].

2.8 Preventing the Transmission of Multidrug-Resistant Bacteria in Humans

Patient-patient transmission has played an important role in the dissemination of MDROs, particularly in healthcare-related settings where high levels of antibiotic use drive high levels of antibiotic resistance. Over the past 50 years, the discipline of infection control has emerged as a means for preventing the transmission of these pathogens.

2.8.1 *Hand Hygiene and Contact Isolation*

Ignaz Semmelweis was among the first to recognize the importance of healthcare workers (HCWs) in spreading infections among hospitalized patients. Semmelweis observed that women whose babies were delivered by students and physicians on an obstetrics ward in Vienna had higher mortality rates from puerperal fever than women whose babies were delivered by midwives. Semmelweis noted that the physicians and students had a disagreeable odor on their hands after working on the autopsy ward; this odor persisted despite washing with soap and water. An antiseptic agent was adopted for hand-washing, and mortality rates subsequently dropped [112]. Oliver Wendall Holmes independently reached a similar conclusion in Boston in 1843, and he encouraged similar measures to limit the spread of puerperal fever [113].

Effective hand hygiene is the most important way to prevent the spread of bacteria within a healthcare setting. HCWs' hands may come in contact with bacteria by touching intact patient skin, infected wounds, medical equipment, or environmental surfaces. If HCWs do not use proper hand hygiene, the contaminated hands can transfer the bacteria to other patients either directly, through patient contact, or indirectly, by touching an inanimate surface that will later come in contact with the patient. The clothing of HCWs and medical equipment can also become contaminated with bacteria and may thereby serve as vectors for transmission from patient to patient.

Several studies provide indirect evidence that HCWs help spread VRE from patient to patient. HCWs caring for patients colonized or infected with VRE acquired the organism on their hands, gowns, and stethoscopes [114, 115]. If VRE persists on an HCW's hands or equipment, transmission to patients could conceivably occur. In one study, proximity to an un-isolated patient with VRE was a significant risk factor for VRE acquisition [116]. In a medical ICU, colonization pressure was the strongest predictor of VRE acquisition [117].

In both of these studies, HCWs were presumably the vectors of VRE transmission. Another study found that having the same nurse as a patient with VRE was a risk factor for VRE acquisition [118].

HCW acquisition of MRSA differs little from that of VRE: 65% of nurses who had performed morning patient-care duties on patients with MRSA in a wound or urine contaminated their nursing uniforms or gowns with MRSA [119].

A program to increase hand hygiene helped reduce rates of VRE [120]. Other studies have reported reduced rates of MRSA transmission coincident with improved compliance with hand hygiene [121–123].

Despite the importance of hand hygiene, overall adherence among HCWs to recommended hand hygiene procedures is typically less than 50% [124]. Poor compliance has been a persistent problem and has not proven easy to correct.

Due to the difficulty in ensuring adequate hand hygiene, other infection-control measures are warranted. Wearing gloves can dramatically reduce hand contamination. In one study, gloves prevented hand contamination in 77% of patient encounters [125]. In another study, universal gloving in an ICU was as effective as universal gloves and gowns in preventing rectal colonization with VRE [126].

The clothing of HCWs can become contaminated when gowns are not worn. As a result, implementation of contact precautions has been a component of controlling several hospital outbreaks of VRE [116, 118, 127], ceftazidime-resistant *K. pneumoniae* [128, 129], carbapenem-resistant *K. pneumoniae* or CRKP [130, 131], and multidrug-resistant *A. baumannii* [132].

In combination with other interventions, contact precautions have also been an important part of reducing rates of VRE [133] and MRSA [134] in endemic settings. Major national guidelines recommend contact isolation for all patients infected or colonized with MDROs [135]. Cohorting of patients and staff has also been effective in controlling transmission of MDROs.

Contact isolation does have its drawbacks. In comparison to un-isolated patients, those in contact isolation are less likely to have documented care [136–138], less likely to be examined by physicians [139], and more likely to experience preventable adverse events [136]. Finding ways to counteract these effects are needed because contact isolation is likely to be used increasingly as drug resistance spreads.

2.8.2 *Environmental Contamination*

The role the environment plays in transmission of MDROs is a topic of ongoing investigation. Both MRSA and VRE can survive for months on dry surfaces [140, 141]. The amount of environmental contamination with MRSA or VRE varies on the body sites at which patients are colonized or infected. In one study, 36% of environmental surfaces in rooms of patients with MRSA-positive wounds or urine were contaminated versus 6% of surfaces in rooms of patients with MRSA at other sites [119]. In another study, patients with diarrhea and heavy stool colonization with MRSA contaminated 59% of surfaces compared to 23% contamination in the rooms of patients with MRSA at other sites [142]. Likewise, 46% of environmental surfaces were contaminated in rooms of VRE-positive patients with diarrhea compared to 15% in VRE-positive patients without diarrhea [118]. Although most studies have focused on inpatient settings, environmental contamination has also been documented in clinics for both MRSA [143] and VRE [144].

Transmission of bacteria via environmental surfaces can occur when HCWs contaminate their hands or gloves by touching infected sites. The transfer of bacteria from environmental surfaces to HCWs' hands has been well documented for MRSA [119, 145] and VRE [145–148]. Transmission can also occur when patients come into direct contact with contaminated medical equipment, such as nebulizers [149] or electronic thermometers [150]. Finally, transmission can occur after contact with contaminated environmental surfaces. In one study, 23% of ICU patients acquired VRE after their room became contaminated [151]. Another study found that admission to a contaminated ICU room was a risk factor for acquiring VRE [152], which implies that improperly cleaned rooms are a source of VRE transmission to patients. Simply by enforcing routine environmental cleaning measures, one study was able to achieve a significant reduction in VRE cross transmission in a VRE-endemic ICU [153]. Another study found that improved attention to environmental cleaning ended an MRSA outbreak on a surgical ward [154]. Recommendations for environmental infection control have been published [155].

Of all the gram-negatives, the importance of environmental transmission is best defined for *A. baumannii. A. baumannii* can survive on dry inanimate surfaces for approximately 1 month [132]. During outbreaks, contamination of environmental surfaces is typically widespread, and medical equipment is often implicated as the source of transmission [56, 156]. Effective environmental cleaning and disinfection of medical equipment is essential for eliminating transmission [132]. In one study, there was a significant correlation between the number of environmental cultures positive for *A. baumannii* and the number of patients colonized or infected with *A. baumannii* [157]. In another study, a change from an open ICU to isolation rooms helped reduce bronchopulmonary acquisition of *A. baumannii* [158].

2.8.3 Active Surveillance

Since many more patients may be colonized than infected with a resistant organism, reliance on clinical cultures may not identify the full reservoir of MDROs. However, the best means to identify this reservoir in a particular setting is unclear. The argument for more intensive screening, known as active surveillance, is that colonized patients can be identified before clinical infection develops or patient-patient transmission occurs. Modeling suggests that active surveillance in the ICU would be useful for reducing VRE transmission [159] and MRSA transmission [160]. Several large studies attest to the benefit of more intensive control strategies that include active surveillance for reducing rates of VRE [133, 161] and MRSA [162–167]. In a large US hospital system, a program of universal active surveillance, contact precautions, hand hygiene, and institutional culture change was associated with a decrease in MRSA transmission and infections [168]. The success of this program is difficult to separate from temporal trends. During an overlapping time period, nine metropolitan areas in the USA saw a decrease in healthcare-associated invasive MRSA infections irrespective of any specific intervention [169].

The Society of Healthcare Epidemiology of America recommends active surveillance for MRSA and VRE [135]. National working groups in the United Kingdom and New Zealand have also recommended targeted active surveillance for MRSA on hospital admission [170, 171]. Several authors, however, have cast doubt on the need for these interventions. In the Netherlands, where overall rates of MRSA infections are low, universal admission screening did not reduce nosocomial MRSA infections [172]. In a cluster-randomized trial of adult ICU patients, existing practice was compared to an intensive MRSA and VRE control strategy, that is, active surveillance plus contact precautions [173]. The incidence density of MRSA and VRE colonization did not differ between the two groups, but the study has been criticized for not using more rapid techniques to identify colonized patients.

Compared to MRSA and VRE, the importance of infection-control measures like active surveillance has been less well defined for multidrug-resistant gram-negatives [174]. Two studies found no benefit to active surveillance and isolation precautions for multidrug-resistant *Enterobacteriaceae* in a non-outbreak setting [175, 176]. Some institutions, however, still pursue aggressive search and destroy policies for these organisms [177]. In an area of high endemicity with CRKP, the implementation of several interventions, including active surveillance, reduced rates of CRKP infections [178]. Active surveillance was also part of a bundled intervention to control an outbreak of CRKP in a long-term acute care hospital, or LTAC [130].

Active surveillance may have a role when other interventions have proven ineffective [179]. Feasibility, the extent of the problem, and local conditions should all guide decision-making. Guidelines tend to promote a one-size-fits-all approach to infection control, but there is empirical evidence to show that there are several ways to achieve the same goal. For example, institutions have reported reduced rates of MRSA even after discontinuing isolation precautions [180] or only with improved hand-washing and gloving [181]. At one institution, a bundle of interventions, not including active surveillance, was successful in reducing VRE infections [182].

2.8.4 Decolonization Strategies

Instead of simply isolating patients who carry multidrug-resistant organisms, some studies have tried to decolonize patients. Theoretically, decolonization should decrease the patient's individual risk of infection and also potentially decrease the risk of transmission.

MRSA decolonization has been attempted with intranasal mupirocin plus topical antiseptics, such as chlorhexadine or triclosan. Attempts at preoperative decolonization have been successful in orthopedic patients (mupirocin and chlorhexadine) [183] and cardiothoracic patients (mupirocin, topical triclosan, and preoperative teicoplanin) [184]. A randomized, controlled trial using mupirocin and chlorhexadine provided strong evidence for preoperative decolonization of *S. aureus* carriers among cardiothoracic patients and weaker evidence for orthopedic patients. The study showed a significant decrease in the number of surgical-site *S. aureus* infections in decolonized patients. However, since the study was done in the Netherlands, the *S. aureus* strains were exclusively methicillin sensitive [185]. A separate study in all surgical patients found no benefit to decolonization, suggesting that it makes sense to focus on certain surgical subspecialties [172]. For nonsurgical patients, decolonization to decrease infection risk has not proven effective with mupirocin [186] or mupirocin plus chlorhexadine [187], but these studies may have been underpowered to detect a difference. In addition, eradicating *S. aureus* carriage for prolonged periods of time is difficult. Although mupirocin is effective in eliminating nasal carriage of *S. aureus* in the short term, studies have found that recolonization with *S. aureus* occurs in over 50% of patients by 3–6 months [188, 189]. Such high rates of recolonization may reflect *S. aureus* reacquisition from environmental or human sources at home or in healthcare settings.

Chlorhexidine sponge baths for ICU patients have been shown to decrease colonization with MRSA and VRE in several studies [190–192]. The role of chlorhexadine in multidrug-resistant gram-negatives is less well defined. Daily chlorhexidine bathing of ICU patients was shown to decrease rates of skin colonization with *A. baumannii* [190, 193] and bloodstream infections with *A. baumannii* [193]. In addition, chlorhexadine baths were part of a bundled intervention that controlled an outbreak of CRKP [130].

A more controversial issue is gut decontamination for multidrug-resistant gram-negatives. Decontamination of the gastrointestinal tract was of limited efficacy in a few small studies in patients colonized with ESBL-*Enterobacteriaceae* [194–196] and CRKP [197]. A cluster-randomized trial from the Netherlands, where antimicrobial-resistance rates are low, showed that selective oral and digestive tract decontamination reduced the rate of highly resistant bacteremia by 63 and 59%, respectively [198]. In this study, topical formulations of tobramycin, colistin, and amphotericin B were used in the oropharynx for oral decontamination and in both the oropharynx and stomach for digestive decontamination. Selective decontamination carries the benefits of reducing the risk of subsequent infection and horizontal patient-patient transmission. If commonly prescribed antibiotics are used for decolonization, however, the patient will be at risk for acquiring other resistant bacteria.

As the prevalence of multidrug-resistant organisms increases, the importance of containing their transmission within healthcare facilities will become increasingly important. The infection-control literature is replete with noncontrolled studies utilizing multiple interventions. As a result, inadequate evidence is often available to provide support for recommendations. In an era of diminishing resources, identifying specifically which interventions are needed will be essential. Furthermore, as the administration of medical care moves out of hospitals and into clinics and other nursing facilities, greater vigilance to infection control in these nontraditional settings will become a greater priority.

2.9 Antibiotic Resistance in Nonhuman Sources

Antibiotic resistance is not limited to humans. Over the past 40 years, there has been increasing concern over the emergence of antibiotic-resistant bacteria in agricultural feedlots and the potential for these bacteria to spread to people.

Antibiotics are used in food animals for a variety of purposes, such as prophylaxis, targeted treatment of sick animals, and growth promotion [199]. As in humans, the use of antibiotics in food animals creates a selective pressure that enables antibiotic-resistant bacteria to emerge and disseminate. Resistant bacteria that develop in food animals can reach humans through a variety of mechanisms, including meat consumption, contact with animal manure, and handling of contaminated meat.

2.9.1 Fluoroquinolone-Resistant Campylobacter and Salmonella

The link between antibiotic use in food animals and antibiotic resistance in humans is strongest for *Campylobacter* and *Salmonella.* Food animals are the primary reservoir for both types of bacteria, and there is a clear temporal association between the introduction of fluoroquinolones in food animals, particularly poultry, and the emergence of fluoroquinolone-resistant *Campylobacter* and *Salmonella* [200].

After approval of fluoroquinolone use for poultry in 1995, the incidence of domestic acquisition of fluoroquinolone-resistant *Campylobacter* infections increased significantly in Minnesota [201]. Molecular subtyping revealed an association between resistant *Campylobacter* strains acquired domestically by humans and strains found in chicken products [201]. The introduction of fluoroquinolone use to poultry farms was also associated with increases in human fluoroquinolone-resistant *Campylobacter* in the Netherlands [202] and Denmark [203]. Since *Campylobacter* is infrequently transferred from person to person in developed countries, antibiotic use in humans is unlikely to explain these increases in resistance.

The emergence of fluoroquinolone resistance in *Salmonella* has paralleled the *Campylobacter* experience. Several large, population-based studies have shown higher hospitalization rates in patients with resistant versus susceptible *Campylobacter* and *Salmonella* infections [204–206].

A US ban on enrofloxacin and sarafloxacin was implemented during 2005. The effects of this ban are not yet understood [207].

The case of *Campylobacter* and *Salmonella* represents direct transfer of resistant bacteria from food animals to humans. Another potential mechanism of spreading resistance from animals to humans is via gene transfer. In a study of retail meat sold in Pittsburgh, USA, and Seville, Spain, the majority of poultry samples contained *E. coli* strains producing ESBL or CMY-type β-lactamases [208]. If these resistance genes are passed on to bacteria in a person's gut, colonization and potentially infection with cephalosporin-resistant *Enterobacteriaceae* could occur.

Studies have shown that antimicrobial-resistance genes can be transferred in the human intestine between *E. coli* of animal and human origin [209, 210]. Although it is unclear how frequently gene transfer occurs under natural conditions, there is some evidence that it is already taking place. In the US population, drug-resistant *E. coli* isolates from humans shared similar phylogenetic and virulence markers with strains from retail poultry, suggesting that poultry was the likely source [211].

2.9.2 Avoparcin and VRE

Avoparcin, an analog of vancomycin, was introduced to European animal husbandry in 1974 as a growth promoter. In growth promotion, subtherapeutic levels of antibiotics are added to animal feed or water to improve daily weight gain and feed utilization [212]. It is postulated that these low levels of antibiotics reduce the bacterial burden in the animal's digestive tract and thereby free up more nutrients for the animal's growth.

After avoparcin's introduction to European livestock, *vanA*-mediated vancomycin resistance emerged among *E. faecium* in Europe. VRE was detected in the liquid manure of animals that received avoparcin as a food additive but not in the manure of animals that did not [213]. Healthy Europeans began to carry VRE in their intestinal tract, and carriage was linked to meat consumption. In a Dutch study, fecal samples were positive for VRE in 0/42 vegetarians and 6/62 (9.7%) meat-eaters [214]. When VRE isolates from food animals were compared to those found in people, indistinguishable genetic elements encoding for vancomycin resistance were identified [215, 216].

Due to concerns about animal-to-human transmission of VRE, avoparcin was banned in all EU countries in 1997. The prevalence of VRE carriage in healthy persons subsequently declined [217]. During the 1990s, the European Union also banned the use of other antibiotics as growth promoters. Denmark, one of the first countries to impose such a ban, experienced a dramatic decrease in antimicrobial resistance in the food animal reservoir. After the ban's implementation, however, Denmark saw an increase in the therapeutic use of certain antibiotics among food animals. There was also some loss in productivity of the livestock industry [218].

The WHO supports a ban on growth promoters, but other countries, including the United States, have not adopted such measures. To avoid the need for growth promotion, alternative feed and management strategies have been proposed [212]. Several agencies, including the WHO, have also called for limiting the use of critically important clinical antibiotics in farm animals [219, 220].

To help guide future policy, the human risk of using antibiotics in food animals must be better quantified. National monitoring programs on nonhuman usage of antibiotics and antimicrobial resistance should be developed. Due to the global movement of people and food products, coordinated international efforts will be needed.

2.10 The Dry Antibiotic Development Pipeline

Antibiotics have a unique feature not shared by virtually any other drug class: Once an antibiotic is released for wide-scale use, its efficacy diminishes. Consider aspirin, one of the oldest drugs. Aspirin is as effective an analgesic today as the first time it was used. The same cannot be said of penicillin. In the 1950s, the use and overuse of penicillin resulted in penicillin resistance. This pattern of use and overuse of antibiotics leading to resistance has been repeated numerous times during the twentieth and twenty-first centuries.

The diminished effectiveness of antibiotics should make them a tempting target by the pharmaceutical industry for continual drug discovery and development, but it has not. New antibiotics have never been easy to find. However, pharmaceutical companies have recently curtailed or eliminated antibiotic discovery. Since the beginning of 2008, the US Food and Drug Administration has approved only two new antibacterial antibiotics, telavancin and ceftaroline.

The withdrawal of pharmaceutical companies' antibiotic discovery is at the heart of the dry pipeline. Drug companies are simply not searching for new antibiotics at a time when they are desperately needed [221].

There are several reasons for this paradox. The decreased efficacy of antibiotics due to development of bacterial resistance affects profitability of antibiotics in a way that no other drug class is affected. The profitability of any drug can be expressed as its "NPV_R": the return in future dollars after adjustment for the investment and any lost income, usually expressed as the number of millions of dollars [222]. While antibiotics can be profitable, big pharma looks at the NPV_R of other drug classes to prioritize its discovery and development. One industry spokesman estimated that antibiotics have an NPV_R of 100 but that oncologic drugs have an NPV_R of 300, neurologic drugs an NPV_R of 720, and musculoskeletal drugs an NPV_R of 1150 [223].

The consolidation from 70 to 12 pharmaceutical companies with only about six working on antibiotic drug discovery has also dramatically affected the pipeline [224]. Much of the antibiotic discovery is now occurring in academic centers and small biotechnology companies.

Marketing also works against pharmaceutical efforts to sell antibiotics since these drugs must be "marketed" to prescribers each time an infection occurs. In contrast, an antihypertensive or lipid-controlling drug usually requires one-time marketing since they are often lifelong agents.

Drug companies often complain about the disincentives of the approval process, although these complaints for the approval of antibiotics may be overstated [225].

Finally, the very existence of antibiotic stewardship programs may be a disincentive to big pharma. Many newer agents are put on "reserve" by these stewardship programs, limiting sales. Even if efforts were made to improve these difficulties, pharmaceutical companies have no guarantee of success since finding new antimicrobial compounds, particularly new classes of antibiotics, has been exceedingly difficult.

2.10.1 Progress on New Antibiotic Agents

Despite all the struggles to find new antibiotics, there are some prospects on the horizon [226]. Many of these agents are variations on older antibiotics such as ceftobiprole, a cephalosporin with activity against MRSA, similar to ceftaroline. Unlike older, available cephalosporins, ceftaroline and ceftobiprole bind to the altered penicillin-binding proteins that led to methicillin resistance in *Staphylococcus aureus* (MRSA). Aside from MRSA activity, ceftobiprole and ceftaroline have spectrums of activity similar to ceftriaxone. Drugs with activity against resistant gram-positive bacteria such as MRSA and VRE include oritavancin and dalbavancin. The latter has limited VRE activity but has an extremely long half-life that allows administration as infrequently as once a week. Both of these drugs are related to a recently FDA-approved antibiotic, telavancin. Tetracycline analogs, macrolide analogs, fluoroquinolone analogs, and oxazolidinone analogs are currently under investigation. Detailed discussion of investigation agents is beyond the scope of this chapter.

Modifications of existing antibiotics to improve their spectrums of activity will likely be of limited benefit to deal with the problem of antibiotic resistance among bacteria since bacteria can adapt quickly to these modifications by changing existing resistance mechanisms. New classes of antibiotics without any existing resistance mechanisms are needed.

High-throughput screening, including the use of combinatorial genomic libraries, has not led to the discovery of an abundance of new antibiotics (or even leads) than were promised a few years ago [227]. Screening possible antibiotic-producing microorganisms is an established method for finding antibiotics that can be traced back to Alexander Fleming's discovery of penicillin. One class, the pleuromutilins, was discovered this way and has been used in agriculture for years. The first member of this class for human use, retapamulin, has been FDA-approved for topical application. These drugs are inhibitors of ribosomal protein synthesis with considerable gram-positive activity, including MRSA and *S. pneumoniae*. Oral and parenteral preparations from this class are under investigation.

For MDR gram-negative bacteria, especially *P. aeruginosa* and Acinetobacter spp., new classes of agents are urgently needed. Several companies are developing analogs of aminoglycosides such as ACHN-490 and SPX-1212. BAL30072 is a novel siderophore sulfactam that has activity against MDR gram-negative bacteria, including those possessing class A carbapenemases or metallo-β-lactamases [228].

The β-lactamase inhibitors best exemplify antibiotics that hamper the resistance mechanism in MDROs. Three compounds, clavulanic acid, sulbactam, and tazobactam, are currently available and effectively inhibit class A β-lactamases. Unfortunately, classes B, C, and D are becoming widely dispersed and are not inhibited by the currently available drugs, producing resistance to most of the currently available ß-lactam antibiotics. A number of β-lactam-derived and non-β-lactam-derived β-lactamase inhibitors are under investigation [229]. The only compound in clinical trials, AVE1330A, now known as NXL 104, is a non-β-lactam inhibitor and has activity against class A, C, and D β-lactamases. NXL 104 is being used in combination with ceftazidime and ceftaroline. Unfortunately, no compounds seem to inhibit class B metallo-β-lactamases.

Other strategies for novel antibiotics include forming hybrid molecules with chemical linkages between two antimicrobial agents such as quinalactams, a combination of a fluoroquinolone and a cephalosporin. Unfortunately, investigational quinalactams had no greater activity than either agent given separately, but the hybrid concept is still under investigation. Peptides with antimicrobial activity such as bactericidal permeability-increasing (BPI) peptide show some promise but have a ways to go before approval by the FDA [230, 231]. Agents that target bacterial virulence mechanisms and using genomics to develop new targets for antibiotic agents represent fruitful areas for research, but the promise of new agents remains a distant one [232, 233].

2.10.2 Rediscovery of Older Agents

The lack of new antibiotics has forced clinicians to revisit agents that fell out of favor, usually because of their toxicity. The polymyxins, especially polymyxin E and colistin, are compounds that have come back into use, even though they are limited by toxicity, particularly nephrotoxicity [234]. Another agent, fosfomycin, which inhibits bacterial cell wall synthesis, has been successfully used to treat multidrug-resistant gram-negative infections with *K. pneumoniae, P. aeruginosa,* and *A. baumannii* [235, 236]. Nitrofurantoin and tetracycline use in urinary tract infections for resistant organisms have also seen resurgence in recent years [237].

2.11 Optimizing Antibiotic Use: A Call to Action

As new antibiotics were discovered, clinicians had alternatives when antibiotic-resistant bacteria appeared. The seemingly never-ending cycle of antibiotic use, antibiotic resistance, new antibiotic use, new antibiotic resistance, and still more new antibiotic use is about to come to a screeching halt.

Clinicians must recognize how perilously close we are to a post-antibiotic era [238]. According to the World Health Organization, antimicrobial resistance is considered 1 of the 3 greatest threats to human health [239]. Climbing out of this predicament will require a coordinated and comprehensive approach. The entire healthcare system will be called upon to participate because antibiotic resistance is threatening every advance that healthcare is making. New surgical procedures and implants, cancer chemotherapy, and transplantation advances will all be lost if patients acquire infections with untreatable bacteria.

The dry pipeline for antibiotics prompted the Infectious Disease Society of America to call for a global commitment to develop new antibacterial drugs [240]. It will be many years, if not decades, until the production of new antibiotics matches the need for new drugs due to antibiotic resistance. We need to find ways to conserve the effectiveness of antibiotics that we currently have [241].

The European Centre for Disease Prevention and Control (EDEC) and the European Medicines Agency (EMA) are actively monitoring antibiotic resistance and antimicrobial use throughout Europe, finding remarkable variations among its member nations in both resistance and use [242]. The findings suggest higher antibiotic resistance and higher antibiotic use in the countries of southern Europe compared with northern Europe.

The CDC has developed strategies for clinicians and the public in its "Get Smart" Program (http://www.cdc.gov/getsmart) and its "Get Smart for Healthcare" Program (http://www.cdc.gov/getsmart/healthcare). The former emphasizes outpatient antibiotic use, while the latter focuses on inpatient antibiotic use.

In recognition of the rapid, worldwide dispersal of antibiotic-resistant microorganisms, officials from the European Union and North America have formed the Transatlantic Task Force on Urgent Antimicrobial Resistance. The task force is focusing on appropriate therapeutic use of antimicrobial drugs in the medical and veterinary communities, prevention of both healthcare- and community-associated drug-resistant infections, and strategies for improving the pipeline of new antimicrobial drugs, which could be better addressed by intensified cooperation.

Finally, to emphasize the global nature of the problem, in 2011, the World Health Organization's World Health Day theme was "The Fight Against Antimicrobial Resistance Must Continue on a Global Scale."

2.12 Antibiotic Stewardship

While international cooperation and national agencies provide surveillance data, guidance, and vital resources in the fight against antibiotic resistance and help in optimizing antibiotic use, change must occur with healthcare providers, both among institutions and individuals. There are only two ways currently to address the problem of antibiotic resistance: Control antibiotic use and limit the spread of resistant pathogens. No one doubts the importance of infection-control practices in limiting the spread of antibiotic-resistant organisms, but optimizing antibiotic use, also known as antibiotic stewardship, remains essential for successful control of the antibiotic resistance. Outcomes of antibiotic stewardship programs essentially focus on decreases in four main measures: antibiotic use, clinical parameters, antibiotic resistance, and costs.

A number of studies support the notion that optimizing antibiotic use will improve an institution's antibiotic resistance and use problems [243–252]. Additional studies emphasize cost savings with the initiation of an antibiotic stewardship program [253–258]. Implementation of an antimicrobial stewardship program in a healthcare facility will have other benefits such as helping to reduce mortality, decreasing the risk of *C. difficile*-associated diarrhea, and producing shorter hospital stays [259, 260].

Despite a number of studies that point toward improvement in optimizing antibiotic use, up to 48% of US institutions do not have stewardship programs [261]. This survey cited a number of barriers, including personnel shortages (55%), financial considerations (36%), opposition from prescribing physicians (27%), and resistance from administration (14%) to establishing antimicrobial stewardship programs.

Starting an antibiotic stewardship program requires careful planning and a multidisciplinary approach [262, 263]. An infectious diseases physician and a clinical pharmacist with infectious diseases training are at the core of the program's membership. The support and collaboration of hospital administration, medical staff leadership, and local providers in the development and maintenance of antimicrobial stewardship programs is essential.

The action plan of an antimicrobial stewardship program is complex and can differ depending upon the problems of an individual institution, although general recommendations have been made [262]. Formulary restriction, prospective audit and feedback of antibiotic use data, development of guidelines for antibiotic use, parenteral to oral antibiotic conversion, streamlining therapy based upon microbiology culture and susceptibility results, and dose optimization are recommendations that have received broad support. Antibiotic cycling has had limited success and has proven difficult to study since compliance with cycling protocols has been challenging [264].

Changing prescribing behavior remains a difficult challenge. For example, formulary restriction does not necessarily prevent the potential overuse of available broad-spectrum antibiotics in routine practice [265]. The mere production of antibiotic use guidelines—the Infectious Disease Society of America has published over 60 guidelines—has not improved antibiotic use in all facilities. Some studies suggest that consultation from an infectious disease consultant is an effective approach but obviously suffers from its resource limitations [266, 267]. One of the most effective strategies is the implementation of computer-assisted decision support for changing provider behavior [251, 268, 269]. However, this strategy is limited by the availability of an electronic medical record, computerized prescriber order entry, and decision support capability. This availability has moved more slowly than anticipated in healthcare institutions and especially in physician practices where only a quarter of larger (>11) physician practices in the USA had a fully functioning electronic medical record (EMR) [270]. For smaller practices, the percentages are even lower.

Any approach to optimizing antibiotic use will need to consider both empiric and targeted use. Empiric antibiotics, that is, drugs prescribed before microbiology results are available, are an important consideration because in nearly 2/3 of treatment courses, microbiology results do not allow targeting antibiotic therapy to a specific pathogen [271]. Once a patient has been treated empirically, targeting, or de-escalation, should occur with treatment tailored to the microbiology and other clinical laboratory results, usually after 72 h. Surprisingly, the frequency of such targeting is quite variable, ranging from 10 to 90% of patients in intensive care units [272]. Future research on rapid microbial diagnosis could help expedite targeting. In two studies, a rapid polymerase chain reaction test to distinguish MRSA from MSSA infections facilitated targeted therapy and was associated with decreased length of stay [273, 274]. Shortening the duration of antibiotic use in certain clinical syndromes, notably ventilator-associated pneumonia, is another important approach to optimizing antibiotic use [275, 276]. Finally, the use of biomarkers such as procalcitonin can help determine if an infection is actually the cause of a patient's condition and has been shown to decrease the duration of antibiotic use in some [277, 278].

2.13 Conclusion

Human medicine has reaped the benefits of antibiotics for the past 80 years, but without urgent action, the utility of these agents will be drastically minimized. To limit the spread of resistance, physicians must use antibiotics judiciously and apply infection-control procedures consistently. These measures alone, however, will not be sufficient. New antibiotics are desperately needed.

To address this emerging crisis, the medical community, governments, pharmaceutical companies, and public health agencies must all work together. Only a coordinated and committed response can slow the rising tide of multidrug-resistant bacteria.

References

1. Klevens RM, Edwards JR, Tenover FC, McDonald LC, Horan T, Gaynes R (2006) Changes in the epidemiology of methicillin-resistant *Staphylococcus aureus* in intensive care units in US hospitals, 1992–2003. Clin Infect Dis 42:389–391
2. Tracy LA, Furuno JP, Harris AD, Singer M, Langenberg P, Roghmann MC (2011) *Staphylococcus aureus* infections in US Veterans, Maryland, USA, 1999–2008. Emerg Infect Dis 17:441–448
3. Yigit H, Queenan AM, Anderson GJ, Domenech-Sanchez A, Biddle JW, Steward CD et al (2001) Novel carbapenem-hydrolyzing beta-lactamase, KPC-1, from a carbapenem-resistant strain of *Klebsiella pneumoniae*. Antimicrob Agents Chemother 45:1151–1161. PMCID: 90438
4. Woodford N, Tierno PM Jr, Young K, Tysall L, Palepou MF, Ward E et al (2004) Outbreak of *Klebsiella pneumoniae* producing a new carbapenem-hydrolyzing class A beta-lactamase,

KPC-3, in a New York Medical Center. Antimicrob Agents Chemother 48:4793–4799. PMCID: 529220
5. Kumarasamy KK, Toleman MA, Walsh TR, Bagaria J, Butt F, Balakrishnan R et al (2010) Emergence of a new antibiotic resistance mechanism in India, Pakistan, and the UK: a molecular, biological, and epidemiological study. Lancet Infect Dis 10:597–602. PMCID: 2933358
6. Moellering RC Jr (2010) NDM-1—a cause for worldwide concern. N Engl J Med 363: 2377–2379
7. Anderson DJ, Kaye KS, Chen LF, Schmader KE, Choi Y, Sloane R et al (2009) Clinical and financial outcomes due to methicillin resistant *Staphylococcus aureus* surgical site infection: a multi-center matched outcomes study. PLoS One 4:e8305. PMCID: 2788700
8. Mauldin PD, Salgado CD, Hansen IS, Durup DT, Bosso JA (2010) Attributable hospital cost and length of stay associated with health care-associated infections caused by antibiotic-resistant gram-negative bacteria. Antimicrob Agents Chemother 54:109–115. PMCID: 2798544
9. Schwaber MJ, Navon-Venezia S, Kaye KS, Ben-Ami R, Schwartz D, Carmeli Y (2006) Clinical and economic impact of bacteremia with extended-spectrum-beta-lactamase-producing *Enterobacteriaceae*. Antimicrob Agents Chemother 50:1257–1262. PMCID: 1426954
10. Sostarich AM, Zolldann D, Haefner H, Luetticken R, Schulze-Roebecke R, Lemmen SW (2008) Impact of multiresistance of gram-negative bacteria in bloodstream infection on mortality rates and length of stay. Infection 36:31–35
11. Davis KA, Stewart JJ, Crouch HK, Florez CE, Hospenthal DR (2004) Methicillin-resistant *Staphylococcus aureus* (MRSA) nares colonization at hospital admission and its effect on subsequent MRSA infection. Clin Infect Dis 39:776–782
12. Boucher H, Miller LG, Razonable RR (2010) Serious infections caused by methicillin-resistant *Staphylococcus aureus*. Clin Infect Dis 51(Suppl 2):S183–S197
13. Cosgrove SE, Sakoulas G, Perencevich EN, Schwaber MJ, Karchmer AW, Carmeli Y (2003) Comparison of mortality associated with methicillin-resistant and methicillin-susceptible *Staphylococcus aureus* bacteremia: a meta-analysis. Clin Infect Dis 36:53–59
14. Mekontso-Dessap A, Kirsch M, Brun-Buisson C, Loisance D (2001) Poststernotomy mediastinitis due to *Staphylococcus aureus*: comparison of methicillin-resistant and methicillin-susceptible cases. Clin Infect Dis 32:877–883
15. Engemann JJ, Carmeli Y, Cosgrove SE, Fowler VG, Bronstein MZ, Trivette SL et al (2003) Adverse clinical and economic outcomes attributable to methicillin resistance among patients with *Staphylococcus aureus* surgical site infection. Clin Infect Dis 36:592–598
16. DiazGranados CA, Zimmer SM, Klein M, Jernigan JA (2005) Comparison of mortality associated with vancomycin-resistant and vancomycin-susceptible enterococcal bloodstream infections: a meta-analysis. Clin Infect Dis 41:327–333
17. DiazGranados CA, Jernigan JA (2005) Impact of vancomycin resistance on mortality among patients with neutropenia and enterococcal bloodstream infection. J Infect Dis 191:588–595
18. Carmeli Y, Eliopoulos G, Mozaffari E, Samore M (2002) Health and economic outcomes of vancomycin-resistant *enterococci*. Arch Intern Med 162:2223–2228
19. Wisplinghoff H, Bischoff T, Tallent SM, Seifert H, Wenzel RP, Edmond MB (2004) Nosocomial bloodstream infections in US hospitals: analysis of 24,179 cases from a prospective nationwide surveillance study. Clin Infect Dis 39:309–317
20. Joseph NM, Sistla S, Dutta TK, Badhe AS, Parija SC (2010) Ventilator-associated pneumonia: a review. Eur J Intern Med 21:360–368
21. Metan G, Sariguzel F, Sumerkan B (2009) Factors influencing survival in patients with multi-drug-resistant *Acinetobacter bacteraemia*. Eur J Intern Med 20:540–544
22. Marchaim D, Gottesman T, Schwartz O, Korem M, Maor Y, Rahav G et al (2010) National multicenter study of predictors and outcomes of bacteremia upon hospital admission caused by *Enterobacteriaceae* producing extended-spectrum beta-lactamases. Antimicrob Agents Chemother 54:5099–5104. PMCID: 2981239

23. Cosgrove SE, Kaye KS, Eliopoulous GM, Carmeli Y (2002) Health and economic outcomes of the emergence of third-generation cephalosporin resistance in *Enterobacter* species. Arch Intern Med 162:185–190
24. Tumbarello M, Spanu T, Sanguinetti M, Citton R, Montuori E, Leone F et al (2006) Bloodstream infections caused by extended-spectrum-beta-lactamase-producing *Klebsiella pneumoniae*: risk factors, molecular epidemiology, and clinical outcome. Antimicrob Agents Chemother 50:498–504. PMCID: 1366869
25. Ibrahim EH, Sherman G, Ward S, Fraser VJ, Kollef MH (2000) The influence of inadequate antimicrobial treatment of bloodstream infections on patient outcomes in the ICU setting. Chest 118:146–155
26. Kumar A, Roberts D, Wood KE, Light B, Parrillo JE, Sharma S et al (2006) Duration of hypotension before initiation of effective antimicrobial therapy is the critical determinant of survival in human septic shock. Crit Care Med 34:1589–1596
27. Shorr AF, Micek ST, Welch EC, Doherty JA, Reichley RM, Kollef MH (2011) Inappropriate antibiotic therapy in gram-negative sepsis increases hospital length of stay. Crit Care Med 39:46–51
28. Sipahi OR (2008) Economics of antibiotic resistance. Expert Rev Anti Infect Ther 6:523–539
29. Daxboeck F, Budic T, Assadian O, Reich M, Koller W (2006) Economic burden associated with multi-resistant gram-negative organisms compared with that for methicillin-resistant *Staphylococcus aureus* in a university teaching hospital. J Hosp Infect 62:214–218
30. Benveniste R, Davies J (1973) Aminoglycoside antibiotic-inactivating enzymes in actinomycetes similar to those present in clinical isolates of antibiotic-resistant bacteria. Proc Natl Acad Sci U S A 70:2276–2280. PMCID: 433717
31. Whitman WB, Coleman DC, Wiebe WJ (1998) Prokaryotes: the unseen majority. Proc Natl Acad Sci U S A 95:6578–6583. PMCID: 33863
32. Wright GD (2010) Antibiotic resistance in the environment: a link to the clinic? Curr Opin Microbiol 13:589–594
33. Wright GD (2007) The antibiotic resistome: the nexus of chemical and genetic diversity. Nat Rev Microbiol 5:175–186
34. D'Costa VM, McGrann KM, Hughes DW, Wright GD (2006) Sampling the antibiotic resistome. Science 311:374–377
35. Brown MG, Balkwill DL (2009) Antibiotic resistance in bacteria isolated from the deep terrestrial subsurface. Microb Ecol 57:484–493
36. Knapp CW, Dolfing J, Ehlert PA, Graham DW (2010) Evidence of increasing antibiotic resistance gene abundances in archived soils since 1940. Environ Sci Technol 44:580–587
37. Cattoir V, Poirel L, Aubert C, Soussy CJ, Nordmann P (2008) Unexpected occurrence of plasmid-mediated quinolone resistance determinants in environmental *Aeromonas* spp. Emerg Infect Dis 14:231–237. PMCID: 2600179
38. Costelloe C, Metcalfe C, Lovering A, Mant D, Hay AD (2010) Effect of antibiotic prescribing in primary care on antimicrobial resistance in individual patients: systematic review and meta-analysis. BMJ 340:c2096
39. Johnson L, Sabel A, Burman WJ, Everhart RM, Rome M, MacKenzie TD et al (2008) Emergence of fluoroquinolone resistance in outpatient urinary *Escherichia coli* isolates. Am J Med 121:876–884
40. Lepper PM, Grusa E, Reichl H, Hogel J, Trautmann M (2002) Consumption of imipenem correlates with beta-lactam resistance in *Pseudomonas aeruginosa*. Antimicrob Agents Chemother 46:2920–2925. PMCID: 127431
41. Carmeli Y, Troillet N, Eliopoulos GM, Samore MH (1999) Emergence of antibiotic-resistant *Pseudomonas aeruginosa*: comparison of risks associated with different antipseudomonal agents. Antimicrob Agents Chemother 43:1379–1382. PMCID: 89282
42. Troillet N, Samore MH, Carmeli Y (1997) Imipenem-resistant *Pseudomonas aeruginosa*: risk factors and antibiotic susceptibility patterns. Clin Infect Dis 25(5):1094–1098
43. Kritsotakis EI, Tsioutis C, Roumbelaki M, Christidou A, Gikas A (2011) Antibiotic use and the risk of carbapenem-resistant extended-spectrum-{beta}-lactamase-producing *Klebsiella*

pneumoniae infection in hospitalized patients: results of a double case-control study. J Antimicrob Chemother 66(6):1383–1391
44. Paterson DL, Ko WC, Von Gottberg A, Mohapatra S, Casellas JM, Goossens H et al (2004) International prospective study of *Klebsiella pneumoniae* bacteremia: implications of extended-spectrum beta-lactamase production in nosocomial Infections. Ann Intern Med 140:26–32
45. Gregory CJ, Llata E, Stine N, Gould C, Santiago LM, Vazquez GJ et al (2010) Outbreak of carbapenem-resistant *Klebsiella pneumoniae* in Puerto Rico associated with a novel carbapenemase variant. Infect Control Hosp Epidemiol 31:476–484
46. Kochar S, Sheard T, Sharma R, Hui A, Tolentino E, Allen G et al (2009) Success of an infection control program to reduce the spread of carbapenem-resistant *Klebsiella pneumoniae*. Infect Control Hosp Epidemiol 30:447–452
47. Monnet DL, Archibald LK, Phillips L, Tenover FC, McGowan JE Jr, Gaynes RP (1998) Antimicrobial use and resistance in eight US hospitals: complexities of analysis and modeling. Intensive Care Antimicrobial Resistance Epidemiology Project and National Nosocomial Infections Surveillance System Hospitals. Infect Control Hosp Epidemiol 19:388–394
48. Jacoby GA, Medeiros AA (1991) More extended-spectrum beta-lactamases. Antimicrob Agents Chemother 35:1697–1704. PMCID: 245253
49. Chang S, Sievert DM, Hageman JC, Boulton ML, Tenover FC, Downes FP et al (2003) Infection with vancomycin-resistant *Staphylococcus aureus* containing the vanA resistance gene. N Engl J Med 348:1342–1347
50. Jacob G, Bush K (2011) ß-lactamase classification and amino acid sequences for TEM, SHV and OXA extended-spectrum and inhibitor resistant enzymes [updated 2011]. Available from www.lahey.org/Studies. Accessed 13 June 2011
51. Ambler RP (1980) The structure of beta-lactamases. Philos Trans R Soc Lond B Biol Sci 289:321–331
52. Bush K, Jacoby GA, Medeiros AA (1995) A functional classification scheme for beta-lactamases and its correlation with molecular structure. Antimicrob Agents Chemother 39:1211–1233. PMCID: 162717
53. Jacoby GA (2005) Mechanisms of resistance to quinolones. Clin Infect Dis 41(Suppl 2): S120–S126
54. Nannini E, Murray BE, Arias CA (2010) Resistance or decreased susceptibility to glycopeptides, daptomycin, and linezolid in methicillin-resistant *Staphylococcus aureus*. Curr Opin Pharmacol 10:516–521
55. Bonomo RA, Szabo D (2006) Mechanisms of multidrug resistance in *Acinetobacter* species and *Pseudomonas aeruginosa*. Clin Infect Dis 43(Suppl 2):S49–S56
56. Maragakis LL, Perl TM (2008) *Acinetobacter baumannii*: epidemiology, antimicrobial resistance, and treatment options. Clin Infect Dis 46:1254–1263
57. Li XZ, Nikaido H (2004) Efflux-mediated drug resistance in bacteria. Drugs 64:159–204
58. Leclercq R (2002) Mechanisms of resistance to macrolides and lincosamides: nature of the resistance elements and their clinical implications. Clin Infect Dis 34:482–492
59. Fournier PE, Vallenet D, Barbe V, Audic S, Ogata H, Poirel L et al (2006) Comparative genomics of multidrug resistance in *Acinetobacter baumannii*. PLoS Genet 2:e7. PMCID: 1326220
60. Peleg AY, Seifert H, Paterson DL (2008) *Acinetobacter baumannii*: emergence of a successful pathogen. Clin Microbiol Rev 21:538–582. PMCID: 2493088
61. McGowan JE Jr (2006) Resistance in nonfermenting gram-negative bacteria: multidrug resistance to the maximum. Am J Med 119(6 Suppl 1):S29–S36; discussion S62-70
62. Hirsch EB, Tam VH (2010) Impact of multidrug-resistant *Pseudomonas aeruginosa* infection on patient outcomes. Expert Rev Pharmacoecon Outcomes Res 10:441–451
63. Zavascki AP, Carvalhaes CG, Picao RC, Gales AC (2010) Multidrug-resistant *Pseudomonas aeruginosa* and *Acinetobacter baumannii*: resistance mechanisms and implications for therapy. Expert Rev Anti Infect Ther 8:71–93

64. Shinefield HR, Ruff NL (2009) Staphylococcal infections: a historical perspective. Infect Dis Clin North Am 23:1–15
65. Kirby WM (1944) Extraction of a highly potent penicillin inactivator from penicillin resistant staphylococci. Science 99:452–453
66. Barber M, Rozwadowska-Dowzenko M (1948) Infection by penicillin-resistant staphylococci. Lancet 2:641–644
67. Jevons MP, Coe AW, Parker MT (1963) Methicillin resistance in staphylococci. Lancet 1:904–907
68. Berglund C, Soderquist B (2008) The origin of a methicillin-resistant *Staphylococcus aureus* isolate at a neonatal ward in Sweden—possible horizontal transfer of a staphylococcal cassette chromosome mec between methicillin-resistant *Staphylococcus haemolyticus* and *Staphylococcus aureus*. Clin Microbiol Infect 14:1048–1056
69. Archer GL, Niemeyer DM (1994) Origin and evolution of DNA associated with resistance to methicillin in staphylococci. Trends Microbiol 2:343–347
70. Wielders CL, Vriens MR, Brisse S, de Graaf-Miltenburg LA, Troelstra A, Fleer A et al (2001) In-vivo transfer of mecA DNA to *Staphylococcus aureus* [corrected]. Lancet 357:1674–1675
71. Barrett FF, McGehee RF Jr, Finland M (1968) Methicillin-resistant *Staphylococcus aureus* at Boston City Hospital. Bacteriologic and epidemiologic observations. N Engl J Med 279:441–448
72. O'Toole RD, Drew WL, Dahlgren BJ, Beaty HN (1970) An outbreak of methicillin-resistant *Staphylococcus aureus* infection. Observations in hospital and nursing home. JAMA 213:257–263
73. Chambers HF (2001) The changing epidemiology of *Staphylococcus aureus*? Emerg Infect Dis 7:178–182. PMCID: 2631711
74. Panlilio AL, Culver DH, Gaynes RP, Banerjee S, Henderson TS, Tolson JS et al (1992) Methicillin-resistant *Staphylococcus aureus* in U.S. hospitals, 1975–1991. Infect Control Hosp Epidemiol 13:582–586
75. Centers for Disease Control and Prevention (CDC) (1999) Four pediatric deaths from community-acquired methicillin-resistant *Staphylococcus aureus*—Minnesota and North Dakota, 1997–1999. MMWR Morb Mortal Wkly Rep 48:707–710
76. Klein E, Smith DL, Laxminarayan R (2009) Community-associated methicillin-resistant *Staphylococcus aureus* in outpatients, United States, 1999–2006. Emerg Infect Dis 15:1925–1930. PMCID: 3044510
77. Stranden AM, Frei R, Adler H, Fluckiger U, Widmer AF (2009) Emergence of SCCmec type IV as the most common type of methicillin-resistant *Staphylococcus aureus* in a university hospital. Infection 37:44–48
78. Liu C, Chambers HF (2003) *Staphylococcus aureus* with heterogeneous resistance to vancomycin: epidemiology, clinical significance, and critical assessment of diagnostic methods. Antimicrob Agents Chemother 47:3040–3045. PMCID: 201119
79. Howden BP, Davies JK, Johnson PD, Stinear TP, Grayson ML (2010) Reduced vancomycin susceptibility in *Staphylococcus aureus*, including vancomycin-intermediate and heterogeneous vancomycin-intermediate strains: resistance mechanisms, laboratory detection, and clinical implications. Clin Microbiol Rev 23:99–139. PMCID: 2806658
80. Satola SW, Lessa FC, Ray SM, Bulens SN, Lynfield R, Schaffner W et al (2011) Clinical and laboratory characteristics of invasive infections due to methicillin-resistant *Staphylococcus aureus* isolates demonstrating a vancomycin MIC of 2 micrograms per milliliter: lack of effect of heteroresistant vancomycin-intermediate *S. aureus* phenotype. J Clin Microbiol 49:1583–1587
81. Centers for Disease Control and Prevention (CDC) (2002) *Staphylococcus aureus* resistant to vancomycin—United States, 2002. MMWR Morb Mortal Wkly Rep 51:565–567
82. Sievert DM, Rudrik JT, Patel JB, McDonald LC, Wilkins MJ, Hageman JC (2008) Vancomycin-resistant *Staphylococcus aureus* in the United States, 2002–2006. Clin Infect Dis 46:668–674

83. Perichon B, Courvalin P (2009) VanA-type vancomycin-resistant *Staphylococcus aureus*. Antimicrob Agents Chemother 53:4580–4587. PMCID: 2772335
84. Robbins WC, Tompsett R (1951) Treatment of enterococcal endocarditis and bacteremia; results of combined therapy with penicillin and streptomycin. Am J Med 10:278–299
85. Calderwood SA, Wennersten C, Moellering RC Jr, Kunz LJ, Krogstad DJ (1977) Resistance to six aminoglycosidic aminocyclitol antibiotics among enterococci: prevalence, evolution, and relationship to synergism with penicillin. Antimicrob Agents Chemother 12:401–405. PMCID: 429925
86. Zervos MJ, Kauffman CA, Therasse PM, Bergman AG, Mikesell TS, Schaberg DR (1987) Nosocomial infection by gentamicin-resistant *Streptococcus faecalis*. An epidemiologic study. Ann Intern Med 106:687–691
87. Leclercq R, Derlot E, Duval J, Courvalin P (1988) Plasmid-mediated resistance to vancomycin and teicoplanin in *Enterococcus faecium*. N Engl J Med 319:157–161
88. Uttley AH, Collins CH, Naidoo J, George RC (1988) Vancomycin-resistant enterococci. Lancet 1:57–58
89. National Nosocomial Infections Surveillance System (2004) National Nosocomial Infections Surveillance (NNIS) System report data summary from January 1992 through June 2004, issued October 2004. Am J Infect Control 32:470–485
90. Ramsey AM, Zilberberg MD (2009) Secular trends of hospitalization with vancomycin-resistant *enterococcus* infection in the United States, 2000–2006. Infect Control Hosp Epidemiol 30:184–186
91. Arias CA, Murray BE (2008) Emergence and management of drug-resistant enterococcal infections. Expert Rev Anti Infect Ther 6:637–655
92. Van der Auwera P, Pensart N, Korten V, Murray BE, Leclercq R (1996) Influence of oral glycopeptides on the fecal flora of human volunteers: selection of highly glycopeptide-resistant *enterococci*. J Infect Dis 173:1129–1136
93. Carmeli Y, Samore MH, Huskins C (1999) The association between antecedent vancomycin treatment and hospital-acquired vancomycin-resistant *enterococci*: a meta-analysis. Arch Intern Med 159:2461–2468
94. Fridkin SK, Edwards JR, Courval JM, Hill H, Tenover FC, Lawton R et al (2001) The effect of vancomycin and third-generation cephalosporins on prevalence of vancomycin-resistant *enterococci* in 126 U.S. adult intensive care units. Ann Intern Med 135:175–183
95. Bonten MJ, Willems R, Weinstein RA (2001) Vancomycin-resistant *enterococci*: why are they here, and where do they come from? Lancet Infect Dis 1:314–325
96. Gaynes R, Edwards JR (2005) Overview of nosocomial infections caused by gram-negative bacilli. Clin Infect Dis 41:848–854
97. Jacoby GA, Medeiros AA, O'Brien TF, Pinto ME, Jiang H (1988) Broad-spectrum, transmissible beta-lactamases. N Engl J Med 319:723–724
98. Monnet DL, Biddle JW, Edwards JR, Culver DH, Tolson JS, Martone WJ et al (1997) Evidence of interhospital transmission of extended-spectrum beta-lactam-resistant *Klebsiella pneumoniae* in the United States, 1986 to 1993. The National Nosocomial Infections Surveillance System. Infect Control Hosp Epidemiol 18:492–498
99. Nordmann P, Cuzon G, Naas T (2009) The real threat of *Klebsiella pneumoniae* carbapenemase-producing bacteria. Lancet Infect Dis 9:228–236
100. Centers for Disease Control and Prevention (CDC) (2009) Guidance for control of infections with carbapenem-resistant or carbapenemase-producing *Enterobacteriaceae* in acute care facilities. MMWR Morb Mortal Wkly Rep 58:256–260
101. Yong D, Toleman MA, Giske CG, Cho HS, Sundman K, Lee K et al (2009) Characterization of a new metallo-beta-lactamase gene, bla(NDM-1), and a novel erythromycin esterase gene carried on a unique genetic structure in *Klebsiella pneumoniae* sequence type 14 from India. Antimicrob Agents Chemother 53:5046–5054. PMCID: 2786356
102. Nordmann P, Poirel L, Toleman MA, Walsh TR (2011) Does broad-spectrum {beta}-lactam resistance due to NDM-1 herald the end of the antibiotic era for treatment of infections caused by Gram-negative bacteria? J Antimicrob Chemother 66:689–692

103. Kallen AJ, Srinivasan A (2010) Current epidemiology of multidrug-resistant gram-negative bacilli in the United States. Infect Control Hosp Epidemiol 31(Suppl 1):S51–S54
104. Kallen AJ, Hidron AI, Patel J, Srinivasan A (2010) Multidrug resistance among gram-negative pathogens that caused healthcare-associated infections reported to the National Healthcare Safety Network, 2006–2008. Infect Control Hosp Epidemiol 31:528–531
105. Quale J, Bratu S, Landman D, Heddurshetti R (2003) Molecular epidemiology and mechanisms of carbapenem resistance in *Acinetobacter baumannii* endemic in New York City. Clin Infect Dis 37:214–220
106. Keen EF, Murray CK, Robinson BJ, Hospenthal DR, Co EM, Aldous WK (2010) Changes in the incidences of multidrug-resistant and extensively drug-resistant organisms isolated in a military medical center. Infect Control Hosp Epidemiol 31:728–732
107. Obritsch MD, Fish DN, MacLaren R, Jung R (2004) National surveillance of antimicrobial resistance in *Pseudomonas aeruginosa* isolates obtained from intensive care unit patients from 1993 to 2002. Antimicrob Agents Chemother 48:4606–4610. PMCID: 529178
108. Lin YC, Chen TL, Ju HL, Chen HS, Wang FD, Yu KW et al (2006) Clinical characteristics and risk factors for attributable mortality in *Enterobacter cloacae* bacteremia. J Microbiol Immunol Infect 39:67–72
109. Deshpande LM, Jones RN, Fritsche TR, Sader HS (2006) Occurrence and characterization of carbapenemase-producing *Enterobacteriaceae*: report from the SENTRY Antimicrobial Surveillance Program (2000–2004). Microb Drug Resist 12:223–230
110. Centers for Disease Control and Prevention (CDC) (2010) Detection of *Enterobacteriaceae* isolates carrying metallo-beta-lactamase – United States, 2010. MMWR Morb Mortal Wkly Rep 59:750
111. Bratu S, Landman D, Alam M, Tolentino E, Quale J (2005) Detection of KPC carbapenem-hydrolyzing enzymes in *Enterobacter* spp. from Brooklyn, New York. Antimicrob Agents Chemother 49:776–778. PMCID: 547228
112. Semmelweis IF, Carter KC (1983) The etiology, concept, and prophylaxis of childbed fever. University of Wisconsin Press, Madison
113. Holmes OW (1974) Classic pages in obstetrics and gynecology. Oliver Wendell Holmes. The contagiousness of puerperal fever. The New England Quarterly Journal of Medicine and Surgery, vol. 1, pp. 503–530, 1842–1843. Am J Obstet Gynecol 119:852
114. Zachary KC, Bayne PS, Morrison VJ, Ford DS, Silver LC, Hooper DC (2001) Contamination of gowns, gloves, and stethoscopes with vancomycin-resistant *enterococci*. Infect Control Hosp Epidemiol 22:560–564
115. Bonilla HF, Zervos MA, Lyons MJ, Bradley SF, Hedderwick SA, Ramsey MA et al (1997) Colonization with vancomycin-resistant *Enterococcus faecium*: comparison of a long-term-care unit with an acute-care hospital. Infect Control Hosp Epidemiol 18:333–339
116. Byers KE, Anglim AM, Anneski CJ, Germanson TP, Gold HS, Durbin LJ et al (2001) A hospital epidemic of vancomycin-resistant *Enterococcus*: risk factors and control. Infect Control Hosp Epidemiol 22:140–147
117. Bonten MJ, Slaughter S, Ambergen AW, Hayden MK, van Voorhis J, Nathan C et al (1998) The role of "colonization pressure" in the spread of vancomycin-resistant *enterococci*: an important infection control variable. Arch Intern Med 158:1127–1132
118. Boyce JM, Opal SM, Chow JW, Zervos MJ, Potter-Bynoe G, Sherman CB et al (1994) Outbreak of multidrug-resistant *Enterococcus faecium* with transferable vanB class vancomycin resistance. J Clin Microbiol 32:1148–1153. PMCID: 263627
119. Boyce JM, Potter-Bynoe G, Chenevert C, King T (1997) Environmental contamination due to methicillin-resistant *Staphylococcus aureus*: possible infection control implications. Infect Control Hosp Epidemiol 18:622–627
120. Larson EL, Early E, Cloonan P, Sugrue S, Parides M (2000) An organizational climate intervention associated with increased handwashing and decreased nosocomial infections. Behav Med 26:14–22
121. Cromer AL, Latham SC, Bryant KG, Hutsell S, Gansauer L, Bendyk HA et al (2008) Monitoring and feedback of hand hygiene compliance and the impact on facility-acquired methicillin-resistant *Staphylococcus aureus*. Am J Infect Control 36:672–677

122. MacDonald A, Dinah F, MacKenzie D, Wilson A (2004) Performance feedback of hand hygiene, using alcohol gel as the skin decontaminant, reduces the number of inpatients newly affected by MRSA and antibiotic costs. J Hosp Infect 56:56–63
123. Pittet D, Hugonnet S, Harbarth S, Mourouga P, Sauvan V, Touveneau S et al (2000) Effectiveness of a hospital-wide programme to improve compliance with hand hygiene. Infection Control Programme. Lancet 356:1307–1312
124. Pittet D (2000) Improving compliance with hand hygiene in hospitals. Infect Control Hosp Epidemiol 21:381–386
125. Olsen RJ, Lynch P, Coyle MB, Cummings J, Bokete T, Stamm WE (1993) Examination gloves as barriers to hand contamination in clinical practice. JAMA 270:350–353
126. Slaughter S, Hayden MK, Nathan C, Hu TC, Rice T, Van Voorhis J et al (1996) A comparison of the effect of universal use of gloves and gowns with that of glove use alone on acquisition of vancomycin-resistant *enterococci* in a medical intensive care unit. Ann Intern Med 125:448–456
127. Boyce JM, Mermel LA, Zervos MJ, Rice LB, Potter-Bynoe G, Giorgio C et al (1995) Controlling vancomycin-resistant *enterococci*. Infect Control Hosp Epidemiol 16:634–637
128. Meyer KS, Urban C, Eagan JA, Berger BJ, Rahal JJ (1993) Nosocomial outbreak of *Klebsiella* infection resistant to late-generation cephalosporins. Ann Intern Med 119:353–358
129. Pena C, Pujol M, Ardanuy C, Ricart A, Pallares R, Linares J et al (1998) Epidemiology and successful control of a large outbreak due to *Klebsiella pneumoniae* producing extended-spectrum beta-lactamases. Antimicrob Agents Chemother 42:53–58. PMCID: 105455
130. Munoz-Price LS, Hayden MK, Lolans K, Won S, Calvert K, Lin M et al (2010) Successful control of an outbreak of *Klebsiella pneumoniae* carbapenemase-producing *K. pneumoniae* at a long-term acute care hospital. Infect Control Hosp Epidemiol 31:341–347
131. Munoz-Price LS, De La Cuesta C, Adams S, Wyckoff M, Cleary T, McCurdy SP et al (2010) Successful eradication of a monoclonal strain of *Klebsiella pneumoniae* during a *K. pneumoniae* carbapenemase-producing *K. pneumoniae* outbreak in a surgical intensive care unit in Miami, Florida. Infect Control Hosp Epidemiol 31:1074–1077
132. Karageorgopoulos DE, Falagas ME (2008) Current control and treatment of multidrug-resistant *Acinetobacter baumannii* infections. Lancet Infect Dis 8:751–762
133. Ostrowsky BE, Trick WE, Sohn AH, Quirk SB, Holt S, Carson LA et al (2001) Control of vancomycin-resistant *enterococcus* in health care facilities in a region. N Engl J Med 344:1427–1433
134. Cooper BS, Stone SP, Kibbler CC, Cookson BD, Roberts JA, Medley GF et al (2004) Isolation measures in the hospital management of methicillin resistant *Staphylococcus aureus* (MRSA): systematic review of the literature. BMJ 329:533. PMCID: 516101
135. Muto CA, Jernigan JA, Ostrowsky BE, Richet HM, Jarvis WR, Boyce JM et al (2003) SHEA guideline for preventing nosocomial transmission of multidrug-resistant strains of *Staphylococcus aureus* and *enterococcus*. Infect Control Hosp Epidemiol 24:362–386
136. Stelfox HT, Bates DW, Redelmeier DA (2003) Safety of patients isolated for infection control. JAMA 290:1899–1905
137. Kirkland KB, Weinstein JM (1999) Adverse effects of contact isolation. Lancet 354:1177–1178
138. Evans HL, Shaffer MM, Hughes MG, Smith RL, Chong TW, Raymond DP et al (2003) Contact isolation in surgical patients: a barrier to care? Surgery 134:180–188
139. Saint S, Higgins LA, Nallamothu BK, Chenoweth C (2003) Do physicians examine patients in contact isolation less frequently? A brief report. Am J Infect Control 31:354–356
140. Boyce JM (2007) Environmental contamination makes an important contribution to hospital infection. J Hosp Infect 65(Suppl 2):50–54
141. Kramer A, Schwebke I, Kampf G (2006) How long do nosocomial pathogens persist on inanimate surfaces? A systematic review. BMC Infect Dis 6:130. PMCID: 1564025
142. Boyce JM, Havill NL, Otter JA, Adams NM (2007) Widespread environmental contamination associated with patients with diarrhea and methicillin-resistant *Staphylococcus aureus* colonization of the gastrointestinal tract. Infect Control Hosp Epidemiol 28:1142–1147

143. Johnston CP, Cooper L, Ruby W, Carroll KC, Cosgrove SE, Perl TM (2006) Epidemiology of community-acquired methicillin-resistant *Staphylococcus aureus* skin infections among healthcare workers in an outpatient clinic. Infect Control Hosp Epidemiol 27:1133–1136
144. Grabsch EA, Burrell LJ, Padiglione A, O'Keeffe JM, Ballard S, Grayson ML (2006) Risk of environmental and healthcare worker contamination with vancomycin-resistant *enterococci* during outpatient procedures and hemodialysis. Infect Control Hosp Epidemiol 27:287–293
145. Bhalla A, Pultz NJ, Gries DM, Ray AJ, Eckstein EC, Aron DC et al (2004) Acquisition of nosocomial pathogens on hands after contact with environmental surfaces near hospitalized patients. Infect Control Hosp Epidemiol 25:164–167
146. Ray AJ, Hoyen CK, Taub TF, Eckstein EC, Donskey CJ (2002) Nosocomial transmission of vancomycin-resistant *enterococci* from surfaces. JAMA 287:1400–1401
147. Tenorio AR, Badri SM, Sahgal NB, Hota B, Matushek M, Hayden MK et al (2001) Effectiveness of gloves in the prevention of hand carriage of vancomycin-resistant *enterococcus* species by health care workers after patient care. Clin Infect Dis 32:826–829
148. Duckro AN, Blom DW, Lyle EA, Weinstein RA, Hayden MK (2005) Transfer of vancomycin-resistant *enterococci* via health care worker hands. Arch Intern Med 165:302–307
149. Schultsz C, Meester HH, Kranenburg AM, Savelkoul PH, Boeijen-Donkers LE, Kaiser AM et al (2003) Ultra-sonic nebulizers as a potential source of methicillin-resistant *Staphylococcus aureus* causing an outbreak in a university tertiary care hospital. J Hosp Infect 55:269–275
150. Livornese LL Jr, Dias S, Samel C, Romanowski B, Taylor S, May P et al (1992) Hospital-acquired infection with vancomycin-resistant *Enterococcus faecium* transmitted by electronic thermometers. Ann Intern Med 117:112–116
151. Bonten MJ, Hayden MK, Nathan C, van Voorhis J, Matushek M, Slaughter S et al (1996) Epidemiology of colonisation of patients and environment with vancomycin-resistant *enterococci*. Lancet 348:1615–1619
152. Martinez JA, Ruthazer R, Hansjosten K, Barefoot L, Snydman DR (2003) Role of environmental contamination as a risk factor for acquisition of vancomycin-resistant *enterococci* in patients treated in a medical intensive care unit. Arch Intern Med 163:1905–1912
153. Hayden MK, Bonten MJ, Blom DW, Lyle EA, van de Vijver DA, Weinstein RA (2006) Reduction in acquisition of vancomycin-resistant *enterococcus* after enforcement of routine environmental cleaning measures. Clin Infect Dis 42:1552–1560
154. Rampling A, Wiseman S, Davis L, Hyett AP, Walbridge AN, Payne GC et al (2001) Evidence that hospital hygiene is important in the control of methicillin-resistant *Staphylococcus aureus*. J Hosp Infect 49:109–116
155. Sehulster L, Chinn RY (2003) Guidelines for environmental infection control in health-care facilities. Recommendations of CDC and the Healthcare Infection Control Practices Advisory Committee (HICPAC). MMWR Recomm Rep 52:1–42
156. Simor AE, Lee M, Vearncombe M, Jones-Paul L, Barry C, Gomez M et al (2002) An outbreak due to multiresistant *Acinetobacter baumannii* in a burn unit: risk factors for acquisition and management. Infect Control Hosp Epidemiol 23:261–267
157. Denton M, Wilcox MH, Parnell P, Green D, Keer V, Hawkey PM et al (2004) Role of environmental cleaning in controlling an outbreak of *Acinetobacter baumannii* on a neurosurgical intensive care unit. J Hosp Infect 56:106–110
158. Mulin B, Rouget C, Clement C, Bailly P, Julliot MC, Viel JF et al (1997) Association of private isolation rooms with ventilator-associated *Acinetobacter baumanii* pneumonia in a surgical intensive-care unit. Infect Control Hosp Epidemiol 18:499–503
159. Perencevich EN, Fisman DN, Lipsitch M, Harris AD, Morris JG Jr, Smith DL (2004) Projected benefits of active surveillance for vancomycin-resistant *enterococci* in intensive care units. Clin Infect Dis 38:1108–1115
160. Chaix C, Durand-Zaleski I, Alberti C, Brun-Buisson C (1999) Control of endemic methicillin-resistant *Staphylococcus aureus*: a cost-benefit analysis in an intensive care unit. JAMA 282:1745–1751

161. Hachem R, Graviss L, Hanna H, Arbuckle R, Dvorak T, Hackett B et al (2004) Impact of surveillance for vancomycin-resistant *enterococci* on controlling a bloodstream outbreak among patients with hematologic malignancy. Infect Control Hosp Epidemiol 25:391–394
162. Chaberny IF, Schwab F, Ziesing S, Suerbaum S, Gastmeier P (2008) Impact of routine surgical ward and intensive care unit admission surveillance cultures on hospital-wide nosocomial methicillin-resistant *Staphylococcus aureus* infections in a university hospital: an interrupted time-series analysis. J Antimicrob Chemother 62:1422–1429
163. Huang SS, Yokoe DS, Hinrichsen VL, Spurchise LS, Datta R, Miroshnik I et al (2006) Impact of routine intensive care unit surveillance cultures and resultant barrier precautions on hospital-wide methicillin-resistant *Staphylococcus aureus* bacteremia. Clin Infect Dis 43:971–978
164. Ellingson K, Muder RR, Jain R, Kleinbaum D, Feng PJ, Cunningham C et al (2011) Sustained reduction in the clinical incidence of methicillin-resistant *Staphylococcus aureus* colonization or infection associated with a multifaceted infection control intervention. Infect Control Hosp Epidemiol 32:1–8
165. Robicsek A, Beaumont JL, Paule SM, Hacek DM, Thomson RB Jr, Kaul KL et al (2008) Universal surveillance for methicillin-resistant *Staphylococcus aureus* in 3 affiliated hospitals. Ann Intern Med 148:409–418
166. Muder RR, Cunningham C, McCray E, Squier C, Perreiah P, Jain R et al (2008) Implementation of an industrial systems-engineering approach to reduce the incidence of methicillin-resistant *Staphylococcus aureus* infection. Infect Control Hosp Epidemiol 29:702–708
167. Rodriguez-Bano J, Garcia L, Ramirez E, Lupion C, Muniain MA, Velasco C et al (2010) Long-term control of endemic hospital-wide methicillin-resistant *Staphylococcus aureus* (MRSA): the impact of targeted active surveillance for MRSA in patients and healthcare workers. Infect Control Hosp Epidemiol 31:786–795
168. Jain R, Kralovic SM, Evans ME, Ambrose M, Simbartl LA, Obrosky DS et al (2011) Veterans Affairs initiative to prevent methicillin-resistant *Staphylococcus aureus* infections. N Engl J Med 364:1419–1430
169. Kallen AJ, Mu Y, Bulens S, Reingold A, Petit S, Gershman K et al (2010) Health care-associated invasive MRSA infections, 2005–2008. JAMA 304:641–648
170. Coia JE, Duckworth GJ, Edwards DI, Farrington M, Fry C, Humphreys H et al (2006) Guidelines for the control and prevention of methicillin-resistant *Staphylococcus aureus* (MRSA) in healthcare facilities. J Hosp Infect 63(Suppl 1):S1–S44
171. Carter A, Heffernan H, Holland D, Ikram R, Morris A, Roberts S et al (2002) Guidelines for the control of methicillin-resistant *Staphylococcus aureus* in New Zealand. New Zealand Ministry of Health. Available from http://www.moh.govt.nz/cd/mrsa. Accessed 13 June 2011
172. Harbarth S, Fankhauser C, Schrenzel J, Christenson J, Gervaz P, Bandiera-Clerc C et al (2008) Universal screening for methicillin-resistant *Staphylococcus aureus* at hospital admission and nosocomial infection in surgical patients. JAMA 299:1149–1157
173. Huskins WC, Huckabee CM, O'Grady NP, Murray P, Kopetskie H, Zimmer L et al (2011) Intervention to reduce transmission of resistant bacteria in intensive care. N Engl J Med 364:1407–1418
174. Harris AD, McGregor JC, Furuno JP (2006) What infection control interventions should be undertaken to control multidrug-resistant gram-negative bacteria? Clin Infect Dis 43(Suppl 2):S57–S61
175. Gardam MA, Burrows LL, Kus JV, Brunton J, Low DE, Conly JM et al (2002) Is surveillance for multidrug-resistant *enterobacteriaceae* an effective infection control strategy in the absence of an outbreak? J Infect Dis 186:1754–1760
176. Thouverez M, Talon D, Bertrand X (2004) Control of *Enterobacteriaceae* producing extended-spectrum beta-lactamase in intensive care units: rectal screening may not be needed in non-epidemic situations. Infect Control Hosp Epidemiol 25:838–841
177. Kola A, Holst M, Chaberny IF, Ziesing S, Suerbaum S, Gastmeier P (2007) Surveillance of extended-spectrum beta-lactamase-producing bacteria and routine use of contact isolation: experience from a three-year period. J Hosp Infect 66:46–51

178. Ben-David D, Maor Y, Keller N, Regev-Yochay G, Tal I, Shachar D et al (2010) Potential role of active surveillance in the control of a hospital-wide outbreak of carbapenem-resistant *Klebsiella pneumoniae* infection. Infect Control Hosp Epidemiol 31:620–626
179. Siegel JD RE, Jackson M, Chiarello L, The Healthcare Infection Control Practices Advisory Committee (2006) Management of multidrug-resistant organisms in healthcare settings [updated 2006]. Available from: http://www.cdc.gov/ncidod/dhqp/pdf/ar/MDROGuideline2006.pdf. Accessed 7 Feb 2011
180. Fazal BA, Telzak EE, Blum S, Turett GS, Petersen-Fitzpatrick FE, Lorian V (1996) Trends in the prevalence of methicillin-resistant *Staphylococcus aureus* associated with discontinuation of an isolation policy. Infect Control Hosp Epidemiol 17:372–374
181. Hartstein AI, LeMonte AM, Iwamoto PK (1997) DNA typing and control of methicillin-resistant *Staphylococcus aureus* at two affiliated hospitals. Infect Control Hosp Epidemiol 18:42–48
182. Brooks S, Khan A, Stoica D, Griffith J, Friedeman L, Mukherji R et al (1998) Reduction in vancomycin-resistant *Enterococcus* and *Clostridium difficile* infections following change to tympanic thermometers. Infect Control Hosp Epidemiol 19:333–336
183. Rao N, Cannella B, Crossett LS, Yates AJ Jr, McGough R 3rd (2008) A preoperative decolonization protocol for *Staphylococcus aureus* prevents orthopaedic infections. Clin Orthop Relat Res 466:1343–1348. PMCID: 2384036
184. Jog S, Cunningham R, Cooper S, Wallis M, Marchbank A, Vasco-Knight P et al (2008) Impact of preoperative screening for methicillin-resistant *Staphylococcus aureus* by real-time polymerase chain reaction in patients undergoing cardiac surgery. J Hosp Infect 69:124–130
185. Bode LG, Kluytmans JA, Wertheim HF, Bogaers D, Vandenbroucke-Grauls CM, Roosendaal R et al (2010) Preventing surgical-site infections in nasal carriers of *Staphylococcus aureus*. N Engl J Med 362:9–17
186. Wertheim HF, Vos MC, Ott A, Voss A, Kluytmans JA, Vandenbroucke-Grauls CM et al (2004) Mupirocin prophylaxis against nosocomial *Staphylococcus aureus* infections in nonsurgical patients: a randomized study. Ann Intern Med 140:419–425
187. Robicsek A, Beaumont JL, Thomson RB Jr, Govindarajan G, Peterson LR (2009) Topical therapy for methicillin-resistant *Staphylococcus aureus* colonization: impact on infection risk. Infect Control Hosp Epidemiol 30:623–632
188. Fernandez C, Gaspar C, Torrellas A, Vindel A, Saez-Nieto JA, Cruzet F et al (1995) A double-blind, randomized, placebo-controlled clinical trial to evaluate the safety and efficacy of mupirocin calcium ointment for eliminating nasal carriage of *Staphylococcus aureus* among hospital personnel. J Antimicrob Chemother 35:399–408
189. Martin JN, Perdreau-Remington F, Kartalija M, Pasi OG, Webb M, Gerberding JL et al (1999) A randomized clinical trial of mupirocin in the eradication of *Staphylococcus aureus* nasal carriage in human immunodeficiency virus disease. J Infect Dis 180:896–899
190. Evans HL, Dellit TH, Chan J, Nathens AB, Maier RV, Cuschieri J (2010) Effect of chlorhexidine whole-body bathing on hospital-acquired infections among trauma patients. Arch Surg 145:240–246
191. Climo MW, Sepkowitz KA, Zuccotti G, Fraser VJ, Warren DK, Perl TM et al (2009) The effect of daily bathing with chlorhexidine on the acquisition of methicillin-resistant *Staphylococcus aureus*, vancomycin-resistant *Enterococcus*, and healthcare-associated bloodstream infections: results of a quasi-experimental multicenter trial. Crit Care Med 37:1858–1865
192. Vernon MO, Hayden MK, Trick WE, Hayes RA, Blom DW, Weinstein RA (2006) Chlorhexidine gluconate to cleanse patients in a medical intensive care unit: the effectiveness of source control to reduce the bioburden of vancomycin-resistant *enterococci*. Arch Intern Med 166:306–312
193. Borer A, Gilad J, Porat N, Megrelesvilli R, Saidel-Odes L, Peled N et al (2007) Impact of 4% chlorhexidine whole-body washing on multidrug-resistant *Acinetobacter baumannii* skin colonisation among patients in a medical intensive care unit. J Hosp Infect 67:149–155

194. Paterson DL, Singh N, Rihs JD, Squier C, Rihs BL, Muder RR (2001) Control of an outbreak of infection due to extended-spectrum beta-lactamase–producing *Escherichia coli* in a liver transplantation unit. Clin Infect Dis 33:126–128
195. Troche G, Joly LM, Guibert M, Zazzo JF (2005) Detection and treatment of antibiotic-resistant bacterial carriage in a surgical intensive care unit: a 6-year prospective survey. Infect Control Hosp Epidemiol 26:161–165
196. Buehlmann M, Bruderer T, Frei R, Widmer AF (2011) Effectiveness of a new decolonisation regimen for eradication of extended-spectrum beta-lactamase-producing *Enterobacteriaceae*. J Hosp Infect 77:113–117
197. Zuckerman T, Benyamini N, Sprecher H, Fineman R, Finkelstein R, Rowe JM et al (2011) SCT in patients with carbapenem resistant *Klebsiella pneumoniae*: a single center experience with oral gentamicin for the eradication of carrier state. Bone Marrow Transplant 46(9):1226–1230
198. de Smet AM, Kluytmans JA, Blok HE, Mascini EM, Benus RF, Bernards AT et al (2011) Selective digestive tract decontamination and selective oropharyngeal decontamination and antibiotic resistance in patients in intensive-care units: an open-label, clustered group-randomised, crossover study. Lancet Infect Dis 11:372–380
199. Prescott JF (2008) Antimicrobial use in food and companion animals. Anim Health Res Rev 9:127–133
200. WHO (1998) Use of quinolones in food animals and potential impact on human health. World Health Organization, Geneva
201. Smith KE, Besser JM, Hedberg CW, Leano FT, Bender JB, Wicklund JH et al (1999) Quinolone-resistant *Campylobacter jejuni* infections in Minnesota, 1992-1998. Investigation Team. N Engl J Med 340:1525–1532
202. Endtz HP, Ruijs GJ, van Klingeren B, Jansen WH, van der Reyden T, Mouton RP (1991) Quinolone resistance in *Campylobacter* isolated from man and poultry following the introduction of fluoroquinolones in veterinary medicine. J Antimicrob Chemother 27:199–208
203. Engberg J, Aarestrup FM, Taylor DE, Gerner-Smidt P, Nachamkin I (2001) Quinolone and macrolide resistance in Campylobacter jejuni and C. coli: resistance mechanisms and trends in human isolates. Emerg Infect Dis 7:24–34. PMCID: 2631682
204. Holmberg SD, Solomon SL, Blake PA (1987) Health and economic impacts of antimicrobial resistance. Rev Infect Dis 9:1065–1078
205. Lee LA, Puhr ND, Maloney EK, Bean NH, Tauxe RV (1994) Increase in antimicrobial-resistant *Salmonella* infections in the United States, 1989–1990. J Infect Dis 170:128–134
206. WHO (2003) Joint FAO/OIE/WHO expert workshop on non-human antimicrobial usage and antimicorbial resistance: scientific assessment. World Health Organization, Geneva
207. Nelson JM, Chiller TM, Powers JH, Angulo FJ (2007) Fluoroquinolone-resistant *Campylobacter* species and the withdrawal of fluoroquinolones from use in poultry: a public health success story. Clin Infect Dis 44:977–980
208. Doi Y, Paterson DL, Egea P, Pascual A, Lopez-Cerero L, Navarro MD et al (2010) Extended-spectrum and CMY-type beta-lactamase-producing *Escherichia coli* in clinical samples and retail meat from Pittsburgh, USA and Seville, Spain. Clin Microbiol Infect 16:33–38
209. Smith HW (1969) Transfer of antibiotic resistance from animal and human strains of *Escherichia coli* to resident *E. coli* in the alimentary tract of man. Lancet 1:1174–1176
210. Trobos M, Lester CH, Olsen JE, Frimodt-Moller N, Hammerum AM (2009) Natural transfer of sulphonamide and ampicillin resistance between *Escherichia coli* residing in the human intestine. J Antimicrob Chemother 63:80–86
211. Johnson JR, Sannes MR, Croy C, Johnston B, Clabots C, Kuskowski MA et al (2007) Antimicrobial drug-resistant *Escherichia coli* from humans and poultry products, Minnesota and Wisconsin, 2002-2004. Emerg Infect Dis 13:838–846. PMCID: 2792839
212. Hardy B (2002) The issue of antibiotic use in the livestock industry: what have we learned? Anim Biotechnol 13:129–147
213. Klare I, Heier H, Claus H, Reissbrodt R, Witte W (1995) vanA-mediated high-level glycopeptide resistance in *Enterococcus faecium* from animal husbandry. FEMS Microbiol Lett 125:165–171

214. Schouten MA, Voss A, Hoogkamp-Korstanje JA (1997) VRE and meat. Lancet 349:1258
215. Jensen LB, Ahrens P, Dons L, Jones RN, Hammerum AM, Aarestrup FM (1998) Molecular analysis of Tn1546 in *Enterococcus faecium* isolated from animals and humans. J Clin Microbiol 36:437–442. PMCID: 104555
216. Stobberingh E, van den Bogaard A, London N, Driessen C, Top J, Willems R (1999) *Enterococci* with glycopeptide resistance in turkeys, turkey farmers, turkey slaughterers, and (sub)urban residents in the south of The Netherlands: evidence for transmission of vancomycin resistance from animals to humans? Antimicrob Agents Chemother 43:2215–2221. PMCID: 89449
217. Klare I, Badstubner D, Konstabel C, Bohme G, Claus H, Witte W (1999) Decreased incidence of VanA-type vancomycin-resistant *enterococci* isolated from poultry meat and from fecal samples of humans in the community after discontinuation of avoparcin usage in animal husbandry. Microb Drug Resist 5:45–52
218. WHO (2002) Impacts of antimicrobial growth promoter termination in Denmark. World Health Organization, Geneva
219. WHO (2007) Critically important antimicrobials for human medicine: categorization for the development of risk management strategies to contain antimicrobial resistance due to non-human antimicrobial use. In: Report of the 2nd WHO expert meeting, Copenhagen, Denmark
220. FDA (2010) The judicious use of medically-important antimicrobial drugs in food-producing animals. The Food and Drug Administration, Washington, DC
221. Wenzel RP (2004) The antibiotic pipeline–challenges, costs, and values. N Engl J Med 351:523–526
222. Stewart JJ, Allison PN, Johnson RS (2001) Putting a price on biotechnology. Nat Biotechnol 19:813–817
223. Projan SJ (2003) Why is big Pharma getting out of antibacterial drug discovery? Curr Opin Microbiol 6:427–430
224. Fox JL (2006) The business of developing antibacterials. Nat Biotechnol 24(12):1521–1528
225. Powers JH (2003) Development of drugs for antimicrobial-resistant pathogens. Curr Opin Infect Dis 16:547–551
226. Moellering RC Jr (2011) Discovering new antimicrobial agents. Int J Antimicrob Agents 37:2–9
227. Payne DJ, Gwynn MN, Holmes DJ, Pompliano DL (2007) Drugs for bad bugs: confronting the challenges of antibacterial discovery. Nat Rev Drug Discov 6:29–40
228. Page MG, Dantier C, Desarbre E (2010) In vitro properties of BAL30072, a novel siderophore sulfactam with activity against multiresistant gram-negative bacilli. Antimicrob Agents Chemother 54:2291–2302. PMCID: 2876421
229. Drawz SM, Bonomo RA (2010) Three decades of beta-lactamase inhibitors. Clin Microbiol Rev 23:160–201. PMCID: 2806661
230. Hancock RE, Chapple DS (1999) Peptide antibiotics. Antimicrob Agents Chemother 43:1317–1323. PMCID: 89271
231. Levin M, Quint PA, Goldstein B, Barton P, Bradley JS, Shemie SD et al (2000) Recombinant bactericidal/permeability-increasing protein (rBPI21) as adjunctive treatment for children with severe meningococcal sepsis: a randomised trial. rBPI21 Meningococcal Sepsis Study Group. Lancet 356:961–967
232. Barrett JF, Hoch JA (1998) Two-component signal transduction as a target for microbial anti-infective therapy. Antimicrob Agents Chemother 42:1529–1536. PMCID: 105640
233. Moir DT, Shaw KJ, Hare RS, Vovis GF (1999) Genomics and antimicrobial drug discovery. Antimicrob Agents Chemother 43:439–446. PMCID: 89141
234. Garnacho-Montero J, Ortiz-Leyba C, Jimenez-Jimenez FJ, Barrero-Almodovar AE, Garcia-Garmendia JL, Bernabeu-Wittel IM et al (2003) Treatment of multidrug-resistant *Acinetobacter baumannii* ventilator-associated pneumonia (VAP) with intravenous colistin: a comparison with imipenem-susceptible VAP. Clin Infect Dis 36:1111–1118

235. Michalopoulos A, Virtzili S, Rafailidis P, Chalevelakis G, Damala M, Falagas ME (2010) Intravenous fosfomycin for the treatment of nosocomial infections caused by carbapenem-resistant *Klebsiella pneumoniae* in critically ill patients: a prospective evaluation. Clin Microbiol Infect 16:184–186
236. Falagas ME, Kanellopoulou MD, Karageorgopoulos DE, Dimopoulos G, Rafailidis PI, Skarmoutsou ND et al (2008) Antimicrobial susceptibility of multidrug-resistant gram negative bacteria to fosfomycin. Eur J Clin Microbiol Infect Dis 27:439–443
237. Cunha BA (2006) New uses for older antibiotics: nitrofurantoin, amikacin, colistin, polymyxin B, doxycycline, and minocycline revisited. Med Clin North Am 90:1089–1107
238. Alanis AJ (2005) Resistance to antibiotics: are we in the post-antibiotic era? Arch Med Res 36:697–705
239. WHO (2001) WHO global strategy for containment of antimicrobial resistance. World Health Organization, Geneva
240. IDSA (2010) The 10 x '20 initiative: pursuing a global commitment to develop 10 new antibacterial drugs by 2020. Clin Infect Dis 50:1081–1083
241. Gaynes RP (2010) Preserving the effectiveness of antibiotics. JAMA 303:2293–2294
242. ECDC (2010) Annual epidemiological report on communicable diseases in Europe 2010. European Centre for Disease Control and Prevention, Stockholm
243. Buising KL, Thursky KA, Robertson MB, Black JF, Street AC, Richards MJ et al (2008) Electronic antibiotic stewardship–reduced consumption of broad-spectrum antibiotics using a computerized antimicrobial approval system in a hospital setting. J Antimicrob Chemother 62:608–616
244. Raymond DP, Pelletier SJ, Crabtree TD, Gleason TG, Hamm LL, Pruett TL et al (2001) Impact of a rotating empiric antibiotic schedule on infectious mortality in an intensive care unit. Crit Care Med 29:1101–1108
245. Cook PP, Catrou P, Gooch M, Holbert D (2006) Effect of reduction in ciprofloxacin use on prevalence of methicillin-resistant *Staphylococcus aureus* rates within individual units of a tertiary care hospital. J Hosp Infect 64:348–351
246. Rahal JJ, Urban C, Horn D, Freeman K, Segal-Maurer S, Maurer J et al (1998) Class restriction of cephalosporin use to control total cephalosporin resistance in nosocomial *Klebsiella*. JAMA 280:1233–1237
247. Bantar C, Sartori B, Vesco E, Heft C, Saul M, Salamone F et al (2003) A hospitalwide intervention program to optimize the quality of antibiotic use: impact on prescribing practice, antibiotic consumption, cost savings, and bacterial resistance. Clin Infect Dis 37:180–186
248. Lipsky BA, Baker CA, McDonald LL, Suzuki NT (1999) Improving the appropriateness of vancomycin use by sequential interventions. Am J Infect Control 27:84–91
249. Mol PG, Wieringa JE, Nannanpanday PV, Gans RO, Degener JE, Laseur M et al (2005) Improving compliance with hospital antibiotic guidelines: a time-series intervention analysis. J Antimicrob Chemother 55:550–557
250. Solomon DH, Van Houten L, Glynn RJ, Baden L, Curtis K, Schrager H et al (2001) Academic detailing to improve use of broad-spectrum antibiotics at an academic medical center. Arch Intern Med 161:1897–1902
251. Evans RS, Pestotnik SL, Classen DC, Clemmer TP, Weaver LK, Orme JF Jr et al (1998) A computer-assisted management program for antibiotics and other antiinfective agents. N Engl J Med 338:232–238
252. Gross R, Morgan AS, Kinky DE, Weiner M, Gibson GA, Fishman NO (2001) Impact of a hospital-based antimicrobial management program on clinical and economic outcomes. Clin Infect Dis 33:289–295
253. Seligman SJ (1981) Reduction in antibiotic costs by restricting use of an oral cephalosporin. Am J Med 71:941–944
254. Woodward RS, Medoff G, Smith MD, Gray JL 3rd (1987) Antibiotic cost savings from formulary restrictions and physician monitoring in a medical-school-affiliated hospital. Am J Med 83:817–823

255. Glowacki RC, Schwartz DN, Itokazu GS, Wisniewski MF, Kieszkowski P, Weinstein RA (2003) Antibiotic combinations with redundant antimicrobial spectra: clinical epidemiology and pilot intervention of computer-assisted surveillance. Clin Infect Dis 37:59–64
256. Fraser GL, Stogsdill P, Dickens JD Jr, Wennberg DE, Smith RP Jr, Prato BS (1997) Antibiotic optimization. An evaluation of patient safety and economic outcomes. Arch Intern Med 157:1689–1694
257. Coleman RW, Rodondi LC, Kaubisch S, Granzella NB, O'Hanley PD (1991) Cost-effectiveness of prospective and continuous parenteral antibiotic control: experience at the Palo Alto Veterans Affairs Medical Center from 1987 to 1989. Am J Med 90:439–444
258. Omidvari K, de Boisblanc BP, Karam G, Nelson S, Haponik E, Summer W (1998) Early transition to oral antibiotic therapy for community-acquired pneumonia: duration of therapy, clinical outcomes, and cost analysis. Respir Med 92:1032–1039
259. Fowler S, Webber A, Cooper BS, Phimister A, Price K, Carter Y et al (2007) Successful use of feedback to improve antibiotic prescribing and reduce *Clostridium difficile* infection: a controlled interrupted time series. J Antimicrob Chemother 59:990–995
260. Valiquette L, Cossette B, Garant MP, Diab H, Pepin J (2007) Impact of a reduction in the use of high-risk antibiotics on the course of an epidemic of *Clostridium difficile*-associated disease caused by the hypervirulent NAP1/027 strain. Clin Infect Dis 45(Suppl 2): S112–S121
261. Pope SD, Dellit TH, Owens RC, Hooton TM (2009) Results of survey on implementation of Infectious Diseases Society of America and Society for Healthcare Epidemiology of America guidelines for developing an institutional program to enhance antimicrobial stewardship. Infect Control Hosp Epidemiol 30:97–98
262. Shlaes DM, Gerding DN, John JF Jr, Craig WA, Bornstein DL, Duncan RA et al (1997) Society for Healthcare Epidemiology of America and Infectious Diseases Society of America Joint Committee on the Prevention of Antimicrobial Resistance: guidelines for the prevention of antimicrobial resistance in hospitals. Clin Infect Dis 25:584–599
263. Drew RH (2009) Antimicrobial stewardship programs: how to start and steer a successful program. J Manag Care Pharm 15:S18–S23
264. Fridkin SK (2003) Routine cycling of antimicrobial agents as an infection-control measure. Clin Infect Dis 36:1438–1444
265. Paskovaty A, Pflomm JM, Myke N, Seo SK (2005) A multidisciplinary approach to antimicrobial stewardship: evolution into the 21st century. Int J Antimicrob Agents 25:1–10
266. Fox BC, Imrey PB, Voights MB, Norwood S (2001) Infectious disease consultation and microbiologic surveillance for intensive care unit trauma patients: a pilot study. Clin Infect Dis 33:1981–1989
267. Dos Santos EF, Silva AE, Pinhati HM, Maia Mde O (2003) Effectiveness of the actions of antimicrobial control in the intensive care unit. Braz J Infect Dis 7:290–296
268. Sintchenko V, Iredell JR, Gilbert GL, Coiera E (2005) Handheld computer-based decision support reduces patient length of stay and antibiotic prescribing in critical care. J Am Med Inform Assoc 12:398–402. PMCID: 1174884
269. Yong MK, Buising KL, Cheng AC, Thursky KA (2010) Improved susceptibility of Gram-negative bacteria in an intensive care unit following implementation of a computerized antibiotic decision support system. J Antimicrob Chemother 65:1062–1069
270. Rao SR, Desroches CM, Donelan K, Campbell EG, Miralles PD, Jha AK (2011) Electronic health records in small physician practices: availability, use, and perceived benefits. J Am Med Inform Assoc 18:271–275
271. Gaynes RP, Gould CV, Edwards J, Antoine TL, Blumberg HM, Desilva K et al (2009) A multicenter study on optimizing piperacillin-tazobactam use: lessons on why interventions fail. Infect Control Hosp Epidemiol 30:794–796
272. Morel J, Casoetto J, Jospe R, Aubert G, Terrana R, Dumont A et al (2010) De-escalation as part of a global strategy of empiric antibiotherapy management. A retrospective study in a medico-surgical intensive care unit. Crit Care 14:R225

273. Bauer KA, West JE, Balada-Llasat JM, Pancholi P, Stevenson KB, Goff DA (2010) An antimicrobial stewardship program's impact with rapid polymerase chain reaction methicillin-resistant *Staphylococcus aureus/S. aureus* blood culture test in patients with *S. aureus* bacteremia. Clin Infect Dis 51:1074–1080
274. Nguyen DT, Yeh E, Perry S, Luo RF, Pinsky BA, Lee BP et al (2010) Real-time PCR testing for mecA reduces vancomycin usage and length of hospitalization for patients infected with methicillin-sensitive *staphylococci*. J Clin Microbiol 48:785–790. PMCID: 2832423
275. Rello J, Vidaur L, Sandiumenge A, Rodriguez A, Gualis B, Boque C et al (2004) De-escalation therapy in ventilator-associated pneumonia. Crit Care Med 32:2183–2190
276. Niederman MS (2006) De-escalation therapy in ventilator-associated pneumonia. Curr Opin Crit Care 12:452–457
277. Reinhart K, Hartog CS (2010) Biomarkers as a guide for antimicrobial therapy. Int J Antimicrob Agents 36(Suppl 2):S17–S21
278. Nobre V, Harbarth S, Graf JD, Rohner P, Pugin J (2008) Use of procalcitonin to shorten antibiotic treatment duration in septic patients: a randomized trial. Am J Respir Crit Care Med 177:498–505

Chapter 3
Multidrug-Resistant Tuberculosis: A Global Challenge

Ignatius W. Fong

3.1 Introduction

It is estimated that more than one-third of the world's population harbor tuberculosis (predominantly latent infection), and the number of new cases continue to grow with almost 10,000,000 in 2010 [1]. Already 36 million people have been treated since the World Health Organization's (WHO) strategy for tuberculosis (TB) control in 1995. There is an inequitable global distribution of the disease with 22 high-burden countries accounting for 80% of active TB cases in the world, and more than one-third in India and China [2]. Many of these countries have social, economic problems with overcrowding, high rates of poverty and unemployment, and inadequate social and healthcare infrastructures. Although Western developed Nations have to a large degree held tuberculosis in check for the past 50 years, due to effective public health systems, there is a real danger of increase due to the emergence of multidrug-resistant TB (MDR-TB) and the ever expanding immigration from high-burden countries.

Failure of developing countries to keep TB under control has been the result of multiple factors including problems with prevention, treatment, and inadequate interventional strategies [2]. The Millennium Development Goal (MDGs) for TB is to ensure the incidence rate is falling by 2015, and targets of reducing by half the 1990 levels of prevalence and mortality by 2015 may be a daunting task, especially for Africa and Eastern Europe, including former Soviet countries. The number of new cases of TB is still rising worldwide and the number in 2010 is the largest of any previous year in history [3]. Increase in the global numbers of TB is responsible for nearly 2,000,000 deaths, mostly in developing countries every year.

I.W. Fong, M.B.B.S., F.R.C.P.C. (✉)
Department of Medicine, University of Toronto, Toronto, ON, Canada

Division of Infectious Diseases, St. Michael's Hospital,
Toronto, ON, Canada
e-mail: fongi@smh.toronto.on.ca

I.W. Fong (ed.), *Challenges in Infectious Diseases*, Emerging Infectious Diseases of the 21st Century 502, DOI 10.1007/978-1-4614-4496-1_3,

New tuberculosis cases are attributed to increase in the world's population (growth rate of 2% per year), which now stands at seven billion people, the ongoing HIV pandemic and partly from the global emergence of MDR-TB and extensively drug-resistant (XDR)-TB.

3.2 Drug-Resistant Tuberculosis

Tolerable and highly effective drugs for treatment of active and latent tuberculosis are the main strategies to control and keep TB under control worldwide. Loss of the primary first-line drugs for treatment due to resistance is a major setback and threatens to inflame the global spread of MDR-TB. Emergence and spread of MDR-TB is a barrier for effective management and control of TB. The WHO target for eliminating TB by 2050 is being threatened by increased prevalence of MDR-TB [4], and this goal will likely be unattainable from the current perspective. The evolution of MDR-TB is mainly attributed to incomplete and inadequate treatment of active disease. Resistance of *Mycobacterium tuberculosis (MTB)* to anti-TB drugs is caused by chromosomal mutations in genes encoding drug targets. MDR-TB (resistant to at least isoniazid [INH] and rifampin [RIF]) evolves through sequential accumulation of mutations in target genes [4], which affect two of the most effective agents against TB. Investigations in recent years have identified the hypervariable regions (area most susceptible to mutations) of the genome [5] and which genes code for drug resistance [6, 7]. The Global Project on Anti-Tuberculosis Drug Resistance has been gathering data since 1994, and updated analysis of drug resistance between 2002 and 2007 was reported in 2009 [8]. Based on this surveillance which generated data from 83 countries and territories from over 90,000 patients, there were approximately 500,000 cases of MDR-TB by 2007, with 27 countries accounting for 86% of the world's burden, and 50% were in India and China alone [8]. In the world, the median prevalence of MDR-TB in new TB cases was 1.6%, and in previously treated cases 11.7%, and accounts for approximately 5% of global TB cases [9]. However, there is wide variation in different countries and regions of the world from 0 to 22% or more. Countries of the former Soviet Union (USSR), followed by some provinces of China, reported the highest rates of MDR-TB [8]. Countries of Western and Central Europe, the Americas, and most of Africa reported the lowest prevalence is of MDR-TB. However, South Africa with an estimated 16,000 cases of MDR-TB ranks fourth on the global scale in absolute numbers [10]. In South Africa, the prevalence of HIV infection and TB appears to be fueling the development of MDR-TB, and more worrisome is the outbreak of extensively drug-resistant (XDR) TB. The estimated coinfection rate of HIV/TB is 70% but may be above 95% in areas such as Johannesburg [10]. There is also evidence that 11 countries in Africa (including Democratic Republic of Congo, Rwanda, Equatorial Guinea, and Senegal, which were not included in the WHO Third Global Report) have MDR-TB rates greater than 2% of all combined TB cases [11]. Hence, prevalence of MDR-TB is likely underreported in Africa.

The United States of America (USA) and Hong Kong have reported substantial reductions in the prevalence of MDR-TB (even more than reduction in all forms of TB), which is related to strong political will and financial commitments to TB control [8]. Whereas, countries such as Russia, Peru, and South Korea have experienced increased prevalence of MDR-TB. This is worrisome as both Peru and South Korea have had long-term implementation of DOTS (directly observed therapy, short course) [8].

Countries of the former USSR have the highest prevalence of MDR-TB with widespread ongoing epidemic for the past 13–15 years [8]. Estonia, however, is the exception, and it has reversed the trend by reducing the number of cases and fatality of MDR-TB as quickly as drug-sensitive TB with good control program [1]. Nine countries of the former USSR have MDR-TB prevalence rates of 6.8–22.3%, with 19.4% in Moldova and 22.3% in Baku, Azerbaijan, but stable or declining in the Baltic countries (Estonia and Latvia) [8].

The prevalence rates of MDR-TB in China are variable with 8 of 31 provinces and two municipalities showing high proportions, second only to countries of the former USSR up to 2007 [8]. In a recent review of MDR-TB across China from 1981 to 2006, the prevalence of MDR-TB in three groups (zones) had showed upward trend with prevalence 2.6–6.2 times greater in 2005 than that in 1985 [12]. These areas had much higher primary multidrug resistance of 4.3% and acquired drug resistance of 27.5%, with an overall MDR-TB prevalence of 9.9%. The top three zones were from the North East to the Southwest of China, with Hebei, Tibet, and Shanxi having extremely high prevalence of MDR-TB [12]. There is some evidence that prevalence rates of MDR-TB had increased from 2000 to 2003 but has been stable after 2004 in Shanghai and averaged about 4% [13]. Accurate rates of MDR-TB for Beijing are not available, as the number of strains tested was relatively small. In the Global Project on Anti-Tuberculosis Drug Resistance (GPDR-TB) [8], only 154 strains were tested, with a MDR-TB rate of 11.7% reported. A large number of isolates ($n = 1{,}967$) were subsequently tested for drug resistance (but a hospital-based study and subject to bias) and reported an overall MDR-TB rate of 19.4%, with 14.9% of the MDR-TB cases being XDR-TB [14]. The overall mean rate for China of MDR-TB in new cases averages 5% and for previously treated cases up to 25.6% [15]. See Fig. 3.1 for global distribution of MDR-TB (WHO, 2011).

The most recent estimate in 2010 of the global burden of MDR-TB supports an increase in the number of prevalent cases of about 650,000 MDR-TB among the world's 12 million cases of TB [16]. However, it is not known yet whether this represents an increase in the prevalent rate.

3.2.1 *Extensively Drug-Resistant (XDR) Tuberculosis*

The term XDR-TB was first developed by the US Centers for Disease Control and Prevention (CDC) in 2005. The present definition includes resistance to INH and

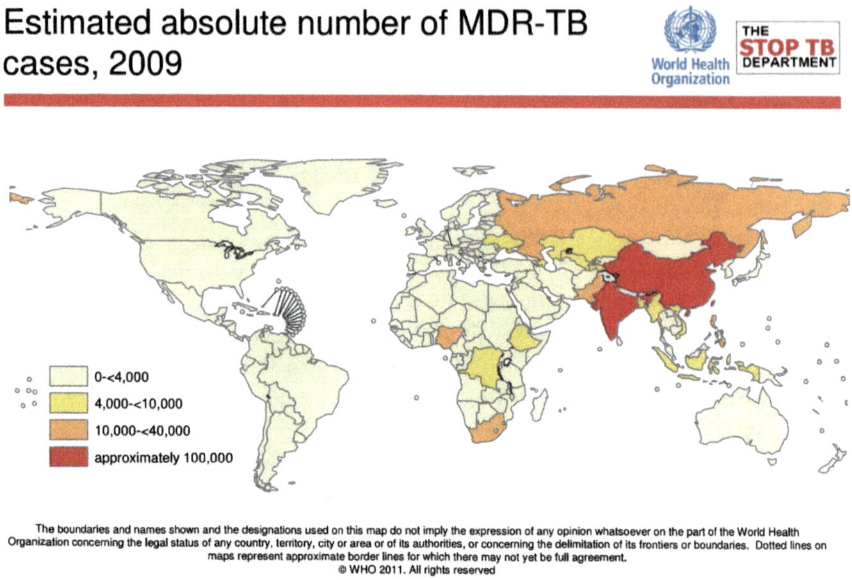

Fig. 3.1 Estimated absolute number of MDR-TB cases, 2009 (NB: Adapted from Ref. [20]. With permission of WHO)

RIF, plus any fluoroquinolone, and one of any three injectable second-line drugs (kanamycin, amikacin, or capreomycin) [17]. XDR-TB presents a huge challenge to treat and carries a high risk of default on treatment, often requiring 6–8 drugs for 24 months or more, and is associated with high failure rate and mortality. Increase prevalence of XDR-TB in various regions of the world is very worrisome and it is a great threat of the global control of TB [18]. The Global Project Surveillance update with data collected up to 2007 reported that 37 countries and territories had cases of XDR-TB, with 308 (8%) of 3,818 MDR-TB cases [8]. More recent surveys had found the highest prevalence rates of XDR-TB cases among MDR-TB tested from former countries of the USSR, China, and South Africa with rates of 10.5–21% [13].

The global burden of XDR-TB may be underestimated as appropriate drugs susceptibility testing of second-line drugs is not available in many regions, and the reproducibility and accuracy of testing are questionable for the gold standard method (agar proportion method on Lowenstein–Jensen media and Middlebrook 7Hll agar). Recently, standardized methods for susceptibility testing of second-line drugs have become available, but the current testing may not be reliable for certain drugs (i.e., cycloserine) [19]. In the latest WHO report, 68 countries had reported at least 1 XDR-TB case by the end of 2010 (Fig. 3.2) [20].

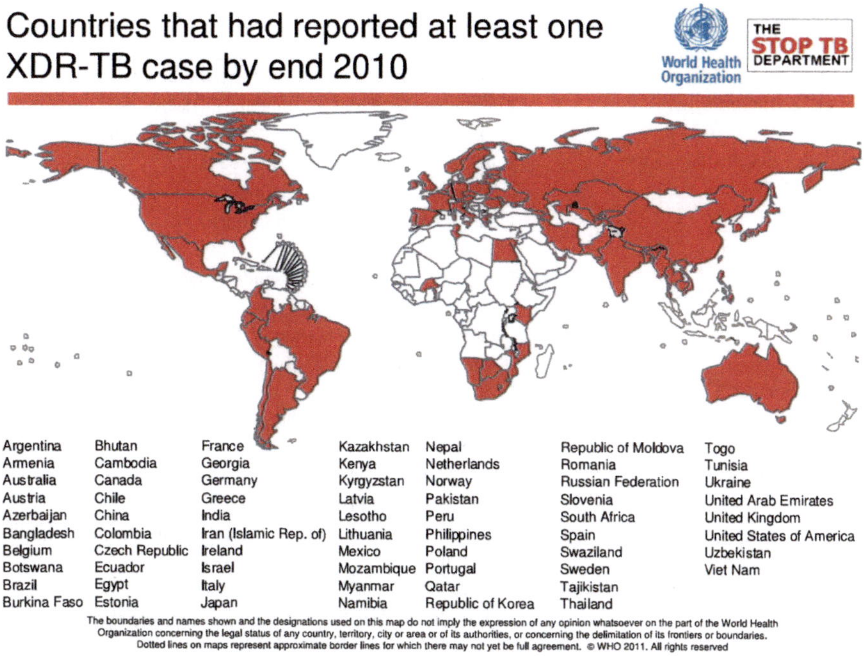

Fig. 3.2 Countries that had reported at least one XDR-TB case by end 2010 (NB: Adapted from Ref. [20]. With permission of WHO)

3.3 Reasons for Emergence of Drug-Resistant TB

Drug-resistant TB was first reported after the introduction of streptomycin monotherapy in 1948 [21]. Standard short-course (6 months) chemotherapy with triple drug combination (INH, RIF, and streptomycin) was developed in the late 1960s and 1970s. This regimen was found to be highly effective that killed naturally occurring single drug-resistant strains and prevented the emergence of multiresistant strains [22, 23]. Standard combination therapy did not necessarily prevent the emergence of drug resistance, even in susceptible strains, especially if patients took the medications erratically or incompletely. Four basic mechanisms for emergence of drug resistance with short-course combination therapy were proposed by Mitchison in 1998 [24], resulting from poor compliance. These included (1) differential bactericidal effects during initial killing, (2) monotherapy during sterilization of the mycobacterium population (resulting from partial compliance), (3) differential subinhibitory drug concentration during regrowth, and (4) differential bacteriopausal effects during regrowth [24].

Table 3.1 Factors in the Development of MDR-TB

Global issues	Regional problems
Variable and inconsistent healthcare infrastructures	Poor public health sector in many regions
	Inadequate social and healthcare infrastructures in resource-poor countries
Lack of reliable diagnostic and disease biomarkers	Capricious manifestation of disease
	Insensitivity of current diagnostic methods
	Delay by several weeks for culture diagnosis
	Host variability to tests
	Poor predictors of disease outcome with bacterial density in sputum
	Imprecise indicators of state of illness with lung pathology
Inadequate protection from vaccine (BCG) for lung TB	Host response variable, often less effective in high-burden countries
	Environmental/genetic variability with disease severity/outcome
Failure of treatment in many patients	Lack of susceptibility testing in many countries and delayed results
	Prolonged multidrug treatment results in default and poor compliance
	Low resources for DOTS
	Emerging MDR-TB/XDR-TB causing treatment failure and increased transmission
Inadequate development programs for new and novel therapy	Lack of highly effective drugs for MDR-TB/XDR-TB
	Poor tolerance and prolonged course with high pill burden results in frequent defaults
HIV pandemic	HIV and TB burden/distribution in same regions
	HIV coinfection results in rapid progression, variable presentation, poor response to treatment
	ART and anti-TB medications, increase pill burden, default and adverse events and IRIS

NB: Partial data and format of the above table were derived from Russell et al. [2]. With permission of the publisher
Abbreviations: *BCG* bacillus Calmette-Guerin, *DOTS* directly observed standardized therapy, *HIV* human immunodeficiency virus, *TB* tuberculosis, *ART* antiretroviral therapy, *IRIS* immune reconstitution inflammatory syndrome

Treatment failure due to multiple causes (most commonly from poor compliance and incomplete treatment) is the primary factor driving the emergence and spread of MDR-TB. Persistence of disease from acquired resistance then allows spread of resistant strains to new subjects (primary resistance). Other factors that have been identified as contributing to treatment failure or spread of resistance include lung cavitatory disease with high bacterial population burden, drug-related adverse events, alcohol abuse, drug abuse, prior history of treatment with anti-TB drugs (the most consistent factor), inadequate resources in high-burden countries (lack of DOTS program), concomitant HIV infection (inconsistent factor), high pill burden with multiple drugs, incarceration, and drug interactions and malabsorption that lead to subtherapeutic levels [4, 25–28] (Table 3.1).

Mathematical models based on population data indicate that the proportion of drug-resistant TB among all cases is driven by three determinants: first, the size of the population infected with TB and the probability of developing active disease with a susceptible strain; second, the size of the population with drug-resistant strains and the chance of developing active infection; third, factors associated with emergence of drug-resistant strains during treatment of initially susceptible strains, and amplification of resistance among those initially infected with drug-resistant strains [29]. The first two determinants are influenced by risk of infection and the immunity of the infected subpopulation (which is affected by the endemic rate of HIV infection and malnutrition), and the third risk factor is largely associated with the mycobacterium population and the treatment regimens (compliance and adherence, quality, and type of drugs and scheduling) [9].

Some models also predict that the future of MDR- and XDR-TB epidemic will depend to a large extent on the transmission efficacy or relative fitness of the drug-resistant MTB strains compared to drug-susceptible strains [30]. However, molecular epidemiological studies have yielded contradicting results. Further work in this area is needed to understand the detail molecular mechanisms and evolutionary forces to drive resistance in this organism. Modeling for the emergence of MDR-TB "hot zones" have found that the future prediction of MDR-TB transmissions requires equal measurements of not only fitness but also amplification probability, case finding, and cure rates [31].

3.3.1 Genetics of MDR-TB

Molecular mechanisms of drug resistance have been elucidated for the major first- and second-line drugs. High rates of transmission of MDR-TB have been associated with MTB complex of Beijing lineage, pointing to the importance of pathogen genetic factors for the epidemiology and outcome [32]. Although Beijing genotype may have selective advantages enabling rapid dissemination, studies from South Africa indicate that the frequency of drug resistance in some Beijing lineages appeared to have been acquired from multiple independent mutations within each cluster of isolates and not clonally derived [33]. Among the numerous genotypes of MTB, there is a common association between Beijing/W strains and resistance. However, the data is inconsistent, some show high frequencies of amplification, some more lethal to experimental mice, but others seem to have low survival or transmissibility [34]. Beijing strains represent about 50% of the strains in East Asia and at least 13% of the strains worldwide. Previous studies have found first-line drug resistance and MDR-TB to be associated with Beijing family in Vietnam, Russia, Taiwan, and elsewhere [34].

The emergence of the Beijing genotype family has been proposed to represent an evolutionary response of MTB to vaccination or antibiotic treatment in recent times [35]. The variability in epidemiological studies on association with virulence and drug resistance may be related to failure to analyze the data on subgroups. The Beijing clade consists of two major groups, so-called typical and atypical Beijing strains that may have different properties. For instance, typical Beijing strains are more frequently from the BCG vaccinated people than non-BCG-vaccinated people (but not the atypical strain), suggesting that BCG vaccination is less protective against typical Beijing strains [35]. The Beijing strains can also be subdivided into four monophyletic subgroups through large-sequence polymorphisms. Compared with other clades (62 clades or lineages by spoligotyping database [36]), the Beijing genotype displayed the largest population increase that has taken place in the past 180 years, and it is one of the most prominent genotypes and appears to be increasing in some areas [34].

Some epidemiological studies have found association of Beijing genotype with drug resistance in certain areas of the world. A high proportion of Beijing strains are found in many countries where greater than 5% of new tuberculosis cases involve MDR-TB (i.e., Azerbaijan, Ukraine, Uzbekistan, Estonia, Latvia, Lithuania, Mongolia, and China) [36]. In a survey of 24 European countries between 2003 and 2007 involving 2,494 MDR-TB isolates, 39% of these cases were attributed to clusters and 84% of these were caused by Beijing isolates [37]; whereas only 6–7% of the susceptible strains in Europe belonged to the Beijing genotype. Several hypotheses have been proposed to explain increased drug resistance in the Beijing family and this includes a higher mutation frequency; some Beijing strains have alterations in so-called putative mutation genes, resulting in altered DNA repair and mutation rate [38].

Genetic studies assessing INH resistance have found more mutations (Kat G315 the most important encoding resistance to INH) among Beijing strains, but the association is less certain for mutations in the rpoB gene, which account for 90% drug resistance to RIF [32]. A significantly higher proportion of the rpoB S531L mutation was found in Beijing genotype strains from Germany and Russia but not in Korea [39]. In a study from Russia, Beijing strains also showed more mutations in the emb B 306 gene encoding ethambutol (EMB) susceptibility [40]. Up to recently, Beijing genotypes have not been associated with other drug-resistant genes such as pncA, gyrA, and rpsL/rrs, which are responsible for resistance to PZA, fluoroquinolone, and streptomycin, respectively [36].

Drug-resistant strains of MTB arise by mutation, and possibly by horizontal gene transfer (although the latter has not been shown for MTB-resistant genes), among mycobacterial species [41]. Numerous gene alterations can confer drug resistance, and hundreds of alleles have been associated with INH resistance, and many of these affect the function of the katG gene, which encodes catalase-peroxidase enzyme required for INH inactivation [42]. INH resistance and the evolution of MDR-TB are complex dynamic processes, and INH-resistant mutation in katG, ahpc, and inhA was associated with RIF resistance, but only katG 315 mutations were associated with EMB resistance [4]. Rifampin resistance is due to mutation in the rpoB gene, which encodes the RNA polymerase B-subunit, and sequencing studies have shown that 90–95% of RIF-resistant MTB isolates have a mutation within 81-bp hotspot region (codons 507–533), most commonly at codons 531, 526, and 513 [7].

In general, drug combinations are an effective way to prevent the development and spread of resistant TB which is very low. The previous models estimated that the probability of 1 resistant mutation arising is low, about 10^{-8} per generation, and the chance of resistant mutations to 2 drugs is exceedingly small (10^{-16} per generation in an initially drug-sensitive MTB) [41]. However, more recent estimates using stochastic birth–death model estimated that the probability of emergence of resistance to the two principle anti-TB drugs before initiation of therapy ranges from 10^{-4} to 10^{-5}, several orders of magnitude higher than previous calculations (1,000–10,000 times higher) [42]. This study suggests that MDR-TB may not be entirely "man-made" (or distinct from functional monotherapy in the presence of combination therapy) and may explain the independent emergence of MDR- and XDR-TB over wide geographical areas.

The basis for selection of XDR-TB would be similar to the mechanisms for MDR-TB outlined above, which involves the selection of bacterial mutants with innate resistance to many chemotherapeutic drugs. Acquired and amplified drug resistance are the primary means of the evolution of XDR-TB. It is believed that the main factor driving the rise and spread of XDR-TB is likely transmitted resistance [43]. There is evidence, however, that clusters of XDR-TB outbreaks are related to clonal strains. The early 1990's MDR-TB outbreak in New York City, associated with HIV epidemic, prisons, and hospitals, was associated within minor sub-lineage of Beijing/W genotype [44]. Furthermore, in the Tugela Ferry outbreak in South Africa, 85% of the 46 isolated XDR-TB strains belonged to the KwaZulu-Natal (KZN) genotype family of strains [45]. Although the KZN family was first associated with resistance to first-line drugs in 1996, accumulated resistance to several second-line drugs occurred within 5 years [46]. However, a molecular epidemiology study across South Africa (but excluding the province of KZN) found seven different genotypes in XDR-TB isolates, of which the Beijing family was the most common [47]. Analysis of MTB strains from Cape Town over 12 years (1993–2004) showed that the incidence of non-Beijing clade remained stable, but Beijing clade cases increased exponentially over time [48]. Also, it has been postulated that mixed infection may accelerate the emergence of drug-resistant strains, and in one study of 109 MDR-TB isolates, there was high frequency of mixed subpopulations, but multiple drug resistance was not linked to a single strain [47].

Molecular analysis of KZN strains of XDR-TB has detected twelve single nucleotide polymorphisms (SNP) with protein-coding mutations [46]. Some of the mutations involves genes associated with antibiotic resistance (i.e., gyrA for fluoroquinolone, rpoB for rifampin), and others involved genes associated with membrane transport or cell wall synthesis (i.e., mmpl 13a), possibly associated with drug target modification or intracellular accumulation, and some uncharacterized genes that could be related to drug resistance. See Table 3.2 for frequency of mutations and target gene conferring drug resistance for MTB [4].

Table 3.2 Molecular basis for MTB drug resistance

Drugs	Gene target	Encoded protein/ RNA products	Major target	Level of resistance
INH	KatG	Catalase/peroxidase	Entire gene	High
INH/EMB	inhA	Enoyl-acyl carrier	Upstream regulatory region	Low
RIF	rpoB	β-Subunit of RNA polymerase	81 bp HSR	High
PZA	pncA	Pyrazinamidase	Several codons	High
EMB	Emb B	Arabinsyl transferase	Several codons	High
EMB	Ini A	INH-inducible gene	Few codons	High
SM	rrs	16srRNA	Several nucleotides	Low
SM	rpsl	Ribosomal protein S12	Codons 43 and 48	High
FQs	gyr A/gyrB	A/B subunits of DNA gyrase	Few codons	High
KAN/AM	rrs	16srRNA	Position 1401 or 1484	High
CAP/VIO	rrs/tlyA	16srRNA/cytotoxin-hemolysin homologue	Several codons	High

Modified from Ahmad and Mokaddas [4]. With permission of the publisher
INHFQs fluoroquinones, *KAN* kanamycin, *AM* amikacin, *CAP* capreomycin, *VIO* viomycin, *HSR* hotspot region, *bp* base pair

3.4 Management of MDR-TB

The management of MDR-and XDR-TB poses considerable challenges in any setting, but greatest for regions or countries with the highest burden of disease where resources are lacking. These challenges include slower rate of case detection (due to inadequate rapid diagnostic tests), that allow prolonged infectiousness and spread of disease. The pervasive problem of inadequate treatment delivery and treatment completion and the need for adequate health infrastructure to address the needs of the poor with tuberculosis are ongoing unresolved issues. Even in the resource-rich countries, the management of MDR-TB is a daunting task, due to delay in susceptibility testing resulting in initial inadequate treatment and need for poorly tolerated second-line and third-line agents for prolonged periods, resulting in poor compliance and incomplete therapy, prolonged isolation in institutions, and exorbitant cost with increased morbidity and mortality. Other concerns in the therapeutics of MDR-TB include the lack of randomized controlled trials and the need for sanctioned standardized therapy. However, by the nature of the disease, standardized treatment may pose certain limitations, due to the number of ineffective second-line or third-line agents, total duration of therapy and isolation, and the variability of the susceptibility of isolates from different areas.

Systematic review and in meta-analysis of 34 clinical reports (mean of 250 patients per report) on treatment outcomes for MDR-TB up to 2008 has been reported [49]. There was considerable heterogeneity between the studies with respect to HIV coinfection (0–76%), previous anti-TB treatment (0–100%), median duration of therapy (11–25 months), and the use of DOTS (47% for the entire duration and another 26% during the intensive phase of therapy). The highest success rate of treatment was observed when at least 18-month duration of therapy was combined with DOT for the entire period (69% versus 58%) [49]. Furthermore, individualized treatment regimens had higher success rate (64%) than standardized regimen (54%), but not statistically significant. Countries with established TB programs and better health infrastructure are more likely to complete successful therapy. Problems face by resource-poor countries are exemplified by the horrific report from KwaZulu-Natal, South Africa, where only 18% of those diagnosed with pulmonary TB completed treatment and only 11% were cured [50]. Unfortunately, clinicians failed to follow national guidelines and 85% of TB cases were diagnosed in the absence of sputum microscopy.

A major obstacle to the treatment of MDR-TB is the lack of highly effective and tolerable drugs since there is the loss of the two most effective agents (INH and RIF). See Table 3.3 for a list of the second-line and third-line agents. In a recent guideline of current principles of therapy for MDR-TB (based mainly on opinions), it was recommended that at least three new anti-TB agents and four when MDR-TB was suspected, for any failing regimen should be implemented. Any first-line agent to which the organism was susceptible should be used plus one newer fluoroquinolone (e.g., moxifloxacin), one injectable anti-TB agent, and one or more second-line oral agents. [51]. Therapy should be daily and not intermittently, and all doses should be directly observed. Other factors include adequate nutrition, emotional and social support, and treatment of concomitant diseases.

In another recent review and recommendation for the most effective treatment of MDR- and XDR-TB, similar guidelines with more specific details were provided [52]. At least four drugs to which the MTB is susceptible should be used, with stepwise selection of five groups of agents on the basis of efficacy, safety, and cost. Among the first group, high-dose INH as an adjunct is recommended (despite the in vitro susceptibility showing some resistance) as well as PZA and EMB (core drugs if known susceptible or as adjuncts if unknown); the second group include the fluoroquinolones of which high-dose levofloxacin is listed as first choice (but there is in vitro evidence that moxifloxacin is more effective); the third group is one of the injectacbles in the following order: capreomycin, kanamycin, and then amikacin; the fourth group in the following order includes prothionamide or ethionamide, cycloserine, and then para-aminosalicylic acid (PAS); and fifth group in the following order includes clofazimine, amoxicillin with clavulanic acid, linezolid, carbapenems, thiacetazone, and then clarithromycin. These guidelines are not evidence based on clinical trials.

An observational study recently reported the results of patients with MDR-TB sequentially assigned one of six "standardized" regimens between 1997 and 2007 [53]. The most effective regimen was given for a minimum of 9 months with gatifloxacin (similar in activity to moxifloxacin), clofazimine, and EMB and PZA, throughout the treatment period, supplemented by prothionamide, kanamycin, and high-dose INH for 4 months during the intense treatment phase, with cure rate of 87.9% ($n=206$). This regimen had manageable side effects with infrequent adverse reactions compared to 221 patients treated with ofloxacin and prothionamide throughout [53]. Adverse events were commonly reported with treatment for

Table 3.3 Drug therapy for MDR-TB (four core drugs[a] + or – additional drugs)

Groups	Drugs	Comments
1. First-line	INH (16–18 mg/kg)	As additional drug, not in WHO guide
	PZA[a]	Core or additional drug if no susceptibility
	EMB[a]	Only if susceptible
2. Fluoroquinolones[a]	Levofloxacin 750 mg/day	If susceptible to ofloxacin
	or moxifloxacin	Resistant to ofloxacin but MIC<2 μg/ml
3. Injectables[a] (one only)		
Aminoglycoside	Kanamycin or amikacin	Streptomycin resistance common and susceptibility test unreliable
or		
Polypeptides (if resistant to aminoglycosides)	Capreomycin or viomycin (less available)	Ototoxic and nephrotoxic
4. Oral second-line drugs[a]		
(>1 agent can be used)	Prothionamide (preferable) or ethionamide	GI intolerance common, hepatitis and psychiatric disorders
	Cycloserine	Neuropsychiatric disorders, risk of seizures with alcohol
	Para-Aminosalicyclic acid	Weak activity, GI side effects
	Thiocetazone	Avoid in HIV subjects; nausea, vomiting, dizziness, rashes with risk of Steven–Johnson syndrome
5. Additional drugs of unclear efficacy		
(cannot be used as core drugs)	Clofazimine	Limited evidence of efficacy, rash, GI side effects, used in leprosy
	Linezolid (300–600 mg/day)	Expensive, myelosuppression, lactic acidosis, peripheral/optic neuropathy, avoid with SSRI
	Clarithromycin or azithromycin	Limited efficacy, GI upset
	Amoxicillin-clavulanic acid	Weak limited activity, diarrhea, rash

NB: The above table was compiled from data obtained from References [51, 52, 90]

INH isoniazid, *EMB* ethambutol, *GI* gastrointestinal, *PZA* pyrazinamide, *SSRI* serotonin reuptake inhibitors ++injectable agents should be use for 6–8 months (intensive phase) with at least three other drugs, and a minimum of three drugs in the continuation phase for at least 21 months (subject to change with new active drugs and further studies)

[a]Core drugs when shown susceptible, otherwise can be use as additional drug

MDR-TB. In one report of 1,027 cases, 79% experienced at least one adverse event, with a median of three events per case (nausea 58%, vomiting 39%, abdominal pain 24%, psychiatric episodes 13%, hepatitis 9%, and renal failure 4%) [54]. Over two-thirds of patients required discontinuation of at least one drug. Analysis of risk factors for defaulters of MDR-TB therapy has found other nondrug factors such as substance abuse, incarceration, substandard housing, later year enrollment, and health district, but severe adverse event in the study of 671 patients did not predict default from therapy [55].

Fluoroquinolones (FLQs or quinolones) are believed to have a significant role to play in the treatment of MDR-TB. A review and meta-analysis of the data on these agents for the treatment of TB has identified 11 trials (1,514 patients) [56]. Ciprofloxacin substitution into first-line regimens led to higher incidence of relapse and sputum culture conversion to positive (thus, this drug should be avoided), and substituting for EMB in first-line regimens led to higher adverse events. Adding or substituting levofloxacin to basic regimens in drug-resistant areas had no effect, and ofloxacin was similar to sparfloxacin. Basically, further trials are needed. Other limitations of quinolones would be the likelihood of the development of resistance by MTB to these agents, similar to what has occurred with other bacterial pathogens worldwide. This dilemma is exemplified in a report from India, where the incidence of MTB resistance to quinolones exponentially increased from 3% in 1996 to 35% in 2004 [57]. Even in developed countries, previous exposure of 10 days of FLQ has been associated with increased of MTB resistance to these agents [58]. Empirical FLQ for the treatment of community acquired pneumonia in Western countries is also associated with longer delays in diagnosis and treatment of TB [59]. On the other hand, increase use of quinolones for MDR-TB has also been associated with the emergence of invasive levofloxacin resistant *Streptococcus pneumoniae* in children in South Africa [60].

Despite the fact that MDR- and XDR-TB are by definition resistant to INH, this may be a relative rather than absolute resistance, and newer guidelines have included high-dose INH for treatment of MDR-TB. The best data has been derived from a randomized small controlled study including 40–42 patients in each group, from India, comparing high-dose INH (16–18 mg/kg versus the standard dose of 5 mg/kg or 300 mg daily), and placebo in addition to second-line drugs [61]. Patients receiving the high-dose INH became sputum negative 2.38 times more rapidly and were 2.37 times more likely of being sputum negative at 6 months. Moreover, these patients had better radiological improvement without increased risk of INH toxicity [61].

In the early years after the global emergence of MDR-TB, successful management was mainly reported from high-income countries with referral hospitals. However, some resource-limited countries with treatment programs or with national services have yielded similar results as in wealthier countries. An analysis of 1,047 MDR-TB cases from Estonia, Latvia, Peru, Philippines, and the Russian Federation, reported successful treatment in 70% of patients, greater in new cases (77%) than previously treated cases (64%) [62]. Moreover, treatment of MDR-TB with second-line drugs in resource-limited countries is highly cost-effective [63]. Besides factors previously mentioned that predisposed to default on treatment, bilateral pulmonary involvement and cavitatory disease greatly reduced the chance of cure of MDR-TB [64].

Others have also found that despite using WHO category 2 regimen, 58% of failures were due to inadequate drug regimen, 42% due to mixed infection or reinfection, and further drug resistance amplification only occurred in 3.4% [65]. In Europe, risk factors for poor treatment outcome of MDR-TB were HIV infection, previous TB treatment, resistance to ofloxacin, and smear positivity at the start of treatment [66]. In worrisome report results of treatment of MDR-TB in a tertiary center in Karachi, Pakistan, admitted for 3–6 months and utilized individualized regimens of 4–6 drugs, successful outcome was only achieved in 39.2 and 41.2% were lost to follow-up during treatment [67]. It is not clear whether or not this result was due to poor public health infrastructure with absence of a DOTS program. It has been a standardized practice in developed countries to institutionalize patients with MDR-TB in respiratory isolation until sputum culture becomes negative, which may take greater than 6–12 weeks. This is very expensive and is a heavy burden on resource-poor countries. There is now evidence that the entire course of treatment can be accomplished in outpatient facilities with high cure rates of 70% in resource-limited settings [68, 69].

3.4.1 Treatment of XDR-TB

XDR-TB has been identified in all regions of the world and provides unique challenges in the management and care with combination of medical and surgical therapy, and is associated with high mortality and adverse reactions to drugs. The cost of hospitalization for one XDR-TB therapy is approximately twice the cost for MDR-TB cases, and in the United States, this averages US$483,000 per patient [70]. Risk factors for XDR-TB have been identified as (1) previous antituberculous therapy (adjusted odds ratio [OR] of 10.5), (2) homelessness (OR 2.73), (3) alcohol abuse (OR 1.8) [71], (4) bilateral cavitatory lung disease (OR 3.4), and (5) prior exposure to second-line injectable drugs (OR 3.6) [72]. By definition, XDR-TB is resistant to the first three groups of anti-TB agents (Table 3.3) and relies on less effective second-line agents and drugs of unclear anti-TB activity. It is also worrisome that MDR-TB isolates have developed efflux pumps genes following exposure to various anti-TB drugs that could result in pan-resistance [73]. Strains from South Korea have also developed polymorphisms associated with cross-resistance to aminoglycosides and capreomycin [74], and cross-resistance between streptomycin, kanamycin, and amikacin is not uncommon in Japan [75]. XDR-TB has emerged in South Africa despite treatment and strict adherence, with evidence of stepwise evolution of drug resistance, suggesting that existing TB control measures were inadequate in the areas with high HIV-coinfected population [76].

Even more alarming is the emergence of totally drug-resistant TB (super extensively drug-resistant strains) which have been reported from Iran with immigrants from Afghanistan, Azerbaijan, Iraq, and some native Iranians [77]. Iran is not even considered a high-burden country for TB, and this underlines the possible dissemination of these super-resistant strains. The outcome of treatment for XDR-TB has generally been poor in both resource-rich countries, as in the United Kingdom (5 of 8 cases died in 3 years) [78], and in poorer nations with high HIV coinfection, such as South Africa, with a mortality of 42% and with only 20% of patients achieving sputum culture conversion [79], and even in countries with low HIV infection such as South Korea, the mortality has been reported in 48% [80]. In the report from South Korea of 176 patients with XDR-TB, poor outcome was associated with previous treatment and cavitatory disease and favorable outcome with the use of linezolid and surgical resection [80]. In a systematic review of XDR-TB published in 2009 [19], treatment success varied from 29.3 to 67% (average of 52%) and the mortality from 7 to 36%. Longer treatment duration, median time to sputum conversion (88–110 days), and median time to culture conversion (60–190 days) were all greater for XDR-TB compared to MDR-TB cases [19]. In a similar review and meta-analysis of 13 observational studies ($n = 560$ patients), 43.7% experienced favorable outcome (cure or treatment completion) and 20.8% died [81]. Use of a later generation FLQ resulted in improved outcome, despite resistance to representative earlier quinolone. Although cross-resistance among all FLQ classes had been documented in vitro [82], the higher level of bactericidal activity of later generation FLQ (i.e., moxifloxacin) may overcome lower-level resistance. Whereas a significant resistance to ofloxacin or ciprofloxacin can be conferred by a single gyrase mutation (>3 μg/ml), two mutations in gyrA or both gyrA and gyrB are required for high-level resistance [83], thus explaining the above results. In the setting of XDR-TB, moxifloxacin (MIC = or <2.0 μg/ml) may be the preferred fluoroquinolone as in a murine model this agent was the most bactericidal followed by sparfloxacin,, levofloxacin, and then ofloxacin [84, 85]. It is of interest that Peru, a country of limited resources and high burden of TB, has achieved one of the highest cure rate (60.4%) in XDR-TB cases using a combination of free individualized therapy, multidrug supervised therapy (average of 5.3, ±1.3 drugs), including cycloserine and a fluoroquinolone, nutritional and psychosocial support, and adverse event management [86].

Observational studies suggest that early pulmonary resection, when feasible, combined with chemotherapy can produce high cure rates with acceptable complications for MDR-TB but more so for XDR-TB [87–89]. The main indications for surgery have been failure of medical treatment (71%), localized disease, persistent cavity with likely relapse (24%), and combined complications, such as severe hemoptysis (5%) in the most recent report [87]. Procedures performed include lobectomy, wedge resection, and pneumonectomies, and favorable outcomes have been as high as 90%. However, appropriate selection of candidates is the key factor (localized disease with good respiratory reserve) and when there is less than four effective drugs available [90]. The duration of treatment for XDR-TB has not been well established, but the WHO recommend a minimum of 18 months after culture conversion to negative, and treatment should be with a minimum of 4–5 effective drugs for at least 18–24 months [43].

3.4.2 HIV Coinfection with MDR- or XDR-TB

The burden of TB and HIV commonly shares the same distribution in developing countries. Moreover, TB is the most common cause of death in HIV-infected subjects in these countries. Sub-Saharan Africa is disproportionately affected as 4 of 5 cases of TB is HIV associated, but worldwide, only 12% of the TB caseload is HIV associated [91].HIV-infected subjects have unique challenges with TB infection and more so with MDR- or XDR-TB strains. HIV-infected patients with active TB can be challenging to diagnose, and a high index of suspicion must be maintained. Although patients with high CD4 cell count presents with typical features, those with advanced disease and low CD4 count often have atypical chest radiographic findings, widespread dissemination, and extrapulmonary disease.

Treating patients with active TB and moderate to severe advanced HIV disease, even for susceptible strains of MTB, is complex and challenging, and the issues are magnified in the context of MDR- and XDR-TB. These patients are required to receive 2 multidrug regimens simultaneously, a 3-drug combination of antiretroviral agents (ART) with pneumocystis pneumonia prophylaxis, and the minimum of 4 or more active TB agents. Thus, the pill burden is high, and chance of adverse events and defaults is increased. Controversial issues have been timing of starting ART in these coinfected patients, because of the concern of the immune reconstitution syndrome (IRIS), drug interactions, and enhanced toxicities. Recent studies have addressed some of these issues. In a randomized multicenter, open label trial from Cambodia (CAMELIA), 661 patients with diagnoses of TB–HIV infection and CD4 cell count equal to or less than 200 cells/μl (25 cells/μl, median count) received ART early (2 weeks after starting anti-TB drugs) or later treatment 8 weeks after [92]. Although there was a significant increase in IRIS in the early group, the risk of death was also significantly less (18% versus 27%) than the later treatment group. Thus, supporting institution of ART earlier rather than later and serious adverse events were similar. A previous trial (SAPIT) had shown improved survival in patients with CD4 cell count less than 500 cells/μl, when ART was initiated during anti-TB therapy [93]. In another recent study of similar design, 807 patients with CD4 cell count <250 cells/μl (median 77 cells/μl), from four continents (Africa, Asia, North America, and South America), were randomized to receive ART within 2 weeks or later, 8–12 weeks after initiation of anti-TB therapy [94]. However, in this trial, earlier ART did not reduce the rate of new AIDS defining illness or death, except in the subgroup of subjects with CD4 cell count less than 50 cells/μl. A third trial published at the same time also addressed the same question, consisting of 642 HIV-infected subjects with confirmed smear-positive TB in South Africa [95]. This trial was an open label, and randomized controlled trial of three groups were performed: (1) sequential-therapy group (ART initiation after completion of anti-TB therapy), (2) early integrated therapy group (ART within 4 weeks of anti-TB drugs, 214 patients), and (3) late integrated therapy group (ART within 4 weeks after completion of the intensive phase of anti-TB treatment). The recent report provided results only from the comparison of groups 2 and 3. All patients had CD4 cell count <500 cells/μl, but the median CD4 cell count was 150 cells/μl. In this trial, early initiation in patients with CD4 cell count less than 50 cells/μl had increased AIDS-free survival, but delayed treatment to the first 4 weeks of continuation phase of anti-TB therapy reduced the risk of IRIS and other adverse events without increasing the risk of AIDS or death in those with higher CD4 cell count [95]. There are some differences between the Cambodian (CAMELIA) study and the Intercontinental and the South African trials that may explain the different results. These included sicker patients with more advanced AIDS in the Cambodian trial with lower CD4 cell count (median 25 cells versus 77 cells and 150 cells/μl) and lower body mass index, resulting in higher overall mortality of 16% versus 6.6% and 7%. However, the majority of patients in all 3 trials had pulmonary TB in the absence of drug resistance; therefore, the patients overall had good prognosis. Albeit the current data support initiating ART in coinfected patients with HIV and tuberculosis earlier (2–4 weeks after anti-TB initiation) in the presence of advanced immunosuppression and delayed institution of ART in those with better preserved immunity (>CD4 100 cells μl) [96]. This may not apply, however, to patients with TB meningitis where intracranial IRIS may be fatal. A previous randomized trial in Vietnam showed initiation of ART within 1 week of starting treatment for TB meningitis did not improve the outcome compared to deferred ART 8 weeks later, but increased the incidence of severe adverse reactions [97].

Drug interaction between current ART and first-line anti-TB drugs is usually known, and adjustments can be easily made, mainly by substituting rifabutin for rifampin and lowering the dose of rifabutin when using a protease inhibitor especially boosted with ritonavir. There is very limited knowledge of drug interaction between antiretrovirals and second-line anti-TB drugs used for MDR-TB strains. Many of these agents were developed many decades ago before the advent of modern pharmacological investigative techniques, and very few drug interaction studies were performed. A recent review, however, has been published to provide some guidelines for potential interactions with second-line anti-TB drugs and antiretroviral agents [98]. A summary of potential drug interactions is summarized in Table 3.4 for these agents. Rifampin and rifabutin that are not listed as MDR-TB are resistant to these agents.

3.5 Meeting the Challenges

Stop TB Partnership was established in 2000 as a global enterprise to enhance political and social actions to stop the global spread of TB [99]. Optimistic targets are to have the prevalence and death rates of the 1990 baseline reduce in half by 2015 and to accomplish a TB-free world by 2050. The latter target appears to be "a pipe dream" from the present viewpoint. To achieve these goals, objectives set forth by the WHO included (1) universal access to high-quality care for all people with TB and thus reduce their suffering and burden; (2) protect and prevent vulnerable population for TB, TB/HIV, and MDR-TB, including promoting human rights for prevention, care, and control of TB; and (3) enhance new tools for diagnosis, monitoring, and treatment to be used globally in a timely and effective manner [99].

Table 3.4 Potential interactions of antiretrovirals and second-line anti-TB drugs

Anti-TB drugs	Protease inhibitors	NNRTI	NRTI
Aminoglycoside/polypeptide	None	None	None
Fluoroquinolones	Moxifloxacin/sparfloxacin	Not likely	Not likely
	Conc. maybe ↓ by ritonavir	Monitor ECG	
Thiomides	Risk of hepatotoxicity with tipranavir/darunavir	Interactions likely risk of hepatotoxicity	Unpredictable
	Avoid liquid ritonavir, alcohol can cause psychosis	Avoid efavirenz/nevirapine	
Cycloserine	Unpredictable; avoid Liquid ritonavir/alcohol risk of seizures	Monitor for psychiatric reactions with efavirenz	Unpredictable
PAS	None likely	None likely	None likely
Clofazamine	May increase level	None likely	Unpredictable
Linezolid	None likely	None likely	None likely but AZT, DDI, D4T can cause added toxicity
Clarithromycin	Conc. ↑ by ritonavir	Conc. ↓ by efavirenz/nevirapine	None
Azithromycin	Conc. ↑ by nelfinavir	None	None
Amoxicillin/clavulanic acid	None likely	None likely	None likely

NB: The above table was derived and modified from Coyne et al. [98]. With permission of the publisher

Conc concentration, *NRTIs* nucleoside reverse transcriptase inhibitors, *NNRTIs* non-nucleoside reverse transcriptase inhibitors, *AZT* zidovudine, *DDI* didanosine, *D4T* stavudine, *PAS* *para*-aminosalicyclic acid

The first goal to achieve universal access to high-quality care for all people with TB involved several components, which poses daunting challenges. Major obstacles to overcome include maintenance of political commitment with adequate and sustained funding for middle- and low-income countries with high burden of TB. All countries had made a commitment to provide adequate domestic and external resources to achieve the Millennium Development Goals relevant to TB. However, these commitments will also change with new governments, development of new disasters that require urgent priorities, and economic hardships. The total cost of the Global Plan for 2006–2015 is estimated as US$56.1 billion, of which US$25.3 billion is currently estimated to be available [99]. However, the remaining US$30.8 billion may be difficult to realize in the near future due to the present global economic downturn and possible looming recession for Europe and North America. A breakdown of the estimated total cost include 80% to support country-level activities especially in Africa (ramp up universal healthcare infrastructure); costs to establish universal DOTS programs (US$28.9 billion); DOTS-Plus and TB/HIV activities would cost about US$5.8 and US$6.7 billion, respectively; and research and development of new tools requires US$9 billion [99]. Currently, there is a network of over 400 committed international organizations, countries, donors from public and private sectors, and government and nongovernmental organizations working together on this Global Plan. To provide universal high-quality care for people with TB requires coordination and collaboration between local, national, and international organizations with a good reporting system in place. Measures for early diagnosis and easy access to proper medical care for the poor, the most disadvantaged, and with the greatest risk for TB are to be implemented. This may involve not only improving medical infrastructure and access but a broader approach for social and economic improvement and education of the public about the manifestations and dangers of TB. Besides improved case finding of active TB expeditiously, the cornerstone of the Global Plan to improve care involves DOTS expansion to all countries and communities and greater implementation of DOTS-Plus for countries with high rates of MDR-TB. The latter requires strict application of DOTS-Plus, careful introduction of second-line drugs, and adequate laboratory support for diagnosis and monitoring to stop the circulation of the resistant strains of MTB. DOTS is a recognized strategy for delivering and improving TB case finding and care. It requires political commitment as well as dedicated public health systems for case detection, with proper microbiology or molecular techniques, insuring patient adherence to treatment, adequate drug supply with short course of chemotherapy, and good reporting and recording system [100]. However, it is estimated that 35% of cases are not receiving DOT services in South East Asia and probably even greater in Africa [99]. Current diagnostic techniques for TB are insensitive (direct microscopy) or slow and cumbersome (culture methods).

New diagnostic tests for rapid diagnosis of smear-negative TB were expected to be implemented in referral laboratories by 2008, but so far, it is not available in most countries of need. Nucleic acid amplification tests (polymerase chain reaction or PCR) show promise for rapid and reliable detection of MTB in sputum and other specimens, with detection of MDR-TB. Several candidate systems have been in development which could be used at the first referral level (district laboratory) and ultimately at the peripheral level. Despite the approval by the US Food and Drug Administration (FDA) of two rapid diagnostic tests for TB in the mid-1990s, utilizing nucleic acid amplification (NAA), these are not widely used except to confirm smear-positive specimens. The Amplified Mycobacterium Tuberculosis Direct (MTD) test (Gen-Probe) and the Amplicor MTB test (Roche Diagnostics) are used mainly by central referral laboratories and have a sensitivity between that of smear and culture, with high specificity for TB but poor negative predictive value for pulmonary and extrapulmonary TB [101]. Moreover, the methods require moderate training, equipment, and are labor intensive, and there is potential for contamination among specimens. The most promising development to date is a sensitive and fully automated commercially available nucleic acid amplification test (NAAT), which was developed mainly for use by outside reference laboratories. The Xpert MTB/RIF assay (Cepheid) is based on real time PCR and molecular beacon technology to detect the presence of MTB nucleic acid and the rpoB gene, associated with RIF resistance, which is present in all MDR-TB [102]. The test requires minimal laboratory expertise, results are available within less than 2 h, and it has been promoted by the WHO even in settings where PCR is difficult to implement [103]. This test was very sensitive and specific for symptomatic patients with pulmonary TB and sputum smear positive (98.2 and 99.2%), and in sputum smear-negative TB, the sensitivity increases from 72.5 to 90.2% with processing of 1 or 3 sputum specimens [103].The Xpert MTB/RIF may not be as sensitive in screening HIV-infected subjects starting ART, as they often lack typical symptoms of cough and fever and may have low concentration of TB bacilli in sputum [104]. This PCR assay has a limit of detection of 131 bacilli/ml of sputum (95% sensitivity), whereas the automated liquid cultures system sensitivity range from 10 to 180 organisms/ml. This assay has also been reported to have lower sensitivity in the rapid diagnosis of extrapulmonary TB, with sensitivity of only 29% from CSF of smear-negative cases of TB meningitis, 63–73% for tissues, lymph nodes, and pleural or pericardial effusions, but up to 86–100% with aspirated pus, synovial, and peritoneal fluids [105]. Despite these limitations, the Xpert MTB/RIF assay would greatly facilitate the rapid diagnosis of TB in most setting where contagion is an issue.

An ideal test for rapid diagnosis of TB should be inexpensive, easily performed without major equipment or technical expertise, and independent of sputum, fluid, or tissue accessibility, such as urine or a blood test. A simple commercial assay is available to detect lipoarabinomannan (LAM) excreted in urine of patients with TB [106]. Moderate sensitivity and high specificity have been found in HIV-infected patients in South Africa, with sensitivities of 67–85% in patients with CD4 cell counts <50 cells/μl (reflecting greater burden of TB bacilli) [107, 108]. This LAM ELISA has produced disappointing results in HIV-uninfected patients with TB [106]. A modification of this assay, using a dip-stick method, is being evaluated, and it would be the ideal test for the rapid diagnosis of TB, if it were confirmed to be sensitive and specific [106].

3.5.1 Prevention of TB

Prevention of primary TB or eradication of latent TB should be a primary objective in any goal to eradicate human TB, but these objectives have received less global attention. Primary prevention with a vaccine (BCG) is largely ineffective in preventing TB, and a more effective vaccine is critically needed. The ability to develop more effective vaccines has been greatly improved with genetic manipulation and compilation of the genome sequence of MTB. In the past decade, there have been ten new preventive TB vaccines that have gone into clinical trials [109]. These vaccines are boosters of BCG prime vaccination. However, novel TB vaccines in clinical trials, based on antigens in early stages of infection recognized by the immune system, do not prevent TB infection but results in control of bacterial growth at a lower level than unvaccinated animals, some of which eventually develop clinical disease [110]. In humans, BCG vaccine can prevent disseminated disease but not establishment of local disease. Active and latent TB appears to involve several different bacterial antigens expressed at various metabolic state (changed gene expression profile), and thus, preventing reactivation may require targeting several different bacterial antigens. The booster vaccines currently in clinical development have been designed to improve BCG efficacy. One such multistage vaccine H56 boosts the effects of BCG to protect primates against active TB and reactivation of latent TB [111]. Thus, clinical development of H56 may produce a significant advance in our ability to prevent TB. Hence, the prospect for development of an effective TB vaccine for commercial use in 5–10 years looks good.

Current efforts to prevent reactivation of latent TB mainly involve recognition of those with latent infection by the TB skin test (TST), absence of clinical disease and a normal chest radiograph, and treatment with INH for 9 months. The HIV epidemic has rendered the TB skin test insensitive in many subjects with impaired immunity. It is also ineffective in detecting latent infection in children who have received BCG vaccination within 10 years because of cross-reactivity, which is a problem in most high-burden countries with TB. The interferon release assays (IGRAs) were designed to replace TST for the diagnosis of latent TB infection. Multiple studies over the past decade have shown that the IGRAs lack the sensitivity to replace the TST and are more expensive [112]. It also suffers from the same insensitivity in severely ill and immunosuppressed patients, and although it could be used in children with suspected active tuberculosis, it is usually unaffordable in these settings of high-burden countries.

The burden of latent TB in the world is huge and although the lifetime risk of active disease is only about 10% for the normal host, it is dramatically increased in HIV infection(about 10% per year), malnutrition, some acute infections (i.e., measles), and other compromised states. Standard treatment with INH reduces the risk of future disease by 75–90%, but the limitations of 9 months of therapy include incomplete compliance. RIF for 4 months may result in better compliance and has been used in contacts of patients with known INH-resistant TB, but fear of rapid development of resistance and lack of large randomized trials limit its usage. A more practical preventive therapy for TB would be a shorter course which could be directly observed to ensure compliance. In a recent open label randomized, multicountry clinical trial involving over 7,700 subjects with latent TB, 9 months of self-administered INH was compared to directly observed once-weekly treatment with INH 900 mg and rifapentine 900 mg (a long acting rifamycin derivative) for 3 months [113]. The efficacy and drug discontinuation adverse events were similar, but treatment completion was greater (82.1%) in the 3-month study regimen than the standard INH group (69.0%). This study was not performed in resource-poor countries with high burden of TB and HIV infection (i.e., such as Africa) and follow-up was only for 33 months. Hence, a similar clinical trial needs to be expedited in these settings with longer follow-up before this regimen can be adopted globally. None of the current or new treatment for latent TB would be expected to be effective for contacts of patients with MDR-TB. There is no known effective treatment or preliminary trials reporting on the management of latent TB with suspected MDR-TB. This is an area that needs to be addressed with future clinical trials of one or more agents for 3–6 months versus placebo or INH alone for patients with suspected latent TB due to MDR-TB, especially in areas of high-burden coinfection with HIV. HIV-coinfected patients with latent TB are at high risk for reactivation especially in those with low CD4 cell count. The insensitivity of the TST to confirm latent TB has been a problem. Moreover, all patients with HIV should be screened for active TB disease even with recent cough and a normal chest radiograph. In South Africa, one-third of patients with culture, sputum-positive TB by active screening had normal chest radiographic findings [114]. Previous guideline for screening for active TB in subjects with cough for 2–3 weeks has been inadequate for HIV-associated TB, and new guideline for HIV-infected subjects include the presence of any 1 of 4 symptoms such as current cough, night sweats, weight loss, or fever [115]. This is estimated to have a sensitivity of 79% and specificity of 50%, and there is some impetus to screen all HIV-infected patients with sputum culture on liquid media for TB even in the absence of symptoms in areas of high endemic TB.

Besides the HIV pandemic, the major fuels for TB are poverty, malnutrition, and overcrowding. Thus, it is most important that these basic chronic social issues be improved or corrected before we can hope to conquer TB. The marked decline in TB incidence in China over the past 10 years may be due more to improvement in these factors secondary to the economic boom than to any public health or medical factors.

3.5.2 New Anti-TB Drugs

Development of new effective drugs for drug-resistant TB is imperative to achieve the global control of TB. More active drugs that can be used in combination for shorter periods; safe and easily available and inexpensive agents are sorely needed. It is dismal that no new anti-TB drug has been marketed for over four decades. Ten new drugs for the treatment of TB are in clinical development and some of these agents are very promising [91]. Diarylquinolines (TMC-207] is a novel ATP synthase inhibitor that is potent against drug-susceptible and drug-resistant strains including MDR-TB [116]. TMC-207 has bactericidal activity similar to that of INH and RIF, and in the phase II randomized trial of newly diagnosed MDR-TB cases, it resulted in significantly higher rate of sputum culture conversion at 2 months when added to an optimized background regimen (48% in the TMC arm versus 9% in the placebo arm) [117]. A larger clinical trial is ongoing to assess the microbiological outcome with the addition of TMC-207 for the 6 months of individualized treatment for MDR-TB [118].

Nitroimidazoles are also a novel class of anti-mycobacterial agents that act on both replicating and non-replicating bacteria, with bactericidal activity against susceptible and drug-resistant MTB strains [116, 118]. Hence, there is a potential of shortening the course of therapy. Two nitroimidazoles are in clinical development. PA-824, a nitroimidazole-oxazine subclass (developed in the USA), has shown good safety and tolerability in adult patients in South Africa and appears to be bactericidal at relatively low doses (200 mg/day or below). OPC-67683, developed in Japan, is a member of the nitroimidazole-oxazole family which is currently being assessed in phase II trials for MDR-TB [118].

Oxazolidinones (linezolid and PNU-100480] are broad-spectrum antibiotics with activity against gram-positive aerobic and anaerobic bacteria as well as mycobacteria. Linezolid which has been approved mainly for the use for resistant Staphylococcus *aureus* (MRSA) and vancomycin-resistant enterococci (VRE) have modest activity against MTB. Retrospective experience with linezolid for treatment of MDR-TB has been mixed with some favorable reports in the USA, but no objective advantages have been found in European countries, due to severe side effects [118]. A reduced dose of 300 mg instead of 600 mg appears to have decreased side effects with retained anti-TB activity, and a phase 2A trial is underway in patients with MDR-TB in South Africa. PNU-100480 is an analog of linezolid developed by Pfizer and it has greater in vitro activity, and in a mouse model, it shortened the time needed to cure TB when added to first-line agents [119]. A phase I clinical trial is in progress.

Ethylenediamines, SQ-109, is a derivative of EMB that appears to have different mechanism of action [116, 118]. In mice, it appears to have improved activity compared to EMB and interacts synergistically with INH and RIF. However, it does seem to have poor oral bioavailability in lower animals, and a phase I dose escalation study is underway. There are several new drugs in preclinical stages of development for TB treatment, and an older antipsychotic agent shows promise for treatment of MDR-TB. Thioridazine, a phenothiazine, has anti-mycobacterium activity in mouse models and has synergistic activity with first-line agents, and it is also active against MDR-TB strains [120]. Thioridazine (Mellaril) was first marketed worldwide for schizophrenia from 1959 for over 40 years but was withdrawn from the world market in 2005 because of concerns of arrhythmia and prolonged Q-T intervals. However, due to the high mortality and morbidity of MDR-TB, it would be ethical to conduct phase 3 trials with this drug in combination with other agents for MDR-TB treatment. Furthermore, this is an established drug previously marketed, and for clinical development for MDR-TB treatment, the duration to obtain approval could be markedly abbreviated. A preliminary report from Argentina has shown promising results with treatment of 14 patients with XDR-TB, treated with thioridazine, moxifloxacin, and linezolid [121]. Other novel approach has been the use of a therapeutic DNA vaccine in combination with standard drugs for MDR-TB, which had shown improvement in mycobacterium load in mice [122].

3.6 Accomplishments of the Global Plan to Stop TB

Significant progress has been made in the past decade to control global TB. It has been estimated that 43 million people were treated on under DOTS, 36 million were cured, and the case fatality rate fell from 8 to 4% between 1995 and 2008 [3]. However, despite this progress, worldwide incidence of TB is falling less than 1% per year [91]. Moreover, the worldwide case detection of TB has stalled around 60% between 1995 and 2008, short of the 70% target. The greatest progress in control of TB has been made in the Western Pacific region (Cambodia, China, the Philippines, and Vietnam), and the South East Asian Region (Bangladesh, India, Indonesia, Myanmar, and Thailand), where case detection is around 65–70%, and DOTS coverage average 65–90% [16]. However, it has been estimated that 35% of cases are still not being managed through existing DOTS services in South East Asia.

The Eastern European region has the lowest level of DOTS coverage (about 46%) and DOTS case detection (about 40%) of all regions, and the regional success (76%) is the second lowest, sub-Saharan Africa with high-burden of HIV being lower at 73% [16]. A recent WHO news release is disturbing as it indicates that MDR- and XDR-TB are spreading at an alarming rate in Eastern Europe [123]. More than 80,000 MDR-TB cases occur each year in the region, and the reported cases of XDR-TB increased sixfold between 2008 and 2009. Although the rates are highest in Eastern Europe and central Asia, many countries in Western Europe have increasing rates of TB and MDR-TB [123]. Also, the overall fatality is about 4–7% for uncomplicated susceptible TB but it rises to above 50% in MDR- and XDR-TB. Some good progress has been made in Africa in the fight against TB. Nine of the 22 TB high-burden countries are in Africa all now have a DOTS program. Although case detection rates have increased to about 50% from 23% in 1995, and the success rate of treatment has remained just about 70%, they are significantly below target (70 and 85%, respectively). Thus, the goal of halving the prevalence and death rates of TB from 1990 levels by 2015 is very unlikely to be achieved in Africa and Eastern Europe.

The barriers to adequate progress and reasons for failure to achieve WHO targets in Eastern Europe are largely related to lack of political will, financial constraints, inadequate laboratory infrastructure, and lack of experience of large-scale and rapid scale-up DOTS and DOTS-Plus. Some of these issues are also common to African Nations, but the greatest challenge appears to be the impact of the HIV epidemic on increasing TB incidence in sub-Saharan Africa. Also, additional factors in Africa include widespread poverty and very weak healthcare systems, poor access to health facilities, substandard laboratories, insufficient staffing of adequately trained personnel, and insufficient links or coordination between national TB and HIV programs [99]. Strategies have been in place to assist resource-poor countries where the number of specialized treatment centers for drug-resistant TB is inadequate. There are five global initiatives dedicated to improve controlling the epidemic of MDR-TB by improving laboratory facilities and assisting in providing second-line-drugs at affordable price [99]. These include (1) Green Light Committee, a joint effort of WHO and Stop TB partnership; (2) Global Laboratory Initiative, a similar joint effort; (3) Global Fund to fight AIDS, Tuberculosis and Malaria, a public and private partnership; (4) UNITAID, a multilateral donor effort; and (5) PEPFAR, President's Emergency Plan for AIDS Relief, the US government program [124].

3.7 Conclusion

There are many remaining unmet challenges to control global TB and this is magnified by MDR-TB and the HIV epidemic. Worrisome reports of MDR-TB still spreading in Eastern Europe up to recently is alarming [123]. It is essential for the world to eradicate MDR-TB in order to have a TB-free world by 2050. Presently, multifarious approach is needed and is being spearheaded by the WHO to conquer global TB. The key components of a medical solution to the global spread of TB and MDR-TB must include development of new potent anti-TB drugs with randomized clinical trials to confirm the most effective regimens, development of a highly effective vaccine, and the availability of affordable rapid and reliable diagnostic tests for TB. Just as important are the nonmedical solutions such as sustained political will, procurement of sufficient funds to support the needed endeavors, including up-scaling of health infrastructures and social basic needs of the underprivileged in resource-poor countries. There are many needs to be met and far to go, but there is hope that 1 day, humanity will defeat and conquer TB, however, probably not by 2050. Moreover, it is important that these new steps or actions be implemented expeditiously as totally drug-resistant TB is now emerging in India (12 cases), and there is a great fear that these strains may spread and produce a global nightmare [125, 126]. A similar trend was also reported in South Africa where 13 of 19 XDR-TB strains were resistant to all eight drugs tested [127].

Despite these alarming trends, there is a recent encouraging report from the WHO that TB disease declined in 2010 for the first time globally to 8.8 million people [9,000,000 in 2005], and the death toll in 2003 fell from 1.8 to1.4 million in 2010 [128]. Significant progress in the fight against TB was noted in China, Brazil, Kenya, and the United Republic of Tanzania. In China alone, the mortality rate from TB fell by nearly 80% to 55,000 people in 2010 compared with 1990 [128].

References

1. Dye C, William BG (2010) The population dynamics and control of tuberculosis. Science 328:856–861
2. Russell DG, Clifton EB 3rd, Flynn J (2010) Tuberculosis: what we don't know can, and does, hurt us. Science 328:852–855
3. World Health Organization (2010) Global tuberculosis control: a short update to the 2009 report (WHO/HTM/TB/2011.16). WHO, Geneva
4. Ahmad S, Mokaddas E (2009) Recent advances in the diagnosis and treatment of multidrug–resistant tuberculosis. Respir Med 103:1777–1790
5. McEvoy CR, van Helden PD, Warren RM, Gey van Pittius NC (2009) Evidence for a rapid rate of molecular evolution at the hypervariable and immunogenic *Mycobacterium tuberculosis* PPE38 gene region. BMC Evol Biol 9:237–258
6. Hazbon MH, Brimacombe M, Bobadilla del Valle M et al (2006) Population genetics study of isoniazid resistant mutations and evolution of multidrug–resistant *Mycobacterium tuberculosis*. Antimicrob Agents Chemother 50:2640–2649
7. Prammananan T, Cheunoy W, Taechamahapun D et al (2008) Distribution of rpoB mutations among multidrug–resistant Mycobacterium (MDR–TB) strains from Thailand and development of a rapid method for mutation detection. Clin Mirobiol Infect 14:446–453
8. Wright A, Zignol M, Van Deun A et al (2009) Epidemiology of antituberculosis drug resistance 2002–07: an updated analysis of the global project on anti-tuberculosis drug resistance surveillance. Lancet 373:1861–1873
9. Chiang CY, Centis R, Migliori GB (2010) Drug–resistant tuberculosis: past, present and future. Respirology 15:413–432
10. Grobush MP (2010) Drug–resistant and extensively drug–resistant tuberculosis in Southern Africa. Curr Opin Pulm Med 16:180–185
11. Amor YB, Nemser B, Singh A, Sankin A, Schluger N (2008) Under reported threat of multidrug–resistant tuberculosis in Africa. Emerg Infect Dis 14:1345–1351
12. Yang XY, Li YP, Mei YW et al (2010) Time and spatial distribution of multidrug–resistant tuberculosis among Chinese people 1981–2006: systematic review. Int J Infect Dis 14:e828–e837
13. Shen X, DeReimer K, Yuan ZA et al (2009) Drug–resistant tuberculosis in Shanghai, China, 2000–2006: prevalence, trends and risk factors. Int J Tuberc Lung Dis 13:253–259
14. Wang D, Yang C, Kuang T et al (2010) Prevalence of multidrug and extensively drug–resistant tuberculosis in Beijing, China: a hospital based retrospective study. Jpn J Infect Dis 63:368–371
15. Migliori GB, Centis R, Lange C, Richardson MD, Sotgiu G (2010) Emerging epidemic of drug–resistant tuberculosis in Europe, Russia, China, South America and Asia: current status and global perspectives. Curr Opin Pulm Med 16:171–179
16. WHO Global tuberculosis control. WHO report (2011). World Health Organization, Geneva. WHO, TB. http://www.who.int/tb/publications/global_report/2011/gtbr11_full.pdf
17. Centers for Disease Control and Prevention (CDC) (2006) Noticed to readers; revised definition of extensively drug–resistant tuberculosis. MMWR Morb Mortal Wkly Rep 55:1176
18. Gandhi NR, Nunn P, Dheda K et al (2010) Tuberculosis 2. Multidrug–resistant and extensively drug–resistant tuberculosis: a threat to global control of tuberculosis. Lancet 35: 1830–1843
19. Sotgiu G, Ferrara G, Matteelli A et al (2009) Epidemiology and clinical management of X DR–TB: systematic review by TBNET. Eur Respir J 33:871–881
20. WHO Global map on X DR–TB (2011). www.who.int./tb/challenges/xdr/xdr-map-November 2011.pdf
21. Medical Research Council (1948) Streptomycin treatment of pulmonary tuberculosis: a Medical Research Council investigation. Br Med J 2(4582):769–782

22. Mitchison DA (1985) The action of antituberculosis drugs in short course chemotherapy. Tubercule 66:219–225
23. Mitchison DA (2005) The diagnosis and therapy of tuberculosis during the past 100 years. Am J Respir Crit Care Med 171:699–706
24. Mitchison DA (1998) How drug resistance emerges as a result of poor compliance during short course chemotherapy of tuberculosis. Int J Tuberc Lung Dis 2:10–15
25. Palaci M, Dietze R, Haddad DJ et al (2007) Cavitatory disease and quantitative sputum bacillary load in cases of pulmonary tuberculosis. J Clin Microbiol 45:4064–4066
26. Drobniewski F, Balanova Y, Ruddy M (2002) Rifampin–and multi–drug–resistant tuberculosis in Russian civilians and prison inmates: dominance of the Beijing strain family. Emerg Infect Dis 8:1320–1326
27. Kimerling ME, Phillips P, Patterson P, Hall M, Robinson CA, Dunlap NE (1998) Low serum antimycobacterial drug levels in non- HIV infected tuberculosis patients. Chest 113: 1178–1183
28. Suarez-Garcia I, Rodriquez-Blanko A, Vidal-Perrez JL, Garcia-Viejo MA, Joraz-Hernandez MJ, Lopez O, Noguerado Ascensio A (2009) Risk factors for multidrug–resistant tuberculosis in a tuberculosis unit in Madrid, Spain. Eur J Clin Microbiol Infect Dis 28:325–330
29. Cohen T, Dye C, Colijin C et al (2009) Mathematical models of the epidemiology and control of drug–resistant TB. Expert Rev Respir Med 3:67–79
30. Borrell S, Gagneux S (2009) Infectiousness, reproductive fitness and evolution of drug–resistant *Mycobacterium tuberculosis*. Int J Tuberc Lung Dis 13:1456–1466
31. Blower SM, Chou T (2004) Modeling the emergence of the "hot zones": tuberculosis and amplification dynamics of drug resistance. Nat Med 10:1111–1116
32. Niemann S, Diel R, Khechinashvilli G, Gegia M, MDivani N, Tang YW (2010) *Mycobacterium tuberculosis* Beijing lineage favors the spread of multidrug–resistant tuberculosis. J Clin Microbiol 48:3544–3550
33. Loeger TR, Feng Y, Chen X et al (2010) The non-clonality of drug resistance in Beijing–genotype isolates of *Mycobacterium tuberculosis* from the Western Cape of South Africa. BMC Genomics 11:670
34. Parwati I, van Crevel R, van Soolingen D (2010) Possible underlying mechanisms for successful emergence of the *Mycobacterium tuberculosis* Beijing genotype strains. Lancet Infect Dis 10:103–111
35. Kremer K, van-der-Werf MJ, Au BK et al (2009) Vaccine–induced immunity circumvented by typical *Mycobacterium tuberculosis* Beijing strains. Emerg Infect Dis 15:335–339
36. Brudey K, Driscoll JR, Rigouts L et al (2006) *Mycobacterium tuberculosis* complex genetic adversity: mining the fourth international spoligotyping database (SpoLDB4) for classification, population genetics and epidemiology. BMC Microbiol 6:23
37. Devaux I, Kremer K, Heersma H, Van Soolingen D (2009) Clusters of multidrug–resistant *Mycobacterium tuberculosis* cases, Europe. Emerg Infect Dis 15:1052–1060
38. Lari N, Rindi L, Bonanni D, Tortoli E, Garzelli C (2006) Mutations in mutT genes of *Mycobacterium tuberculosis* isolates of Beijing genotype. J Med Microbiol 55:599–603
39. Park YK, Shin S, Ryu S et al (2005) Comparison of drug resistance genotypes between Beijing and non-Beijing family strains of *Mycobacterium tuberculosis* in Korea. J Microbiol Methods 63:165–172
40. Mokrousov I, Otten T, Vyshnevskiy B, Narvskaya O (2002) Detection of embB301 mutations in ethambutol–susceptible clinical isolates of *Mycobacterium tuberculosis* from Northwestern Russia: implications for genotype resistance testing. J Clin Microbiol 40:3810–3813
41. Dye C (2009) Doomsday postponed? Preventing and reversing epidemics of drug–resistant tuberculosis. Nat Rev Microbiol 7:81–87
42. Colijn C, Cohen T, Garnesh A, Murray M (2011) Spontaneous emergence of drug–resistance in tuberculosis before and during therapy. PLoS One 6:e18327
43. Jassal M, Bishai WR (2009) Extensively drug–resistant tuberculosis. Lancet Infect Dis 9:19–30
44. Bifani PJ, Mathema B, Liu Z et al (1999) Identification of W variant outbreak of *Mycobacterium tuberculosis* via population based molecular epidemiology. JAMA 282:2321–2327

45. Gandhi NR, Moll A, Sturm AW (2006) Extensively drug–resistant tuberculosis as a cause of death in patients co-infected with tuberculosis and H IV in a rural area of South Africa. Lancet 368:1575–1580
46. Pillay W, Sturm AW (2007) Evolution of the extensively drug–resistant FIS/LAM 4/KZN strain of Mycobacterium tuberculosis in Kwa-Zulu–Natal, South Africa. Clin Infect Dis 45:1409–1414
47. Mlambo CK, Warren RM, Poswa X, Victor TC, Duse AG, Marias E (2008) Genotypic diversity of extensively drug–resistant tuberculosis (XDR–TB) in South Africa. Int J Tuberc Lung Dis 12:99–104
48. van der Spuy GD, Kremer K, Ndabambi SI et al (2009) Changing *Mycobacterium tuberculosis* population highlights clade–specific pathogenic characteristics. Tuberculosis 89: 120–125
49. Orenstein EW, Basu S, Shah WS et al (2009) Treatment outcomes among patients with multidrug–resistant tuberculosis: systematic review and meta-analysis. Lancet Infect Dis 9:153–161
50. Loveday M, Thomson L, Chopra M, Ndela Z (2008) A health systems assessment of the Kwa-Zulu–Natal tuberculosis programme in the context of increasing drug resistance. Int J Tuberc Lung Dis 12:1042–1047
51. Albanna AS, Menzies D (2011) Drug–resistant tuberculosis: what are the treatment options? Drugs 171:815–825
52. Caminero JA, Sotgiu G, Zumla A, Migliori GB (2010) Best drug treatment for multidrug–resistant and extensive drug–resistant tuberculosis. Lancet Infect Dis 10:621–629
53. Van Deun A, Many AK, Salim MA, Das PK, Sarker MR, Daru P, Reider HL (2010) Short, highly effective, and inexpensive standardized treatment of multidrug–resistant tuberculosis. Am J Resp Crit Care Med 182:684–692
54. Bloss E, Kuksa L, Holtz TH, Riekstina V, Skripconoku V, Kammerer S, Leimane V (2010) Adverse events related to multidrug–resistant tuberculosis treatment, Latvia, 2000–2004. Int J Tuberc Lung Dis 14:275–281
55. Franke MF, Appleton SC, Bayona J et al (2008) Risk factors and mortality associated with default from multidrug–resistant tuberculosis. Clin Infect Dis 4–6:1844–1851
56. Ziganshina LE, Squire SB (2008) Fluoroquinolones for treating tuberculosis. Update of Cochrane Database Syst Rev 2005. Cochrane Database Syst Rev CD004795
57. Agrawal D, Udwaha ZF, Rodriquez C, Mehta A (2009) Increasing incidence of fluoroquinolone–resistant *Mycobacterium tuberculosis* in Mumbai, India. Int J Tuberc Lung Dis 13:79–83
58. Devassia RA, Blackham A, Gebretsadik T et al (2009) Fluoroquinolone resistance in *Mycobacterium tuberculosis*: the effect and duration and timing of fluoroquinolone exposure. Am J Resp Crit Care Med 180:365–370
59. Chen TC, Lu PL, Lin CY, Lin WR, Chen YH (2011) Fluoroquinolones are associated with delayed treatment and resistance in tuberculosis: systematic review and meta-analysis. Int J Infect Dis 15:e211–e216
60. von Gottberg A, Klugman KP, Cohen C et al (2008) Emergence of levofloxacin – non-susceptible *Streptococcus pneumoniae* and treatment for multidrug–resistant tuberculosis in children in South Africa: a cohort observational surveillance study. Lancet 371:1108–1113
61. Katiyar SK, Bihari S, Prakash S, Mamtani M, Kulkarni H (2008) A randomized controlled trial of high-dose isoniazid adjuvant therapy for multidrug–resistant tuberculosis. Int J Tuberc Lung Dis 12:139–145
62. Nathanson E, Lambregts-van Weesenbeek C, Rich ML et al (2006) Multidrug–resistant tuberculosis management in resource–limited settings. Emerg Infect Dis 12:1389–1397
63. Resch SC, Salomon JA, Murray M, Weinstein MC (2006) Cost effectiveness of treating multi–resistant tuberculosis. PLoS Med 3:e241
64. Siqiueira HR, Freitas FA, Oliveira DN, Barreto AM, Dalcolmu MP, Albano RM (2009) Clinical evolution of a group of patients with multidrug–resistant TB treated at a referral center in the city of Rio de Janeiro, Brazil. Tisilogia 35:54–62

65. Matthys F, Rigout S, Sizaire V et al (2009) Outcomes of chemotherapy with WHO category II regimen in a population with high prevalence of drug-resistant tuberculosis. PLoS One 4:e7954
66. Kliiman K, Altraja A (2009) Predictors of poor treatment outcome in multi–and extensively drug–resistant pulmonary TB. Eur Respir J 33:1085–1094
67. Rao NA, Irfan M, Mahfooz Z (2009) Treatment outcome of multidrug–resistant tuberculosis in a tertiary care hospital in Karachi. J Pak Med Assoc 59:694–698
68. Malla P, Kanitz EE, Akhtar M et al (2009) Ambulatory -based standardized therapy for multi–drug resistant tuberculosis: experience from Nepal, 2005–2006. PLoS One 4:e8313
69. Heller T, Lessells RJ, Wallrauch CG et al (2010) Community–based treatment for multidrug–resistant tuberculosis in rural Kwa Zulu-Natal, South Africa. Int J Tuberc Lung Dis 14: 420–426
70. Centers for Disease Control and Prevention (CDC) (2009) Plan to combat extensively drug–resistant tuberculosis: recommendation of the Federal Tuberculosis Task Force. Morbid Mortal Wkly Rep 58(RR–3):1–43
71. Kliiman K, Altraja A (2009) Predictors of extensively drug–resistant pulmonary tuberculosis. Ann Intern Med 150:766–775
72. Shin SS, Keshavjee S, Gelmanova IY et al (2010) Development of extensive drug–resistant tuberculosis during multidrug–resistant tuberculosis treatment. Am J Respir Crit Care Med 182:426–432
73. Gupta AK, Kotach VM, Chauhan DS, Sharma R, Singh M, Venkatesan K, Sharma VD (2010) Microarray analysis of efflux pump genes in multidrug–resistant *Mycobacterium tuberculosis* during stressed induced by common anti-tuberculosis drugs. Microb Drug Resist 16:21–28
74. Via LE, Cho SN, Hwang S et al (2010) Polymorphisms associated with resistance to aminoglycosides and capreomycin in *Mycobacterium tuberculosis* from South Korean patients with drug-resistant tuberculosis. J Clin Microbiol 48:402–411
75. Sugarwara I, Zhang J, Li C (2009) Cross-resistance of *Mycobacterium tuberculosis* isolates among streptomycin, kanamycin and amikacin. Indian J Exp Biol 47:520–522
76. Calver AD, Falmer AA, Murray M et al (2010) Emergence of increased resistance and extensively drug–resistant tuberculosis despite treatment adherence, South Africa. Emerg Infect Dis 16:264–271
77. Yelayati AA, Masjedi MR, Farnia P, Tabarsi P, Ghanavi J, Ziafarifi AH, Hoffner SC (2009) Emergence of new forms of totally drug–resistant tuberculosis bacilli: super extensively drug-resistant tuberculosis or totally drug–resistant strains in Iran. Chest 132:420–425
78. Abubakar I, Moore J, Drobniewski F et al (2009) Extensively drug–resistant tuberculosis in the UK: 1995–2007. Thorax 64:512–515
79. O'Donnell MR, Padayatchi N, Master I, Osburn G, Horsburg CR (2009) Improved early results for patients with extensively drug–resistant tuberculosis and HIV in South Africa. Int J Tuberc Lung Dis 13:855–861
80. Jeon DS, Kim DH, Kang HS et al (2009) Survival and predictors in non-HIV infected patients with extensively drug–resistant tuberculosis. Int J Tuberc Lung Dis 13:594–600
81. Jacobson KR, Tierney DB, Jeon CY, Mitnick CD, Murray MB (2010) Treatment outcomes among patients with extensively drug–resistant tuberculosis: systematic review and meta-analysis. Clin Infect Dis 51:6–14
82. Devasia RA, Blackman A, May C et al (2009) Fluoroquinolone resistance in *Mycobacterium tuberculosis*: an assessment of MGIT 960, MODS, and nitrate reductase assay and fluoroquinolone cross–resistance. J Antimicrob Chemother 63:1173–1178
83. Ginesberg AS, Grosset JH, Bishai WR (2003) Fluoroquinolones, tuberculosis and resistance. Lancet Infect Dis 3:432–442
84. Shandil RK, Jayaram R, Kaur P et al (2007) Moxifloxacin, ofloxacin, sparfloxacin, and ciprofloxacin against *Mycobacterium tuberculosis*: evaluation of in vitro and pharmacodynamic indices that best predict in vivo efficacy. Antimicrob Agents Chemother 51: 576–582

85. Poissy J, Aubry A, Fernandez C et al (2010) Should moxifloxacin be used for the treatment of extensively drug–resistant tuberculosis? An answer from a murine model. Antimicrob Agents Chemother 54:4765–4771
86. Mitnick CD, Shin SS, Seung KJ et al (2008) Comprehensive treatment of extensively drug–resistant tuberculosis. N Engl J Med 359:563–574
87. Kang MW, Kim HK, Choi YS, Kim K, Shim YM, Koh WJ, Kim J (2010) Surgical treatment for multidrug–resistant and extensively-drug resistant tuberculosis. Ann Thorac Surg 89:1597–1602
88. Somocurcio JG, Sotomayer A, Shin S, Portilla S, Valcarcel M, Guerra D, Furin J (2007) Surgery for patients with drug–resistant tuberculosis: Report of 121 cases receiving community—based treatment in Lima, Peru. Thorax 62:416–421
89. Shiraishi Y, Katsuragi N, Kita H, Toisha M, Onda T (2008) Experience with pulmonary resection for extensively drug–resistant tuberculosis. Interact Cardiovasc Thorac Surg 7:1075–1078
90. WHO (2008) Guidelines for the programmatic management of drug–resistant tuberculosis an emergency update (WHO/Htm/TB/2008. 402). World Health Organization, Geneva
91. Lawn SD, Zumla AI (2011) Tuberculosis. Lancet 378:57–72
92. Blanc FX, Sok T, Laureilland D et al (2011) Earlier versus later start of antiretroviral therapy in HIV–infected adults with tuberculosis. N Engl J Med 365:1471–1481
93. Abdool Karim SS, Naidoo K, Grobler H et al (2010) Timing of initiation of antiretroviral therapy. N Engl J Med 362:697–706
94. Havlier D, Kendall MA, Ive P et al (2011) Timing of antiretroviral therapy for HIV–1 infection and tuberculosis. N Engl J Med 365:1482–1489
95. Abdool Karim SS, Naidoo K, Grobler A et al (2011) Integration of antiretroviral therapy with tuberculosis treatment. N Engl J Med 365:1492–1501
96. Torok ME, Farrar JJ (2011) When to start antiretroviral therapy in HIV–associated tuberculosis. N Engl J Med 365:1538–1540
97. Torok ME, Yen NT, Chau TT et al (2011) Timing of initiation of antiretroviral therapy the human immunodeficiency virus (HIV)–associated tuberculous meningitis. Clin Infect Dis 52:1374–1383
98. Coyne KM, Pozniak AL, Lamorde M, Boffito M (2009) Pharmacology of second–line antituberculous drugs and potential for interactions with antiretroviral agents. AIDS 23: 437–446
99. WHO (2010) The global plan to stop TB, 2011–2015 (WHO/HTM/STB/2010.2.).World Health Organization, Geneva
100. Ralph AP, Anstey NM, Kelly PM (2009) Tuberculosis into the 2010's: is the glass half full? Clin Infect Dis 49:574–583
101. Dorman SE (2010) New diagnostic tests for tuberculosis: bench, bedside, and beyond. Clin Infect Dis 50(S3):S173–S177
102. Boehme CC, Nabeta P, Hillemann D et al (2010) Rapid molecular detection of tuberculosis and rifampin resistance. N Engl J Med 363:1005–1015
103. WHO Roadmap for rolling out Xpert MTB/RIF for rapid diagnosis of TB and MDR–TB. http//www.who.int./tb/laboratory/roadmap–xpert-mtb-rifipds. Accessed Dec 2010
104. Lawn SD, Wood R (2011) Tuberculosis in antiretroviral treatment services in resource limited settings: addressing the challenges of screening and diagnosis. J Infect Dis 204:S1159–S1167
105. Vadwai V, Boehme C, Nabeta P et al (2011) Xpert MTB/RIF: a new pillar in diagnosis of extrapulmonary tuberculosis? J Clin Microbiol 49:2540–2545
106. Peter J, Green C, Hoelscher M, Mwaba P, Zumla A, Dheda K (2010) Urine for the diagnosis of tuberculosis: current approaches, clinical applicability, and new developments. Curr Opin Pulm Med 16:262–270
107. Lawn SD, Edwards DJ, Kranzer K, Vogt M, Bekker LG, Wood R (2009) Urine lipoarabinomannan assay for tuberculosis screening for antiretroviral therapy, diagnostic yield and association with immune reconstitution disease. AIDS 23:1875–1880

108. Dheda K, Davids V, Lenders L et al (2010) Clinical utility of a commercial LAM–ELISA assay for TB diagnosis in HIV–infected patients using urine and sputum samples. PLoS One 5:e9848
109. Kaufman SH (2011) Fact and fiction in tuberculosis vaccine research: 10 years later. Lancet Infect Dis 11:633–640
110. Orme IM (2006) Pre-clinical testing of new vaccines for tuberculosis: a comprehensive review. Vaccine 24:2–19
111. Lin PL, Dietrich J, Tan E et al (2012) The multistage vaccine H56 boosts the effects of BCG to protect cynomolgus macaques against active tuberculosis and reactivation of latent *Mycobacterium tuberculosis* infection. J Clin Invest 122:303–314
112. Herrera V, Perry S, Parsonnet J, Banaei N (2011) Clinical applications and limitations of interferon-γ release assays for the diagnosis of latent tuberculosis infection. Clin Infect Dis 52:1031–1037
113. Sterling TR, Villarino E, Borisov AS et al (2011) Three months of rifapentine and isoniazid for latent tuberculosis infection. N Engl J Med 365:2155–2166
114. Dawson R, Masuka P, Edwards DJ et al (2010) Chest radiograph reading and recording system: evaluation for tuberculosis screening and patients with advanced HIV. Int J Tuberc Lung Dis 14:52–58
115. World Health Organization (2010) Guidelines for intensified tuberculosis case–finding and isoniazid preventive therapy for people living with HIV in resource constrained settings. WHO, Geneva. http11 whqlibdoc.who.int.publications/2011/9789241500708-eng-pdf. Accessed Dec 2010
116. Lienhardt C, Vernon A, Raviglione MC (2010) New drugs and new regimens for the treatment of tuberculosis: review of the drug development pipeline and implications for national programmes. Curr Opin Pulm Med 16:186–193
117. Diacon AH, Pym A, Grobusch M et al (2009) The diarylquinoline TMC207 for multidrug–resistant tuberculosis. N Engl J Med 360:2397–2405
118. Ma Z, Lienhardt C, McIlleron H, Nunn AJ, Wang X (2010) Global tuberculosis drug development pipeline: the need and the reality. Lancet 375:2100–2109
119. Williams KN, Brickner SJ, Stover CK et al (2009) Addition of PNU–100480 to first–line drugs shortens the time needed to cure murine tuberculosis. Am J Respir Crit Care 180:371–376
120. van Soolingen D, Hernandez-Pando R, Orozco H et al (2010) The antipsychotic thioridazine shows promising therapeutic activity in a mouse model of multidrug–resistant tuberculosis. PLoS One 5:e12640
121. Abbate E, Vescovo M, Natiello M et al (2012) Successful alternative treatment of extensively drug–resistant tuberculosis in Argentina with a combination of linezolid, moxifloxacin and thioridazine. J Antimicrob Chemother 67:473–477
122. Liang Y, Wu X, Zhang J et al (2011) Treatment of multi-drug resistant tuberculosis in mice with DNA vaccines alone or in combination with chemotherapeutic drugs. Scand J Immunol 74:42–46
123. Kelland K (2011) Risky tuberculosis spreading at an alarming rate in Europe: World Health Organization. Reuters Ltd, 14 Sept 2011
124. Chakroborty A (2011) Drug–resistant tuberculosis: an insurmountable epidemic? Inflammopharmacology 19:131–137
125. Udwadia ZF, Amale RA, Ajbani KK, Rodriques C (2011) Totally drug–resistant tuberculosis in India. Clin Infect Dis. doi:10,1093/CID 1 cir 889
126. Lowenberg S (2012) India reports cases of totally drug–resistant tuberculosis (World report). Lancet 379:205
127. Shah NS, Richardson J, Moodley P et al (2011) Increasing drug resistance in extensively drug–resistant tuberculosis, South Africa. Emerg Infect Dis 17:510–513
128. Selyukh A (2011) World tuberculosis cases decline for first-time ever: WHO. Reuters Health

Part II
Challenges in Developing Countries

Chapter 4
Urbanization and Infectious Diseases: General Principles, Historical Perspectives, and Contemporary Challenges

Raquel Reyes, Roy Ahn, Katherine Thurber, and Thomas F. Burke

4.1 Background

In 2009, a major demographic line was crossed: for the first time in history, the majority of the world population lived in cities rather than in towns and countryside (Fig. 4.1). This shift has been occurring over the past 100 years, with the most rapid rate of urban growth occurring over in the latter half of the twentieth century. Urban centers in the more developed regions of the world (i.e., North America, Australia, New Zealand, and Europe) experienced earlier growth in the 1920s–1950s, and since then, the rapid rate of urban growth has been concentrated in the cities and towns of developing nations [1].

According to the United Nations Population Division, the urban areas of the world are expected to absorb the entirety of the projected world population growth through 2050. The majority of this growth is expected to occur in less developed regions and countries such that by mid-century, 54% of the world's urban population will be concentrated in Asia and 20% in Africa. China and India together are

R. Reyes, M.D., M.P.A. (✉)
Division of Global Health, Department of Emergency Medicine,
Massachusetts General Hospital, Boston, MA, USA

Harvard MGH Medicine & Pediatrics Program, Departments of Internal
Medicine and Pediatrics, Massachusetts General Hospital,
Boston, MA, USA
e-mail: rreyes1@partners.org

R. Ahn, M.P.H., Sc.D. • K. Thurber, A.B. • T.F. Burke, M.D.
Division of Global Health, Department of Emergency Medicine,
Massachusetts General Hospital, Boston, MA, USA

I.W. Fong (ed.), *Challenges in Infectious Diseases*, Emerging Infectious Diseases of the 21st Century 502, DOI 10.1007/978-1-4614-4496-1_4,

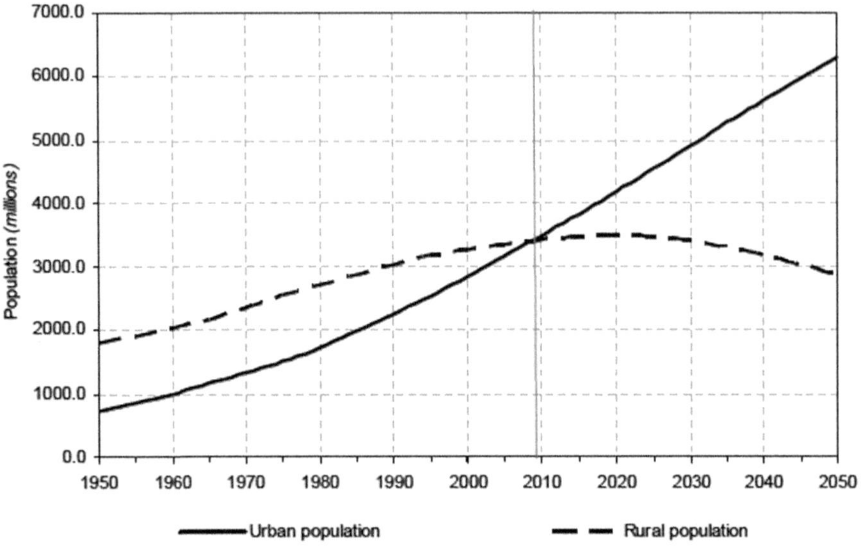

Fig. 4.1 Urban and rural populations of the world, 1950–2050. *Source*: United Nations Department of Economic and Social Affairs, Population Division. World Urbanization Prospects: The 2009 Revision. New York 2010. Reprinted with permission of the United Nations

expected to account for approximately one-third of the increase in the world urban population in this timeframe [1] (Fig. 4.2).

This chapter will use the term "urbanization" to refer to this demographic shift. Urbanization is the result of migration from rural to urban locales as well as the imbalance between death and fertility rates in urban and rural locales—that is, the proportionally higher ratio of births vs. deaths in cities compared to countryside. It is important to recognize, however, that "urban" and therefore "urbanization" are terms that are not easily fixed. The United Nations Statistics Division recognizes that "because of national differences in the characteristics which distinguish urban from rural areas, the distinction between urban and rural population is not amenable to a single definition applicable to all countries" [2]. Nevertheless, for the purposes of this discussion, we will use the term "urbanization" to refer most basically to the demographic shift from less densely populated localities to more densely populated localities. Additional assumptions regarding the implications of urbanization will be explicitly addressed throughout this chapter.

The effect of urbanization on health trends, morbidity, and mortality are numerous. In more developed countries and industrialized centers, for example, violent crimes, drug abuse, and motor vehicle accidents are more common health problems than in rural areas. Environmental pollutants in industrialized centers across the spectrum of more and less developed nations have a deleterious impact on health.

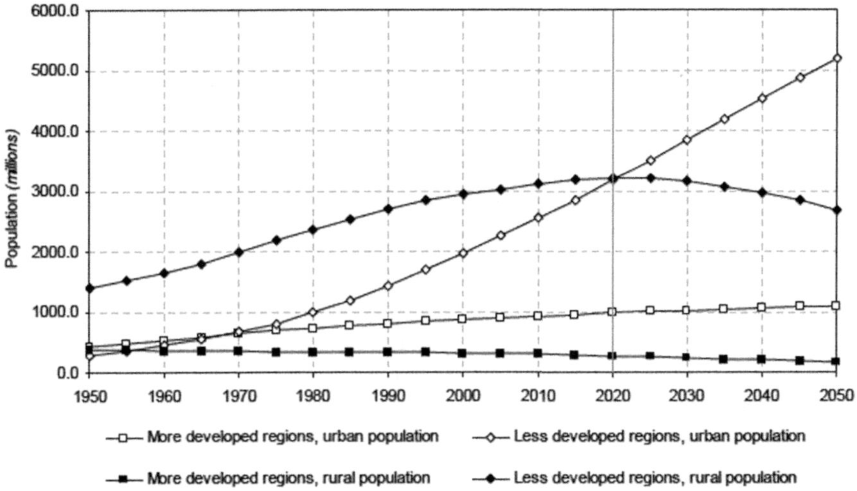

Fig. 4.2 Urban and rural populations by development group, 1950–2050 *Source*: United Nations Department of Economic and Social Affairs, Population Division. *World Urbanization Prospects: The 2009 Revision*. New York 2010. Reprinted with permission of the United Nations

Rapid growth of urban centers with poor urban planning and little capacity to meet the needs of a rapidly growing population often leads to the development of slums and shantytowns. Sanitation and waste removal, safe drinking water, secure housing, and access to adequate nutrition are other important challenges of urbanization. This chapter focuses on the infectious diseases implications of urbanization, which interrelate with the other health concerns listed above.

Along with war and famine, infectious diseases have been a leading cause of death and disability in developing societies for as long as history has been recorded. The field of modern medicine emerged around the study of infections, understanding their transmission, and developing ways to treat them with antibiotics as well as to prevent them with vaccines.

Infectious diseases, by definition, persist and thrive depending on how and how easily they are transmitted, as well as how easily they evolve over time in response to medical intervention. Infectious diseases are propagated via different forms of exposure, including exposure of an uninfected individual to the infected droplets, feces, or bodily fluids of another individual or exposure of an uninfected host to the blood or saliva of an infected vector. In the case of skin flora that can lead to serious infections, the exposure may be touch alone. With greater contact between infected and uninfected individuals, the opportunity for infections to spread increases. Urbanization necessarily provides more opportunity for contact and exposure and therefore has great implications for the transmission and the evolution of infectious diseases around the world.

Drawing on both historical and contemporary perspectives, this chapter will discuss urbanization as it pertains to epidemics and pandemics, specific considerations for developing countries, and implications of urbanization and infectious disease in more developed countries.

4.2 Urbanization, Epidemiology, Epidemics, and Pandemics

Among the most intuitive manifestations of the interrelatedness of population density and infectious diseases are epidemics and pandemics. Throughout recorded history, epidemics have changed the world and influenced the trajectory of nations as well as science, medicine, and health. From plague to smallpox to more recent outbreaks of influenza and SARS, population trends influence and are influenced by infectious disease. The next section lays a basic framework for understanding the importance of shifting population demographics to epidemics and pandemics through a brief review of critical epidemiological principles, followed by historical and contemporary case examples of epidemics and pandemics.

4.2.1 Emergence of the Field of Epidemiology

The field of epidemiology was born of the desire to understand how disease is spread and propagated, particularly during times of epidemics. The Centers for Disease Control defines epidemiology as "the study of the distribution and determinants of health-related states or events in specified populations, and the application of this study to the control of health problems" [3]. The recognition of the importance of population characteristics to spread of disease has informed the field of epidemiology from the outset, and modern epidemiologists develop statistical and mathematical models that incorporate population characteristics to predict disease transmission and evolution as well as to anticipate possible interventions to control them.

4.2.2 Mathematics of Epidemics

The field of epidemiology has bourgeoned significantly since its origin in the early 1900s, and the mathematics involved can be extremely complex. Several variables are basic to the mathematics of epidemics [3, 4]. Models for describing epidemics are based upon the reproductive rate of a given disease—that is, the number of individuals infected directly by the primary case (the first infected person) during the time when she/he is infectious. The reproductive rate is itself determined by the attack rate of the disease (i.e., the risk of transmission in any given encounter), as well as the number of encounters the primary case would have, on average, during the infectious period of the disease. In other words, the greater the population density, the greater the number of encounters and the greater the reproductive rate. There are other factors that determine how a disease will be spread, including acquisition of immunity during an outbreak, existing immunity, the rate at which infected and susceptible individuals enter and leave the community, as well as the different types of encounter required for disease spread (i.e., via droplets, fecal-oral route, vectors, etc.). Population density is one of the most basic variables that affects the duration and impact of an epidemic.

Another important factor, particularly when considering the implications of urbanization, is the rate of entry and exit from the community. A significant proportion of the increase in urban population is due to the migration of people from rural areas to urban areas. As we will discuss in more detail further on this chapter, this can allow for the importation of diseases that were formerly confined to rural areas to urban centers where there may be increased opportunity to spread. This can also allow for increased opportunity to spread if, due to lack of prior exposure, migrants to a given area are more susceptible to a disease that is endemic to that area. In addition, as globalization continues and travel increases among the major cities both nationally and internationally, diseases can be propagated between and among urban centers. This can lead to farther-reaching—even worldwide—outbreaks of disease. Historically, travel by boat or train has enabled the transmission of endemic diseases to novel populations, causing outbreaks of diseases such as measles and smallpox and contributing to the decimation of native peoples. More recently, however, air travel has expedited the movement of airborne pathogens [5]. Viruses can now travel across the world within 24 hours, rather than within days. This statistic becomes even more powerful when considered together with the fact that more than one billion individuals worldwide travel by airplane each year [6, 7].

Another important factor in the mathematics of disease spread, as mentioned above, is the level of susceptibility in a given community. Once a certain level of immunity against a given disease is achieved, either through the conferring of immunity to infected individuals who survive an exposure or through vaccination, the reproductive rate is necessarily reduced as the risk of transmission in a given encounter is decreased. Limits to the spread of disease and the propagation of an epidemic occur when enough individuals in a community are immune to the disease such that the likelihood of an infected individual encountering a susceptible individual is very low. This is the basis for the concept of "herd immunity." The level of immunity required to prevent or interrupt a disease outbreak varies depending on the pathogen. Vaccination programs, which are discussed next, aim to reduce the percentage of individuals susceptible to a given disease and, ideally, achieve high enough rates of immunity to eradicate it.

4.2.3 Vaccines

Edward Jenner is credited as the inventor of the vaccine against smallpox (derived from cowpox lesions) in the late 1700s, although several sources credit a Chinese

Buddhist nun with the earliest recorded practice (as early as the year 1,000) of inoculating people with smallpox for protection from the disease through use of ground scabs inhaled intranasally [8]. Inoculation, also called variolation, was likely also practiced in Africa, Turkey, and India long before the 1700s when the practice became more common in England and the rest of Europe and ultimately led to modern vaccination [9]. Louis Pasteur was the next to develop a successful vaccine, against rabies, in 1885. The late 1800s and 1900s subsequently saw the development of vaccines against plague (1897); cholera (1917); typhoid (1917); diphtheria (1923); pertussis (1926), tuberculosis (BCG, 1927); tetanus (1927); yellow fever (1935); influenza (1945); polio (1955); measles (1963); combined measles, mumps, and rubella (1971); hepatitis B (1982); *Haemophilus influenzae* type B (1990); varicella (1995); hepatitis A (1995); and rotavirus (1998) [10, 11].

The success of vaccination programs is exemplified by the end of smallpox; the last indigenous case of smallpox occurred in 1977 in Somalia, and in 1980, the Global Health Assembly declared smallpox eradicated. Other successes include the elimination of wild-type polio from most countries in the world. In 2003, measles was declared to no longer be endemic in the Americas [12].

The importance of vaccination to the prevention of epidemics cannot be overstated. To maintain these successes moving forward, vaccination programs will have to be expanded to meet the needs of a growing population. Failure to do so will likely lead to resurgence of vaccine-preventable diseases, as in the recent urban outbreaks of yellow fever in several West African cities including Abidjan, Ivory Coast (2001 and 2008), Dakar, Senegal (2002), and Bobo-Dioulasso, Burkina Faso (2004). These outbreaks were likely catalyzed by lower vaccination rates in conjunction with increasing population density and overcrowding conditions favorable for the *Aedes* spp. mosquitoes that carry the virus [13]. Even in developed countries like the USA, vaccination remains an issue. Measles resurged in Southern California between 1988 and 1990, predominantly in urban young adults and children under 5 years of age who had not yet been vaccinated. Outbreaks occurred within schools, colleges, detention facilities, and other institutions in urban areas. In order to control these outbreaks, schools required immediate immunization of non-immunized children and many re-immunization programs were launched [14]. Finally, vaccination is not only a key to prevention of epidemics but is also a cornerstone of curtailing the spread of disease during epidemics and pandemics.

4.2.4 Case Examples of Pandemics

To illustrate the principles described above, the following section describes pandemics from the fourteenth century to the twenty-first century, including plague, Spanish flu, severe acute respiratory syndrome (SARS), and modern influenza pandemics. The critical role and context of the urban environment in each of these historical and contemporary pandemics is also described.

4.2.4.1 Plague

The plague has been responsible for numerous outbreaks and three pandemics in recorded history, most infamously, perhaps, during the fourteenth century in Europe where it was subsequently referred to as "The Black Death." Most estimates are that 50–75 million people worldwide, including about one-third to one-half of all fourteenth century Europeans, succumbed to the plague [15]. The plague was transmitted along trade routes by fleas carried on vermin and other animals infected with different biovars of the bacillum *Yersinia pestis*. There has been some debate over the exact numbers of the infected, and even whether *Yersinia pestis* was the true, sole pathogen responsible [16, 17], but it is widely agreed that "The Black Death" changed European history.

Transmission of plague is dependent on the interaction among vectors (fleas) and hosts (rats, humans, other animals). Although most plague is transmitted in the bubonic form, evolution to pneumonic plague can lead to direct transmission from person to person. Early globalization, such as trade routes from China along the Silk Road into Europe and from seaport to seaport, allowed for the rapid propagation of plague, with up to thousands of people newly infected every day [18]. Recognition of the importance of the migration of traders and their wares into urban centers of trade and industry led to early attempts at outbreak control including quarantines, movement restriction, and closure of ports to ships coming from affected countries [18]. The risk of spread from rats to humans is now known to be related to the population density of rats, the level of flea infestation per rat, as well as the level of bacteria in both the rats and their fleas [19–21]. Although the epidemiology and ecology of ancient plague are certainly more complex than this, the importance of early urbanization in early plague pandemics is clear if not clearly understood.

4.2.4.2 "Spanish" Influenza

The Spanish influenza pandemic of 1918–1919 killed millions of people worldwide, with recent estimates as high as 50 million and some evidence to suggest that urban areas had higher mortality [22]. By that point in history, the field of epidemiology was taking shape. Alongside improved ability to identify microscopic pathogens as well as greater understanding of pathogen transmission and immunologic defense mechanisms, there was greater focus on public health interventions. The influenza vaccine would not be developed until 1945, however, and quarantine was still the mainstay of prevention during influenza outbreaks [23].

Non-pharmacologic interventions to reduce transmission of influenza were based on reducing points of contact among infected and noninfected individuals. These interventions included "social distancing" policies such as closings of schools, churches, and theaters, as well as prohibitions on large public gatherings. Recent analyses of historical data have demonstrated that such interventions, when implemented early, were associated with approximately 50% lower peak death rates and lower cumulative excess mortality [24]. The duration of these interventions also had an effect; when cities relaxed these restrictions, the epidemic returned with a rebound in morbidity and mortality [24–26]. Another study used mathematical models to demonstrate that the number of infected individuals to which a healthy individual is exposed also may correlate with mortality—that is, the greater the exposure, the more severe the illness and the higher the case fatality rate [27]. These studies have led many public health experts to argue in favor of a multipronged approach including early, sustained non-pharmacologic interventions alongside use of antivirals and vaccine development in the event of another influenza pandemic.

4.2.4.3 Severe Acute Respiratory Syndrome (SARS)

Severe acute respiratory syndrome (SARS) was the first worldwide outbreak of the new millennium and perhaps the most impressive demonstration of the interrelatedness of urbanization, globalization, and viral spread. SARS is now known to be caused by a novel coronavirus, thought most likely to have been carried in animals prior to introduction to humans. The first people infected with SARS lived outside of the city of Guangzhou, China. It was subsequently spread from an infected patient to hospital staff, one of whom traveled to Hong Kong and stayed in a hotel where he infected 16 other people, who then went on to carry it to other hospitals and other countries around the world. In Hong Kong, nearly half of SARS infections were acquired in health centers [28]. In Toronto, health centers were also epicenters of nosocomial spread [29, 30].

The SARS pandemic began outside of a major city, was brought to a major city, and from there was spread to other major cities around the world. As was highlighted above in reference to the bubonic plague, globalization and urbanization tend to go hand in hand. In modern times, international travel via aircraft allows for transmission from one major urban center to other major urban centers across the world within hours, catalyzing the process and allowing regional epidemics to become global pandemics within a matter of weeks or even days.

4.2.4.4 Avian and Swine Influenza

Earlier in this chapter, the epidemiology and lessons learned during the 1918 influenza outbreak were reviewed. This section will briefly discuss the ways that urbanization influences modern outbreaks of influenza. As with SARS, such factors include rapid spread via infected droplets in crowded centers (including health facilities), increased international travel, and animal to human to human transmission. Shifting animal demographics related to urbanization may also play a role in the evolution of viral outbreaks.

Influenza strains infect a variety of birds, both wild and domestic. Although relatively little is understood regarding the mechanisms by which cross-species transmission occurs, infected poultry, pigeons, and swine tend to play a role in the outbreak of novel strains of influenza that can subsequently cause significant morbidity and mortality among humans [31]. H5N1 Avian influenza is now epidemic among poultry and likely some migratory birds as well. When H5N1 is transmitted to humans, the route appears to be via direct contact with infected birds rather than via contact with other infected humans. This explains why the H5N1 virus did not become epidemic or pandemic among people. In the era of urbanization and globalization, however, once genetic reassortment does allow for efficient human to human transmissibility, a handful of infections can lead to a worldwide pandemic.

The most recent H1N1 influenza pandemic, for example, was caused by an influenza virus that was a reassortment among human, avian, and swine strains of the virus [32, 33]. The index case was in Mexico, and the virus rapidly spread from there throughout the world via air travel. Unlike seasonal flu, such influenza pandemics are rare. There were only three influenza pandemics in the twentieth century, in 1918, 1957, and 1968. This is because in order for an influenza virus to cause a pandemic, three conditions must be met: first, the viral strain must be antigenically novel such that the population has little or no preexisting immunity; second, the strain must be transmitted to humans; and third, the strain must be efficiently transmitted from person to person [34, 35]. Once these conditions are met, particularly in the age of urbanization and globalization, worldwide spread occurs rapidly. As with SARS, all of the index cases in the early weeks of the H1N1 pandemic of 2009–2010 could be traced to air travel from the index city [36].

Changing human population dynamics also influence animal population dynamics. In more remote and rural areas, localized farming is common. As populations shift, however, large agribusinesses are developed in order to supply urban populations with meat, poultry, and produce. As a consequence, animals are often kept in crowded conditions that may allow for rapid transmission of disease. These large animal farms are also points of multiple, sustained contact between humans and birds or swine, which may increase the opportunity for viral mutation to take place. Similarly, transport of live animals to large markets in urban centers can be a potential point of ignition.

4.3 Urbanization and Specific Infectious Diseases

Urbanization affects the spread of infectious diseases in both developed and developing countries, in wealthy enclaves as well as informal settlements. However, as the World Health Organization has described, disease threats disproportionately affect the urban poor and socioeconomic gradients are evident across many diseases [37]. The following section provides examples of major diseases—that is, those that affect large numbers of people—with a special emphasis on these diseases' impacts on urban residents. It is intended to provide an overview of selected diseases and evidence of their importance in the age of urbanization; however, it does not purport to provide exhaustive coverage of infectious diseases related to urbanization, which are numerous and varied. Furthermore, it is important to note that these diseases affect all countries, regardless of countries' stages of economic development.

4.3.1 Water and Sanitation-Related Diseases

Approximately one-third of the world's population lacks access to clean water, and nearly 40% lacks access to "improved sanitation facilities" for safe disposal of human waste [38]. While people living in rural areas have the least access to clean water and adequate sanitation, urban dwellers, especially those in developing countries, still face major water and sanitation challenges. For example, sanitation rates differ substantially between urban areas of developing countries (71%) and urban areas of developed countries (100%) [38]. Furthermore, some health experts posit that urbanization will bring wild animals—and their waste—into closer contact with drinking supplies for humans, thereby increasing the risk for waterborne zoonotic infectious diseases [39].

According to the World Health Organization, nearly two million diarrhea-related deaths are reported each year [38]. Fecal matter in water consumed by households can lead to diseases such as cholera, cryptosporidiosis, giardiasis and typhoid, among others [40]. The urban slum environment is fertile ground for these diseases, due in large part to overcrowded housing conditions, lack of availability of treated water, and lack of adequate sanitation facilities. Cholera outbreaks, for example, have been reported in urban slums in various parts of the world, ranging from Kolkata, India, and Jakarta, Indonesia, to Nairobi, Kenya, and Kampala, Uganda [41, 42]. Specific studies have implicated factors such as the construction of pit latrines in close proximity to wells (from which people draw their drinking water) in the fecal contamination of water sources [43]. Similarly, researchers investigating a 2007 typhoid outbreak in a West Bengal, India, slum suggested that *Salmonella typhi* bacteria in the fecal matter from victims were carried via open sewage drains, which then contaminated nearby unchlorinated drinking water sources [44].

Several studies have examined the water storage practices of urban residents in resource-poor areas. A study of the Parque Universitario slum in Fortaleza, Brazil, found a higher likelihood of fecal matter presence in household tap water stored in clay pots rather than in capped plastic bottles. The authors posit several explanations for the modes of transmission of fecal matter in these "wide mouth" clay pots: "scooping with contaminated hands in the container, manually clearing blocked filters and inadvertently contaminating [water storage] vessels during cleaning" [45]. Overall, it is notable that 30% of the water samples in the study contained fecal material.

Strategies to reduce the incidence of waterborne infectious diseases are numerous and varied. The World Health Organization has adopted a "household water treatment and safe storage" (HWTS) framework for preventing diarrheal disease. Water treatment techniques include the use of bleach, chlorine, and filters and the boiling of water, among other simple, cheap methods [46]. In terms of water storage, a study of urban dwellers in South India found that the practice of storing water in brass containers significantly decreased the presence of *E. coli* compared to other types of storage containers [47]. Other scientists have argued for a holistic approach to addressing the water and sanitation needs of slums. A study in Ahmedabad, India, demonstrated that "slum upgrading" could significantly reduce incidents of waterborne illness. Slum upgrading was defined as creating "connections to a water supply for individual households, underground sewage for individual households, toilets for individual households, storm water drainage, stone paving of internal and approach roads, solid waste management, and street lighting" [48].

Reducing diarrheal illness related to urbanization will require not only addressing the current problems borne of rapid migration with virtually no urban planning—that is, "slum upgrading"—but also curtailing the development of slums in the first place.

4.3.2 Vector-Borne Diseases

As demographics shift from rural to urban, and as urban centers increasingly encroach on adjacent deserts, forests, and fields, human hosts may be newly exposed to diseases spread by fleas (plague), flies (leishmaniasis), mosquitoes (malaria, yellow fever, dengue, Japanese encephalitis), and ticks (Lyme, Babesia). When migrants from rural areas bring livestock with them to urban centers (often in slums or shantytowns on the outskirts of cities), vector ecology is also affected.

For example, over the latter half of the last century, the incidence and worldwide distribution of dengue has been increasing [49]. Dengue is spread by the same *Aedes* spp. mosquitoes that also carry yellow fever. Interestingly, dengue fever, in contrast to many of the other vector-borne illnesses, is primarily an urban problem. The *Aedes* mosquitoes live in and around houses. When a dengue epidemic occurs, it begins in cities and spreads centrifugally outward to neighboring city areas, suburbs, and towns [50]. The increasing incidence of dengue and dengue hemorrhagic fever has been tied to population growth, urbanization, and poor urban planning leading to poor water sanitation and human solid waste reservoirs for the mosquitoes that transmit the infection (e.g., tires, plastic containers) [13, 49].

Other vector-borne illnesses such as yellow fever and leishmaniasis have also been affected by urbanization. As discussed earlier, the recent epidemics of yellow fever in West Africa are most likely due to a combination of inadequate vaccination coverage, increasing population density, as well as the environmental factors just described that allow for proliferation of *Aedes* spp. mosquitoes. A combination of shifting population dynamics, deforestation, and expansion of nonimmune human populations into endemic areas has been correlated with increased transmission of visceral leishmaniasis around the world [51].

Finally, we turn our attention to malaria. The problem of resistant malaria is described elsewhere in this book. The remainder of this section discusses the impact of urbanization on malaria.

Malaria, which is a vector-borne disease caused by selected *Plasmodium* species, is a leading global killer, especially of children. In Africa, 20% of all child deaths are due to malaria [52]. According to the World Health Organization, there were nearly 250 million cases of malaria in 2008, in 100 countries [53]. However, the majority of the estimated one million deaths due to malaria each year occur in Africa [54].

Data from sub-Saharan Africa suggests an increased risk for malaria in rural areas when compared with urban areas. For example, the *Plasmodium falciparum* entomological inoculation rate, defined as the number of "infective bites per person per annum," [55] is considerably lower in sub-Saharan African urban areas than in rural ones [56]. There may be several reasons for this. First, unlike for *Aedes* spp. mosquitoes, urban areas are inhospitable environments for *Anopheles* mosquito development, the major vectors of the *Plasmodium* parasites that cause malaria [57]. City pollution is thought to inhibit larval development of *Anopheles* mosquitoes [58]. In addition, city dwellers have increased access to insecticide-treated nets (ITNs). Urban residents have a rate of ITN use three times higher than that of rural residents in sub-Saharan Africa. Finally, urban residents live in closer proximity to health-care facilities compared to their rural counterparts, affording them greater access to treatment for malaria once infected [54].

Nevertheless, malaria remains a major urban health concern. Malaria experts have estimated that 200 million city dwellers in Africa are at risk for malaria [59]. Some experts note that characteristics of rapid urban development (e.g., open wells, poor sanitation in slum areas) may provide opportunities for water to pool and, consequently, for malarial vectors to breed [55, 60]. This may be especially true among poorer sections of cities: urban malaria prevalence rates in Africa have been shown to be inversely correlated with individuals' socioeconomic status [61]. Furthermore, there is an emerging concern that many city residents lack sufficient immunity to malaria [58] and that urban children in endemic countries who regularly visit rural areas may be at increased risk for malarial anemia [62]. In cities where farming activities exist, so, too, does the potential for the urban environment to support anopheline mosquito development [58]. Lastly and particularly concerning is recent evidence from slum areas in sub-Saharan African cities that suggests that various *Anopheles* species are beginning to adapt to polluted city water sources [13, 57, 58].

4.3.3 Respiratory Infections: Highlight on Tuberculosis

The epidemic and pandemic potential of viral respiratory infections such as influenza and SARS in the age of urbanization and globalization was reviewed previously. This section focuses on the bacterial airborne disease tuberculosis (TB), which is caused by *Mycobacterium tuberculosis*. 1.7 million people died from TB in 2009; 85% of all global TB cases occurred on the African and Asian continents [63]. TB is also an urbanization and health issue; high rates of TB have been reported in large cities throughout the world [64, 65], prompting concerns of possible urban TB epidemics in the future as more people migrate into cities [64].

Experts posit various explanations for the proliferation of TB in urban settings. First, overcrowding is known to be positively correlated with the incidence of TB [64, 66]. For example, one study of neighborhoods in Harare, Zimbabwe, found that living in a home with two or more people per room was a significant risk factor for TB [67].

Dubbed by WHO as a "disease of poverty," the urban poor are particularly at risk for TB infection due not only to overcrowding but also to higher rates of underlying malnutrition and comorbidities including HIV [66, 68]. One study in Mexico documented that neighborhoods with low socioeconomic status (SES) had higher TB morbidity and mortality rates compared to higher SES neighborhoods [69].

Numerous other studies underscore the dilemma of poor urban dwellers who, due to lack of knowledge about TB and lack of access to quality health-care services, often remain undiagnosed or, once diagnosed, are not able to complete TB treatment [68, 70, 71]. A recent study of 106 private physicians in Mumbai found that these physicians prescribed more than 60 different treatment regimens for TB, and less than 10% of these physicians prescribed regimens meeting the study authors' definition of a "correct prescription" for TB drug treatment [72].

The dangers of TB are compounded by the emergence of multidrug-resistant TB (MDR-TB) and extensively drug-resistant TB (XDR-TB), discussed in detail elsewhere in this book. MDR-TB accounted for 440,000 cases worldwide in 2008 [63]. MDR-TB has been reported in many large cities, such as Mumbai, Sao Paulo, and Shanghai [13, 71, 73, 74] and in smaller numbers, XDR-TB cases have been documented in many cities around the world [75, 76]. New York City alone reported 19 cases of XDR-TB between 1993 and 2006 [77]. Data from Mumbai, India, found much higher rates of MDR-TB in Mumbai, compared to rural areas of India [78]. In China, there is concern that workers from rural areas infected with TB are migrating to the cities in search of work, consequently transmitting TB and possibly contributing to TB drug resistance [71, 79] There is concern that these Chinese migrants are neither seeking nor receiving appropriate, timely TB treatment [80]. The case fatality rate associated with MDR-TB is much higher than for nonresistant TB, especially if left untreated. Researchers studying TB in a poor section of Sao Paolo, Brazil, for example, reported a 60% mortality rate among the non-HIV-infected MDR-TB patients in the study sample [74].

4.3.4 HIV/AIDS (and Other Sexually Transmitted Infections)

HIV/AIDS is by far the most widespread epidemic in the world, with the greatest morbidity and mortality. A chapter in this book focuses on the HIV pandemic; this section will briefly highlight some ways that urbanization may impact on the propagation and evolution of the virus.

HIV is distinct from the other examples discussed in this chapter in that it is transmitted via infected bodily fluids—that is, through blood exposure, sexual exposure, and during pregnancy, delivery, and breastfeeding—rather than via droplets, vectors, or fecal-oral contamination, which are perhaps more intuitively and directly related to urbanization. Urbanization may, however, influence behaviors that affect the risk of acquiring HIV, including alcohol and drug use as well as sexual behavior. Migrants to urban centers are often young people who are separated from their families and traditional social structures. In addition, the disparity

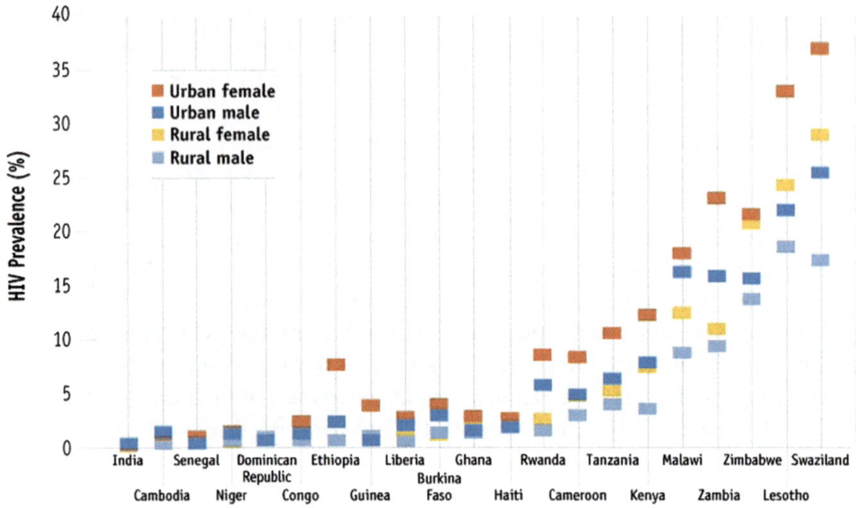

Fig. 4.3 HIV prevalence by gender and area of residence 2003–2008. *Source*: WHO calculations based on data from Demographic and Health Surveys (DHS) 2003–2008. Reprinted with permission from WHO

between the rich and poor in urban environments can be stark. Migrants are typically seeking opportunity, coming to the city from a less privileged socioeconomic background. The confluence of these factors may lead to higher-risk behaviors.

According to the U.N., there were 2.6 million new cases of HIV infection in the world in 2009, and 1.8 million of these new cases were in sub-Saharan Africa alone [81]. In many sub-Saharan African countries, such as Zambia and Kenya, HIV prevalence rates among 15–49 year olds are higher in urban areas than in rural areas [82] (Fig. 4.3).

Considerable attention has been paid to the issue of high-risk sexual behaviors among workers who migrate to cities in search of work [13, 83, 84]. Much of this literature focuses on Asian countries. In China, where an estimated 140 million migrants reportedly exist, studies have described risky sexual practices and poor knowledge about HIV among male migrant workers [85], and even among migrant workers' school-aged children [86]. A study of male taxi drivers from rural Bangladesh who migrated for work to the capital, Dhaka, reported that approximately 60% of respondents had recently engaged in sex with commercial sex workers without using condoms [87]. Several studies of commercial sex workers in cities of India have documented the elevated risk of HIV infection among this population [88]. The phenomenon of young women and girls migrating to cities, becoming engaged in commercial sex work, and contracting HIV is well documented. A recent study of 287 Nepalese women and girls who had been sex-trafficked into urban brothels in India and then returned to Nepal revealed a 38% HIV-positive rate among these victims [89]. Seventeen of these women and girls were also found to have TB [90]. It appears that sexual behaviors of migrant workers will help fuel the spread of HIV in cities—but also in the rural communities to which these workers will return.

Similar factors likely contribute to the transmission of HIV in sub-Saharan Africa, which has seen an impressive redistribution of populations and rise of rural-to-urban migration. Between 1960 and 1980, the crude population density more than doubled across sub-Saharan Africa and there was a nearly tenfold increase in the number of cities with populations exceeding 500,000 [91].

Linkages between urban slums/informal settlements and HIV have been described in the literature. In Kenya, an analysis of the Nairobi Cross Sectional Slum Survey found that slum residents who had either migrated from economically poor rural villages or from other slums were more likely to engage in risky behaviors with respect to HIV/AIDS (i.e., condom use and number of sexual partners) than other slum residents [83]. These findings are consistent with a recent study of five African cities—Accra, Dar es Salaam, Harare, Kampala, and Nairobi—which reported that living in a slum predicted riskier sexual behaviors [92]. Some researchers have posited that in migrating from rural areas to cities, individuals no longer find themselves bound to traditional values, resulting in increased promiscuity and an increased vulnerability to HIV infection [93].

Finally, when discussing HIV and urbanization, it is important to consider opportunistic infection and comorbidities. Tuberculosis infection tends to be both more severe and more difficult to treat among patients with HIV. Opportunistic infections, including infections with molds and fungus, may be influenced by movement between rural and urban environments. The high-risk sexual behaviors that lead to HIV transmission also place individuals at risk of acquiring other sexually transmitted infections, including syphilis. Additionally, because injection drug use has primarily been an urban health issue, urbanization may lead to an increase in injection drug use and thus further the spread of HIV. Injection drug use with shared needles can transmit many other viruses in addition to HIV. Approximately one in five injection drug users (approximately 16 million worldwide) is HIV-positive [94]. HIV also increases the risk of hepatitis C virus (HCV)—almost a third of individuals with HIV are co-infected with HCV [95, 96].

These trends are not only a problem of the developing world. During the early stages of the HIV epidemic in the United States, for example, the first patients diagnosed with HIV and those at highest risk were white men who had sex with men living in urban areas. The HIV epidemic in the USA continues to be primarily an urban problem, with more than 80% of HIV diagnoses occurring in major metropolitan areas [97].

4.4 Conclusions and Future Directions

The world's population continues to grow exponentially, and more people are living in cities and megacities. This population growth, coupled with the interconnectedness of the entire world, has significant implications for disease. This chapter described major infectious disease threats in the urban environment, past and present, and illustrated several mechanisms by which urbanization can affect the epidemiology of infectious diseases (Table 4.1).

Urbanization disproportionately impacts the poor. Hence, not only "slum upgrading" but also prevention of slums will be important in order to mitigate the harmful effects of rapid urbanization. Further development of health systems in parallel with improved housing, sanitation, and access to clean water is necessary. Anticipating continued growth and expansion should prompt governments to dedicate additional resources to urban planning. Vaccination, monitoring and reporting of new cases, and ring chemoprophylaxis are critical for curtailing epidemics and pandemics. Disease surveillance systems and systems for communication and reporting are crucial [98]. Rapid innovations in information technology may inform the development of such systems.

Systems for epidemic response also must be strengthened. Rapid, early detection and diagnosis are keys to addressing any disease outbreak. Clinical diagnostic algorithms must be identified early and health providers educated about them, as laboratory diagnostic tools often take time to become available and affordable. Health-care workers should be targeted to receive treatment and prophylaxis as soon as possible. The manufacture and distribution of sufficient quantities of vaccine, treatment, and chemoprophylaxis during outbreaks is also a major challenge. Finally, processes for effective coordination of efforts among agencies involved in epidemic response must be developed in advance.

In terms of future directions, three topics merit further consideration on the urbanization and global health agenda: (1) bioterrorism, (2) nosocomial infections and the development of resistant organisms, and (3) noninfectious diseases (i.e., chronic diseases) in urbanizing areas. First, there is a need to address the looming threat of bioterrorism, which capitalizes on the epidemiologic principles discussed in this chapter. Four diseases are recognized to have significant bioterrorism potential in urban settings. This chapter has discussed two disease agents—plague and smallpox virus—which can spread from person to person. The other two are anthrax (spores) and botulism (toxin), which are not spread from person to person but could cause mass infection and death if released in aerosolized form into a crowded area or, in the case of botulinum toxin, into the food supply. Outbreak preparedness requires identification of vaccines and treatments for these potential threats, developers who would be able to produce vaccines and treatments should need arise, and a sophisticated system of targeted, efficient diagnosis, isolation, treatment, and, where necessary, vaccination, to curtail further spread.

Second, to the extent that urbanization influences the development of medical centers and affects the use of broad-spectrum antibiotics, nosocomial infections such as *Clostridium difficile* and resistant organisms such as methicillin-resistant *Staphylococcus aureus* (MRSA) and vancomycin-resistant *Enterococcus* (VRE) bear mentioning. MRSA is now found fairly widely in the community and may be more common in urban residents compared to rural residents [99]. Less common but of great concern is the emergence of vancomycin-resistant *Staphylococcus aureus* (VRSA). Only a few cases of VRSA have been reported in the USA to date [100],

Table 4.1 Influences of urbanization on selected infectious diseases.

Infection	Influences of migration, urbanization, and globalization	
	Less developed areas	More developed areas
Diarrheal illness		
Cholera Salmonella including typhii *E. coli* Cryptosporidia	Rapid increase in slums leads to poor access to clean water and sanitation. Diarrheal disease is still the most common cause of death in children under 5 years.	Reliance on large agribusinesses can lead to wide-spread outbreaks of food-borne illness.
Vector-borne		
Leishmaniasis Yellow fever Dengue Malaria Rickettsial	Migrants from rural areas bring livestock with them to urban centers, influencing vector ecology. *Aedes* mosquitoes thrive in urban environments; *Anophales* mosquitoes do not. Rapid increases in population density can overwhelm vaccination programs, decrease herd immunity, and render a population more susceptible to outbreaks. Access to prevention, diagnosis, and treatment is greater in urban areas. Urban centers increasingly encroach on adjacent wilderness, bringing human hosts into closer contact with vectors.	
Sexually-transmitted & blood-borne		
HIV Syphilis Hepatitis B and C	Migrants separated from their social networks may have higher rates of risk-taking behaviors, leading to higher rates of acquisition and transmission of STIs. STIs are prevalent among commercial sex-workers. Access to prevention, diagnosis and treatment is higher in urban areas.	Higher-risk behaviors including IVDU and MSM are more prevalent in urban areas.
Respiratory/droplet		
Influenza SARS	Rapid increases in population density can overwhelm vaccination programs, decrease herd immunity, and render a population more susceptible to outbreaks. Air-travel connects urban centers around the world and can facilitate spread of highly contagious illness in minimal time.	

(continued)

Table 4.1 (continued)

Infection	Influences of migration, urbanization, and globalization	
	Less developed areas	More developed areas
Tuberculosis	Rapid increase in population density can lead to overcrowding, poor housing, and lack of ventilation. Lack of access to diagnosis and treatment can lead to development of MDR-TB.	As population increases, incarceration and homelessness increase, both of which are risk factors for TB. Immigration and globalization bring diseases from the developing world to the developed world.
Bioterrorism		
Plague (*Yersinia pestis*) Smallpox	Highly-contagious infections can spread rapidly among a non-immune population, facilitated by high population density.	
Anthrax	Inhalation of anthrax spores could cause mass morbidity and mortality if released in a crowded urban center.	
Botulism	Mass reliance on large agribusiness could allow for significant morbidity and mortality if *C. botulinum* were released into the canned food supply.	
Nosocomial & drug resistant bacteria		
C. difficile MRSA VRE ESBL organisms VRSA	Large medical centers with access to broad-spectrum antibiotics tend to be located in urban centers. Broad-spectrum antibiotic use can lead to the development of resistant organisms.	

but they highlight the importance of judicious use of antibiotics as well as adherence to contact precaution protocols for hospitalized patients with suspected or confirmed resistant bacterial colonization.

Finally, it is important to acknowledge that a growing proportion of the global burden of disease is noncommunicable. Pollution, trauma, violence, and obesity all are major causes of death and disability that are on the rise with urbanization and globalization. Cardiovascular disease has been the leading cause of morbidity and mortality in both the developed and the developing world for the past 15 years [101]. This in part is due to improved control of infectious diseases and increasing lifespan (i.e., people are living long enough for cardiovascular disease to become salient) coupled with persistent, relatively higher rates of cigarette smoking in the developing world. More research in all aspects of chronic disease and urbanization processes need further elucidation.

Overall, urban centers pose great challenges in terms of disease, but they also present unique opportunities for health promotion and disease prevention. For example, the concentration of human and financial resources in cities can translate into greater capacity to carry out health campaigns in order to reduce the risk of transmission of diseases like HIV/AIDS and TB. Access to health education, condoms, disease diagnosis and treatment also may be greater in the urban centers compared to rural areas.

Urban centers have the potential to bring together a critical mass of people from multiple disciplines and sectors (e.g., medicine, health, economics, engineering, sociology, social work, architecture), harness collective knowledge, and foster an environment that promotes the development of innovative, integrative solutions to health problems. Ultimately, such holistic solutions are desperately needed to address the world's emerging urbanization and health threats.

Acknowledgments The authors wish to thank the following individuals for research and editorial assistance: Genevieve Purcell, Kathryn Tindell, Emily deRedon, Kathryn Conn, and Christine Cho.

References

1. United Nations, Department of Economic and Social Affairs, Population Division (2010) World urbanization prospects: the 2009 revision: highlights, New York
2. United Nations, Department of Economic and Social Affairs, Statistics Division (2010) Methods and classifications, population density and urbanisation, standards and methods, concepts and definitions, paras. 2.81–2.88 [Internet]. [cited 2011 Sept 8]. Available from: http://unstats.un.org/unsd/methods.htm
3. Principles of epidemiology in public health practice: an introduction to applied epidemiology and biostatistics, 3rd edn [Internet]. U.S. Department of Health and Human Services Centers for Disease Control and Prevention (CDC) Office of Workforce and Career Development, Atlanta, GA; [cited 2011 Feb 26]. Available from: http://www.cdc.gov/training/products/ss1000/ss1000-ol.pdf

4. Giesecke J (2007) Mathematical models for epidemics. In: Nelson KE, Williams CM (eds) Modern infectious disease epidemiology: theory and practice, 2nd edn. Oxford University Press Inc, New York, pp 200–214
5. Fenner F (1971) Infectious disease and social change: part 2. Med J Aust 1:1099–1102
6. Mangili A, Gendreau MA (2005) Transmission of infectious disease during commercial air travel. Lancet 365:989–996
7. Ward BJ, Plourde P (2006) Travel and sexually transmitted infections. J Travel Med 13:300–317
8. Plotkin SL, Plotkin SA (2008) A short history of vaccination. In: Plotkin SA, Orenstein WA, Offit PA (eds) Vaccines, 5th edn. Elsevier, China, pp 1–16
9. Riedel S (2005) Edward Jenner and the history of smallpox and vaccination. Proc (Bayl Univ Med Cent) 18:21–25
10. U.S. Department of Health and Human Services Centers for Disease Control and Prevention. Vaccines and immunizations [Internet]. Centers for Disease Control and Prevention, Atlanta, GA; 2011 Sept 1. Available from: http://www.cdc.gov/vaccines/default.htm
11. Orenstein WA, Pickering LK, Mawle A, Hinman AR, Wharton M (2010) Immunization. In: Mandell GL, Bennet JE, Dolin R (eds) Principles and practice of infectious disease, 7th edn. Churchill Livingstone Elsevier, Philadelphia, pp 3917–3946
12. The College of Physicians of Philadelphia (2011) The history of vaccines [Internet] [cited 2011 Sept 8]. Available from: http://www.historyofvaccines.org
13. Alirol E, Getaz L, Stoll B, Chappuis F, Loutan L (2011) Urbanisation and infectious diseases in a globalised world. Lancet Infect Dis 11:131–141
14. Dales LG, Kizer KW, Rutherford GW, Pertowski CA, Waterman SH, Woodford G (1993) Measles epidemic from failure to immunize. West J Med 159:456–464
15. Herlihy D, Cohn SK Jr (1997) The Black Death and the transformation of the West. Harvard University Press, Cambridge, MA
16. Cohn SK Jr (2008) Epidemiology of the Black Death and successive waves of plague. Med Hist Suppl 27:74–100
17. Prentice MB, Rahalison L (2007) Plague. Lancet 369:1196–1207
18. Sloan AW (1973) History of medicine: medical and social aspects of the great plague of London in 1665. S Afr Med J 47:270–276
19. Dennis DT, Mead PS (2010) Yersinia species, including plague. In: Mandell GL, Bennett JE, Raphael Dolin R (eds) Principles and practice of infectious diseases, 7th edn. Elsevier, Philadelphia, p 2943
20. Tikhomirov E (1999) Epidemiology and distribution of plague. In: Plague manual: epidemiology, distribution, surveillance and control. WHO, Geneva, pp 11–37
21. Gage KL (1999) Plague surveillance. In: Plague manual: epidemiology, distribution, surveillance and control. WHO, Geneva, pp 135–166
22. Johnson NP, Mueller J (2002) Updating the accounts: global mortality of the 1918–1920 “Spanish” influenza pandemic. Bull Hist Med 76:105–115
23. Nelson KE, Williams CM (2007) Early history of infectious disease: epidemiology and control of infectious diseases. In: Infectious disease epidemiology: theory and practice. Jones and Bartlett Publishers Inc, Sudbury, pp 3–23
24. Hatchett RJ, Mecher CE, Lipsitch M (2007) Public health interventions and epidemic intensity during the 1918 influenza pandemic. Proc Natl Acad Sci U S A 104:7582–7587
25. Morse SS (2007) Pandemic influenza: studying the lessons of history. Proc Natl Acad Sci U S A 104:7313–7314
26. Markel H, Lipman HB, Navarro JA et al (2007) Nonpharmaceutical interventions implanted by US cities during the 1918–1919 influenza pandemic. JAMA 298:644–654
27. Paulo A, Correia-Neves M, Domingos T, Murta A, Pedrosal J (2010) Influenza infectious dose may explain the high mortality of the second and third wave of 1918–1919 influenza pandemic. PLoS One 5:e11655
28. Yuen KY, Wong SSY, Malik Peiris JS (2010) The severe acute respiratory syndrome. In: Fong IW, Alibek K (eds) New and evolving infections of the 21st century. Springer, New York, pp 163–193

29. Affonso DD, Andrews GJ, Jeffs L (2004) The urban geography of SARS: paradoxes and dilemmas in Toronto's health care. J Adv Nurs 45:568–578
30. Svoboda T, Henry B, Shulman L et al (2004) Public health measures to control the spread of the severe acute respiratory syndrome during the outbreak in Toronto. N Engl J Med 350:2352–2361
31. de Jong MD (2010) Avian influenza viruses and pandemic influenza. In: Fong IW, Alibek K (eds) New and evolving infections of the 21st century. Springer, New York, pp 327–359
32. The Writing Committee of the World Health Organization (WHO) Consultation on Human Influenza A/H5 (2005) Avian influenza A (H5NI) infections in humans. N Engl J Med 353:1374–1385
33. Belshe RB (2005) The origins of pandemic influenza – lessons from the 1918 virus. N Engl J Med 353:2209–2211
34. Guan Y, Vijaykrishna D, Bahl J, Zhu H, Wang J, Smith GJ (2010) The emergence of pandemic influenza viruses. Protein Cell 1:9–13
35. Taubenberger JK, Morens DM (2010) Influenza: the once and future pandemic. Public Health Rep 125(Suppl 3):16–26
36. Khan K, Arino J, Hu W et al (2009) Spread of a novel influenza A (H1N1) virus via global airline transportation. N Engl J Med 361:212–214
37. World Health Organization (2008) Our cities, our health, our future: acting on social determinants for health equity in urban settings. World Health Organization Centre for Health Development, Kobe
38. World Health Organization and United Nation Children's Fund Joint Monitoring Programme for Water Supply and Sanitation (JMP) (2008) Progress on drinking water and sanitation: special focus on sanitation. UNICEF/WHO, New York/Geneva
39. Expert Meeting Group Report (2004) Expert consensus. In: Cotruvo JA, Dufour A, Rees G et al (eds) Waterborne zoonoses: identification, causes and control. IWA Publishing on behalf of World Health Organization, London, pp 3–16
40. Moe CL (2004) What are the criteria for determining whether a disease is zoonotic and water related? In: Cotruvo JA, Dufour A, Rees G et al (eds) Waterborne zoonoses: identification, causes and control. IWA Publishing on behalf of World Health Organization, London, pp 27–45
41. Kigotho AW (1998) Cholera hits east African cities. Lancet 351:45
42. Deen JL, von Seidlein L, Sur D et al (2008) The high burden of cholera in children: comparison of incidence from endemic areas in Asia and Africa. PLoS Negl Trop Dis 2:e173
43. Kimani-Murage EW, Ngindu AM (2007) Quality of water the slum dwellers use: the case of a Kenyan slum. J Urban Health 84:829–838
44. Bhunia R, Hutin Y, Ramakrishnan R, Pal N, Sen T, Murhekar M (2009) A typhoid fever outbreak in a slum of South Dumdum municipality, West Bengal, India, 2007: evidence for foodborne and waterborne transmission. BMC Public Health 9:115
45. Copeland CC, Beers BB, Thompson MR et al (2009) Faecal contamination of drinking water in a Brazilian shanty town: importance of household storage and new human faecal marker testing. J Water Health 7:324–331
46. International Network to Promote Household Water Treatment and Safe Storage (2007) Combating waterborne disease at the household level. World Health Organization, Geneva
47. Brick T, Primrose B, Chandrasekhar R, Roy S, Muliyil J, Kang G (2004) Water contamination in urban south India: household storage practices and their implications for water safety and enteric infections. Int J Hyg Environ Health 207:473–480
48. Butala NM, Vanrooyen MJ, Patel RB (2010) Improved health outcomes in urban slums. Soc Sci Med 71:935–940
49. Gubler DJ (1998) Epidemic dengue and dengue hemorrhagic fever: a global public health problem in the 21st century. In: Scheld WM, Armstrong D, Hughes JM (eds) Emerging infections I. ASM Press, Washington, DC, pp 1–14
50. Vazquez-Prokopec GM, Kitron U, Montgomery B, Horne P, Ritchie SA (2010) Quantifying the spatial dimension of dengue virus epidemic spread within a tropical urban environment. PLoS Negl Trop Dis 4(12):e920

51. Desjeux P (2004) Leishmaniasis: current situation and new perspectives. Comp Immunol Microbiol Infect Dis 27:305–318
52. Roll Back Malaria. Children and malaria [Internet]. World Health Organization; [cited 2011 June 23]. Available from: http://www.rollbackmalaria.org/cmc_upload/0/000/015/367/RBMInfosheet_6.htm
53. World Health Organization (2010) Malaria fact sheet No. 94 [Internet]. World Health Organization, Geneva; [cited 2011 Apr 14]. Available from: http://www.who.int/mediacentre/factsheets/fs094/en/
54. Hay SI, Guerra CA, Tatem AJ, Atkinson PM, Snow RW (2005) Urbanization, malaria transmission and disease burden in Africa. Nat Rev Microbiol 3:81–90
55. Kallander K, Nsungwa-Sabiiti J (2009) Home-based management of malaria in the era of urbanisation. Lancet 373:1582–1584
56. Tatem AJ, Guerra CA, Kabaria CW, Noor AM, Hay SI (2008) Human population, urban settlement patterns and their impact on *Plasmodium falciparum* malaria endemicity. Malar J 7:218
57. Kasili S, Odemba N, Ngere FG, Kamanza JB, Muema AM, Kutima HL (2009) Entomological assessment of the potential for malaria transmission in Kibera slum of Nairobi, Kenya. J Vector Borne Dis 46:273–279
58. Robert V, Macintyre K, Keating J, Trape JF, Duchemin JB, Warren M, Beier JC (2003) Malaria transmission in urban sub-Saharan Africa. Am J Trop Med Hyg 68:169–176
59. Keiser J, Utzinger J, CladasdeCastro M, Smith TA, Tanner M, Singer BH (2004) Urbanization in sub-Saharan Africa and implications for malaria control. Am J Trop Med Hyg 71(Suppl 2):118–127
60. Tiwari S, Ghosh SK, Ojha VP, Dash AP, Raghavendra K (2010) Reduced susceptibility to selected synthetic pyrethroids in urban malaria vector *Anopheles stephensi*: a case study in Mangalore city, South India. Malar J 9:179
61. Klinkenberg E, McCall PJ, Wilson MD, Akoto AO, Amerasinghe FP, Bates I et al (2006) Urban malaria and anaemia in children: a cross-sectional survey in two cities in Ghana. Trop Med Int Health 11:578–588
62. Siri JG, Wilson ML, Murray S, Rosen DH, Vulule JM, Slutsker L, Lindblade KA (2010) Significance of travel to rural areas as a risk factor for malarial anemia in an urban setting. Am J Trop Med Hyg 82:391–397
63. World Health Organization (2010) Global tuberculosis control: WHO report 2010. World Health Organization, Geneva
64. Lonnroth K, Jaramillo E, Williams BG, Dye C, Raviglione M (2009) Drivers of tuberculosis epidemics: the role of risk factors and social determinants. Soc Sci Med 68:2240–2246
65. Wood R, Liang H, Wu H et al (2010) Changing prevalence of tuberculosis infection with increasing age in high-burden townships in South Africa. Int J Tuberc Lung Dis 14:406–412
66. Hargreaves JR, Boccia D, Evans CA, Adato M, Petticrew M, Porter JDH (2011) The social determinants of tuberculosis: from evidence to action. Am J Public Health 101:654–662
67. Corbett EL, Bandason T, Cheung YB et al (2009) Prevalent infectious tuberculosis in Harare, Zimbabwe: burden, risk factors and implications for control. Int J Tuberc Lung Dis 13:1231–1237
68. David AM, Mercado SP, Becker D, Edmundo K, Mugisha F (2007) The prevention and control of HIV/AIDS, TB and Vector-borne diseases in informal settlements: challenges, opportunities and insights. J Urban Health 84:65–74
69. Alvarez-Hernandez G, Lara-Valencia F, Reyes-Castro PA, Rascon-Pacheco RA (2010) An analysis of spatial and socio-economic determinants of tuberculosis in Hermosillo, Mexico, 2000–2006. Int J Tuberc Lung Dis 14:708–713
70. Suganthi P, Chadha VK, Ahmed J et al (2008) Health seeking and knowledge about tuberculosis among persons with pulmonary symptoms and tuberculosis cases in Bangalore slums. Int J Tuberc Lung Dis 12:1268–1273
71. Wang W, Wang J, Zhao Q, Darling ND, Yu M, Zhou B, Xu B (2011) Contribution of rural-to-urban migration in the prevalence of drug resistant tuberculosis in China. Eur J Clin Microbiol Infect Dis 30:581–586

72. Udwadia ZF, Pinto LM, Uplekar MW (2010) Tuberculosis management by private practitioners in Mumbai, India: has anything changed in two decades? PLoS One 5:e12023
73. Karande S, Bavdekar SB (2002) Children and multidrug-resistant tuberculosis in Mumbai (Bombay), India. Emerg Infect Dis 8:1360–1361
74. Telles MA, Ferrazoli L, Waldman EA et al (2005) A population-based study of drug resistance and transmission of tuberculosis in an urban community. Int J Tuberc Lung Dis 9:970–976
75. Hasan R, Jabeen K, Ali A et al (2010) Extensively drug-resistant tuberculosis, Pakistan. Emerg Infect Dis 16:1473–1475
76. Zhao M, Li X, Xu P et al (2009) Transmission of MDR and XDR tuberculosis in Shanghai, China. PLoS ONE 4:e4370
77. Centers for Disease Control and Prevention (2007) Extensively drug-resistant tuberculosis—United States, 2003–2006. MMWR Morb Mort Wkly Rep 56:250–253
78. Almeida D, Rodrigues C, Udwadia ZF, Lalvani A, Gothi GD, Mehta P, Mehta A (2003) Incidence of multi-drug resistant tuberculosis in urban and rural India and implications for prevention. Clin Infect Dis 36:e152–e154
79. Tang S, Squire SB (2005) What lessons can be drawn from tuberculosis (TB) control in China in the 1990s? An analysis from a health system perspective. Health Policy 72:93–104
80. Long Q, Li Y, Wang Y et al (2008) Barriers to accessing TB diagnosis for rural-to-urban migrants with chronic cough in Chongqing, China: a mixed methods study. BMC Health Serv Res 8:202
81. Joint United Nations Programme on HIV/AIDS (UNAIDS) (2010) UNAIDS report on the global AIDS epidemic 2010. UNAIDS, Geneva
82. UNAIDS (2008) Report on the global AIDS epidemic. UNAIDS, Geneva
83. Greif MJ, Nii-Amoo Dodoo F (2011) Internal migration to Nairobi's slums: linking migrant streams to sexual risk behavior. Health Place 17:86–93
84. Zulu EM, Nii-Amoo Dodoo F, Chika-Ezeh A (2002) Sexual risk-taking in the slums of Nairobi, Kenya, 1993–98. Popul Stud (Camb) 56:311–323
85. Li L, Morrow M, Kermode M (2007) Vulnerable but feeling safe: HIV risk among male rural-to-urban migrant workers in Chengdu, China. AIDS Care 19:1288–1295
86. Li S, Huang H, Cai Y, Xu G, Huang F, Shen X (2009) Characteristics and determinants of sexual behavior among adolescents of migrants workers in Shangai (China). BMC Public Health 9:195
87. Roy T, Anderson C, Evanas C, Rahman MS (2010) Sexual risk behaviour of rural-to-urban migrant taxi drivers in Dhaka, Bangladesh: a cross-sectional behavioural survey. Public Health 124:648–658
88. Sarkar K, Bal B, Mukherjee R, Niyogi SK, Saha MK, Bhattacharya SK (2005) Epidemiology of HIV infection among brothel-based sex workers in Kolkata, India. J Health Popul Nutr 23:231–235
89. Silverman JG, Decker MR, Gupta J, Maheshwari A, Willis BM, Raj A (2007) HIV prevalence and predictors of infection in sex-trafficked Nepalese girls and women. JAMA 298:536–542
90. Dharmadhikari AS, Gupta J, Decker MR, Raj A, Silverman JG (2009) Tuberculosis and HIV: a global menace exacerbated via sex trafficking. Int J Infect Dis 13:543–546
91. Quinn TC (1994) Population migration and the spread of types 1 and 2 human immunodeficiency viruses. Proc Natl Acad Sci U S A 91:2407–2414
92. Greif MJ, Nii-Amoo Dodoo F, Jayaraman A (2011) Urbanisation, poverty and sexual behaviour: the tale of five African cities. Urban Stud 48:947–957
93. Buve A, Bishikwabo-Nsarhaza K, Mutangadura G (2002) The spread and effect of HIV-1 infection in sub-Saharan Africa. Lancet 359:2011–2017
94. Vlahov D, Robertson AM, Strathdee SA (2010) Prevention of HIV Infection among injection drug users in resource-limited settings. Clin Infect Dis 50(Suppl 3):S114–S121
95. Fleming CA, Crave DE, Thornton D, Tumilty S, Nunes D (2003) Hepatitis C virus and human immunodeficiency virus coinfection in an urban population: low eligibility for interferon treatment. Clin Infect Dis 36:97–100

96. Shepard CW, Finelli L, Alter MJ (2005) Global epidemiology of hepatitis C virus infection. Lancet 5:558–567
97. Centers for Disease Control and Prevention (2008) Cases of HIV infection and AIDS in urban and rural areas of the United States, 2006. HIV AIDS Surveill Supplemental Report [serial online] [cited 2011 Jun 20] 13. Available from: http://www.cdc.gov/hiv/topics/surveillance/resources/reports/2008supp_vol13no2/default.htm
98. Patel RB, Burke TF (2009) Global health: urbanization—an emerging humanitarian disaster. New Engl J Med 361:741–743
99. Anwar MS, Jaffery G, Rehman Bhatti KU, Tayyib M, Bokhari SR (2004) *Staphylococcus aureus* and MRSA nasal carriage in general population. J Coll Physicians Surg Pak 14(11):661–664
100. Chang S, Sievert DM, Hageman JC et al (2003) Infection with vancomycin-resistant *Staphylococcus aureus* containing the vanA resistance gene. N Engl J Med 348:1342–1347
101. Pearson T (1999) Cardiovascular disease in developing countries: myths, realities, and opportunities. Cardiovasc Drugs Ther 13:95–104

Chapter 5
Challenges in Enteric Epidemics: Barometers of Inadequate Water and Sanitation

Luther A. Bartelt and Richard L. Guerrant

Abbreviations

AIDS	Acquired immunodeficiency syndrome
APOE	Apolipoprotein E
cAMP	Cyclic adenosine monophosphate
CFR	Case fatality rate
CTC	Cholera treatment center
CTU	Cholera treatment unit
CTX	Cholera toxin
DALY	Daily adjusted life years
EAEC	Enteroaggregative *E. coli*
ICDDR-B	International Centre for Diarrhoeal Disease Research Bangladesh
IDP	Internally displaced population
IHR	International health Regulations
MSPP	Ministère de la Santé Publique et de la Population
PAHO	Pan American Health Organization
PEM	Protein energy malnutrition
ORS	Oral rehydration solution
ORT	Oral rehydration therapy
RO-ORS	Reduced-osmolar oral rehydration solution

L.A. Bartelt, M.D., D.T.M. & H. (✉)
Divisions of Infectious Disease and Gastroenterology and the Center for Global Health, University of Virginia, Charlottesville, VA, USA
e-mail: luther.bartelt@gmail.com

R.L. Guerrant, M.D.
The Center for Global Health, University of Virginia, Charlottesville, VA, USA

I.W. Fong (ed.), *Challenges in Infectious Diseases*, Emerging Infectious Diseases of the 21st Century 502, DOI 10.1007/978-1-4614-4496-1_5,

SSH	Sea surface height
SST	Sea surface temperature
TCP	Toxin-coregulated pilus
VBNC	Viable but non-culturable
UN	United Nations
WHO	World Health Organization

5.1 Introduction

Infectious diarrheal illnesses, markers of inadequate water and sanitation systems, rank among the leading causes of morbidity and mortality worldwide, disproportionately so in low-income countries and among children [1–3]. Following the recognition of water as a vehicle for enteric pathogen transmission, a sanitary revolution swept across Europe and North America, reducing the burden to primarily sporadic outbreaks of limited extent [4–6]. For the majority of the world's population, however, the health benefits of clean water and "flush" toilets are far from reach. The most recently headlined barometer of inadequate water and sanitation came roaring out of deplorable sanitary conditions in earthquake-devastated Haiti in October 2010. In a matter of 8 weeks, an introduced cholera epidemic (caused by *Vibrio cholerae* O1) surged through the Haitian population, causing an astonishing 121,518 cases where the disease had not existed for decades [7, 8]. The use of intravenous and oral rehydration therapy (ORT) for patients with rapid dehydration kept the epidemic case fatality rate (CFR) to 2.1% and was a reminder of the simple yet vital importance of fluid resuscitation [8]. Shown to be effective in 80% of cholera cases as well as for other acute diarrheal diseases, ORT has likely saved more than 40 million lives since its advent in the 1960s and thus has made more contributions to reducing mortality due to cholera and other diarrheal illnesses globally than any other therapy [9]. Yet, 2.6 billion people (42% of the world's population) remain at risk of life-threatening diarrheal illness simply for lack of clean water and sanitation [4, 10]. Moreover, morbidity due to epidemic and endemic infectious diarrhea may actually be increasing [2]. Contributing to the overall burden of diarrheal disease is the recently recognized long-term deleterious sequelae of enteropathogens on impaired early childhood development and associations with malnutrition even in the absence of loose stools [11]. The myriad potential of enteric pathogens to viciously ravage susceptible populations, as well as to stealthily rob at-risk children of their maximum potential, poses one of the greatest challenges of the twenty-first century.

The etiological agents of infectious diarrhea are diverse. With some regional variation, the most common enteric pathogens include the Enterobacteriaceae (toxigenic strains of *Escherichia coli*, *Campylobacter* sp., *Shigella* sp., *Salmonella* sp. (including typhoid), and *Vibrio* sp.), protozoal parasites (*Cryptosporidium* sp., *Giardia lamblia,* and *Entamoeba histolytica*), and viruses (*Rotavirus*, *Norovirus*, and *Enterovirus* (including polio)) [12]. Though transmitted through shared waterborne vehicles, each pathogen occupies a unique environmental niche. Some pathogens, such as

Cryptosporidium and *Giardia*, are ubiquitous worldwide and have zoonotic potential via mammalian reservoirs [13]. Others, such as *Salmonella typhi*, have exclusively human reservoirs and can persist chronically in asymptomatic carrier hosts [14]. The vibrios, a group of gram-negative bacilli that includes *Vibrio cholerae* O1 and O139, the infectious agent of cholera, are capable of surviving for long periods in the environment, even amid unfavorable conditions, through transformation into dormant states [15].

The lessons learned from cholera highlight the challenges faced when confronting enteric illnesses. Cholera was among the first recognized waterborne pathogens. Once a leading cause of mortality in Europe and North America, its near elimination from industrialized countries in the late nineteenth century heralded one of the greatest modern public health achievements. Yet, in the twenty-first century, cholera plagues millions worldwide and kills hundreds of thousands every year. Recently, dynamic cholera occurrences have afflicted impoverished communities and sociopolitical refugees. Global concerns have escalated following the emergence of more virulent strains, the recognition of increasing antimicrobial resistance, potential increased environmental reservoirs subsequent to climate change, and broadening human migration and travel patterns. Fears of potential pandemic spread are woven into social hysteria surrounding cholera outbreaks. Compounding pervasive public health obstacles in low-income countries are complex sociopolitical and natural disasters that further disrupt precarious water-sanitation infrastructures. Innovative environmental and climatological investigations have dramatically improved our understanding of cholera dynamics, and expensive therapeutic advances have improved survival, but all of these technologies remain controversial in the face of the ongoing "silent humanitarian crisis" of inadequate water and sanitation. This chapter therefore emphasizes *V. cholerae*, as a prototypic enteric illness for understanding the socioeconomic disparities of infections in impoverished communities, the challenges underlying waterborne disease transmission, the dynamic interplay between pathogen and the environment, and the obligatory multifaceted response from the health-care and scientific community. Interlaced throughout the discussion are examples of challenges of other enteric pathogens, followed by a commentary discussion regarding the cumulative effects of enteric illnesses on the future of at-risk populations.

5.2 Cholera: A Prototype for Enteric Infections

Vibrio cholerae (serotypes O1 and O139), a facultative gram-negative bacterium with both human and environmental stages, is the enteric agent of cholera. Its victims suffer characteristic voluminous watery diarrhea ("rice-water" stools) that, when severe, can cause fatal dehydration and electrolyte abnormalities [15]. Though the potent cholera toxin (CTX) causes profound fluid and electrolyte losses, the host intestine shows no histological changes. Molecular studies have demonstrated that CTX binds the apical enterocyte membrane GM1-ganglioside receptor leading to irreversible adenylate cyclase activation and subsequently increased mucosal cAMP levels. Chloride (Cl^-) channels inserted into the apical membrane of crypt cells then stimulate active Cl^- secretion, and electroneutral NaCl absorption is inhibited. Villous cells also demonstrated decreased activity of apical membrane Na^+/H^+ and $Cl^-/HCO3^-$ exchange. Glucose-stimulated Na^+ absorption, however, is unaltered [16]. Other proteins of *V. cholerae*, such as *Vibrio cholerae* cytolysin, form anion channels on the apical membrane triggering an outward flux of chloride [17]. Combined, these ion-channel alterations result in dramatic ion and fluid shifts leading to profound watery diarrhea and electrolyte abnormalities [18]. The molecular complexities of this mechanism, including dependence on platelet-activating factor, phospholipase A_2, and prostaglandin concentrations, are still being clarified [16].

The primary genetic determinants of *V. cholerae* virulence include the presence of *ctxAB*, *tcp*, and *toxR* [19]. Their protein by-products, CTX, toxin-coregulated pilus (TCP), and ToxR, respectively, interact to promote toxin acquisition and production. CTX-encoding genes are carried on prophages (CTXϕ) and are present in all pathogenic *V. cholerae* [20]. These phages also carry the SXT element that harbors antibiotic resistance [21]. TCP tethers bacterial cells together and enhances virulence in vivo. ToxR is a CTXϕ receptor that mediates phage incorporation and thus regulates toxigenicity as well [22].

Toxigenic *V. cholerae* is highly transmissible and is one of the few bacterial diseases able to cause abrupt severe epidemics with true pandemic potential. It is also capable of remaining endemic once introduced into a suitable environment. Consequently, cholera has been one of the most academically scrutinized and publicly feared pathogens. Medical historians debate whether cholera emerged as a new infectious agent in the early nineteenth century, or if it had existed in ancient populations in the Indian subcontinent and the Middle East centuries prior [23]. Since first described by Thomas Sydenham in 1817, at least seven pandemics of cholera have swept globally, affecting every continent. The first six occurred between 1817 and 1923. Each were caused by the classical biotype of *Vibrio cholerae* O1 and originated in areas of the Indian subcontinent where cholera remains endemic [15]. Early pandemics generally lasted for about 10–12 years and spread across Asia with variable extension to Europe and the Americas [24]. Owing to improved municipalized water quality and modern sanitation, the disease appeared to be contained for almost 40 years. In 1961, a sporadic case of a new strain, *V. cholerae* O1, El Tor biotype, was identified in Egypt [15]. During that same year, an outbreak of the El Tor biotype spread globally, originating from the Celebes Islands of Indonesia rather than the Indian subcontinent. This current pandemic of cholera is characterized by seasonal outbreaks in endemic regions of Asia [25], a persistent presence with high mortality rates in Africa [26, 27], epidemics among displaced populations following natural disasters and refugees seeking sociopolitical asylum [28, 29], emerging environmentally derived atypical strains such as *V. cholerae* O139 in Bangladesh in 1992, the evolution of hybridized variants with long-term environmental survivability and concomitantly more virulent toxins [20], and increasing multidrug resistance. Cholera, therefore, is at once both an ancient scourge and an emerging infectious disease.

The reasons for why cholera remains such a problem today are multifactorial, and a detailed review of these factors exemplifies common features of enteric infections. Without question, the persistence of ongoing cholera and other enteric pathogen transmission is due to the inadequate water-sanitation systems and impoverished living conditions of afflicted communities. Biological mechanisms that propagate *V. cholerae* O1 and O139 pathogenicity, such as increased virulence following infection and the persistence in an environmental reservoir, are also important to disease spread. Environmental factors related to climate change, likely through associations with planktonic blooms, have a profound influence on vibrio populations. Finally, human behavior and migration patterns, increasingly common in the twenty-first century, may facilitate introduction of *V. cholerae* into new or previously low-risk communities.

5.2.1 Epidemiology

5.2.1.1 Current Epidemiology

While massive cholera outbreaks peak public interest, the global prevalence of cholera is greatly underappreciated [30]. According to the World Health Organization (WHO), in 2009, there were 221,226 cases of cholera, including 4,946 deaths, with a global case fatality rate (CFR) of 2.24% [31, 32]. Although rates had decreased between 1999 and 2004, a resurgence has occurred over the past 5 years. Between 2008 and 2009, there was a 16% increase in prevalence [31]. The vast majority of the 45 countries reporting cholera during the same time were restricted to Africa, with a few reported cases in Asia (Fig. 5.1). Africa represents between 94 and 98% of the reported annual cases globally since 2000 [31]. In contrast, Europe, North America, and South America have reported only sporadic cases, almost all of which were imported. Only rare cases of local acquisition occurred in the United States, where *V. cholerae* is endemic in the Gulf Coast and causes sporadic infections from undercooked shellfish [33]. In 2009, Europe and Canada reported no local cases, and Australia and Japan reported no cases of either imported or autochthonous disease [31].

Although International Health Regulations (IHR) have mandated official notification of cholera outbreaks by all WHO member states since 1969, adherence is far from universal, and case reporting may be as low as 1% [34]. Underreporting due to stigmatization and fear of economic consequences through sanctions is common. In particular, cases in South Asia are vastly underrepresented. In some endemic countries such as Bangladesh, more than two million cases of acute watery diarrhea occur without an identified pathogen, many of which would be tabulated as cholera if specifically identified. Cholera there may cause illness in two out of every thousand of the population each year, and rates may be even higher in some subregions [31, 35]. Even when governmental statistics are reported, they may be incomplete and patchy. In India, annualized incidence rates in Kolkata slums are 6.2/1,000 for children 2–4 years old and 8.6/1,000 for children less than two; however, incidence

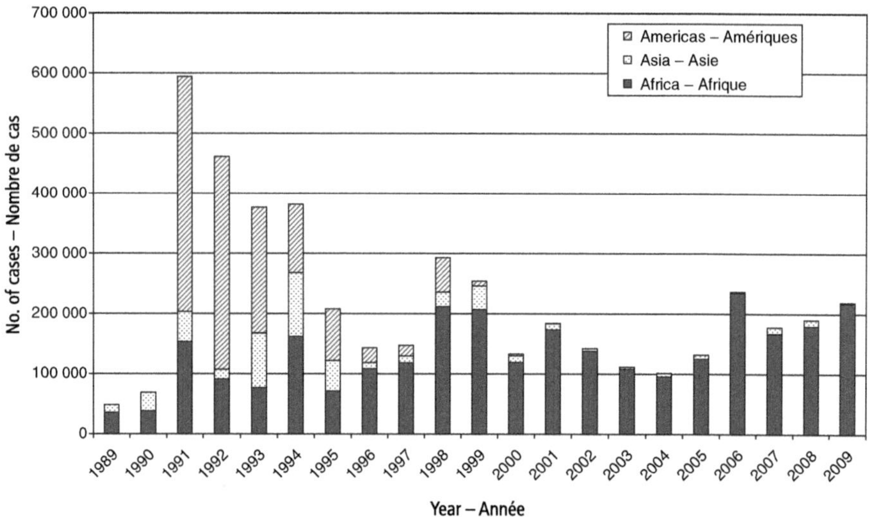

Fig. 5.1 Number of reported cholera cases to the WHO by year and continent, 1989–2009 [31]. Reprinted with permission from WHO

rates are entirely unknown in rural parts of the country [36]. Among these rural households (two-thirds of India's total population of 1.15 billion), only 28% use piped drinking water and only 26% have access to proper sanitation. The attack rates in epidemics are also underestimated [37]. Among 68 outbreaks in India between 1997 and 2006, the actual number affected was six times greater than the WHO reported and occurred over a much broader geographic area than initially thought [38]. Between 2000 and 2004, three countries did not report any cases of cholera, yet each experienced outbreaks in 2005: The Gambia (214 cases and 13 deaths, CFR 6.1%), Mauritania (4,132 cases and 70 deaths, CFR 1.7%), and Sao Tome (1,966 cases and 33 deaths, CFR 1.7%). Similarly, in 2006, Angola and Sudan both experienced profound epidemics with a combined 44,718 cases, none of which were reported to the WHO [26]. Thailand has not reported cholera since 1994, yet epidemics have occurred in the southern part of the country, and *V. cholerae* was isolated from 5.4% of cases of bacterial diarrheal disease among hospitalized children in Bangkok between January 1995 and December 2000 [34]. A review of cases reported online to The Program for Monitoring Emerging Diseases (ProMED) found that while 66% of outbreaks occurred in Africa between 1995 and 2005, 16.8% were in Southeast Asia (defined as South and Southeastern Asia) [39]. Inconsistencies in disease terminology likely accounts for 500,000–700,000 cases of cholera "misclassified" as "acute watery diarrhea" [31, 40]. One multinational survey utilizing specific diagnostic testing found that *V. cholera* represented 0.6% of all cases of endemic diarrhea, suggesting an annual incidence of 11 million from endemic cholera alone, excluding outbreaks [41]. After accounting for the aforementioned underreported cases, the WHO estimates an annual global prevalence of to 3–5 million with 100,000–130,000 deaths [37].

The current pandemic is characterized by a global geographical shift toward higher prevalence in Africa. During the first several years of the seventh pandemic, officially reported cases in Africa represented only 20% of the global total. Unlike the continents affected by pre-seventh pandemics, when the disease reached sub-Saharan Africa in 1970, it remained entrenched and dramatically increased to represent 94% of all cases between 2000 and 2005 [26, 42–44]. The emergence of cholera in Africa was through two major routes. One originated in Western countries of Sierra Leone, Liberia, Guinea, Nigeria, and other coastal countries and the other in the Middle East extending to Eastern African countries of Djibouti, Somalia, and Ethiopia [45]. Since then, epidemics have since been recognized across the entire continent [10, 45–69]. In Beira, Mozambique, children less than two have rates of 6.2/1,000, similar to Kolkata [37]. The attack rate during outbreaks across all subregions of Africa is disproportionately large [39]. A recent crisis in Zimbabwe accounted for 31% of all the cases from Africa in 2009 (CFR, 4.3%) [27]. Ongoing outbreaks in 2009 were also reported in Zimbabwe, Democratic Republic of the Congo, Ethiopia, Kenya, Mozambique, Nigeria, South Africa, and Sudan [31].

V. cholerae O1 (biotype El Tor, serotype Ogawa) has recently spread rapidly throughout Haiti. Despite no infectious disease outbreaks reported through the first 8 months following the catastrophic 7.0 Richter-scale earthquake on January 12, 2010, within 1 month after the onset of the outbreak on October 21, 2010, all provinces were affected. During the first 2 months, 121,518 cases had been reported, 63,711 patients were hospitalized, and there were 2,591 deaths; the case fatality rate (CFR) was 2.1% with a peak at 9% [7, 70]. Within months, imported cases in the Dominican Republic, Florida, Massachusetts, and Venezuela had occurred [8, 70]. Improved municipal water and sanitation systems helped to quell further spread; however, many communities remain vulnerable. Surprisingly, Haiti was one of two (the other Uruguay) countries spared from disease after the seventh pandemic first struck South America in 1991. Up to one million cases were projected in Haiti alone in 2011, and further spread of disease will be an ongoing concern for several years [71].

The pattern of indiscriminate infection across all age groups in Haiti by what was most likely a single clone is characteristic of outbreaks in non-endemic settings [72]. Epidemics in endemic regions display a different pattern. In endemic regions like India and Bangladesh, poor sanitation coupled with environmental conditions favor vibrio growth. In these regions, cholera predominately affects children aged 2–15 and has low rates of secondary transmission, high rates of asymptomatic carriage, and a relatively low CFR [38]. Seasonal peaks correspond to the warm seasons before and after monsoonal rains [73]. The first peak occurs during the spring with a larger second peak in the fall. Onset of epidemics coincides with the warmest water temperatures and drier weather [74]. Simultaneous outbreak foci occur, typically with a sporadic beginning relatively close to water sources without apparent interconnectedness [75]. Secondary outbreaks quickly follow with spatial-temporally clustered spikes but are often short-lived [73]. Whether these patterns represent increased human-human contact following adverse weather events, increased water contamination, or an environmentally driven increase in presence and/or pathogenicity of vibrios remains unclear [76]. Epidemics in traditionally

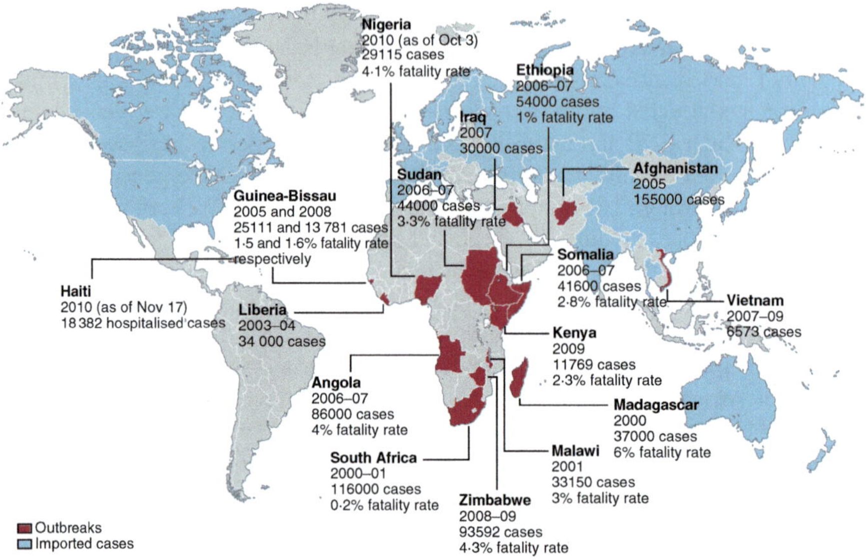

Fig. 5.2 Major outbreaks of cholera since 2000: selected outbreaks in red, with associated case atality rates (where reported). Countries with imported cases between 2004 and 2009 are in blue [77]. Reprinted with permission from WHO

non-endemic locations such as occurred in Peru, Brazil, sub-Saharan Africa, and Haiti typically affect all age groups, usually emerge from a single point source, and have low asymptomatic rates and relatively higher mortality rates.

5.2.1.2 Case Fatality Rate Trends

During the past 3 years, the WHO reported between 177,963 and 237,000 cholera cases including 4,031 deaths. During the first 6 months of 2009, however, there were more than 98,000 cases and 4,000 deaths [37]. The internationally recognized benchmark case fatality rate (CFR) for cholera is <1% [77]. Economic disparities associate with a higher CFR. During an outbreak in 1991, in Peru, an overall CFR of 0.34% was reported, yet it exceeded 3% in the poor highlands and jungle regions [76]. Although having decreased 17% from the previous year, there were exceptionally high average mortalities in Africa in 2009: 217,333 cases, including 4,883 deaths (CFR, 2.25) [31]. Between 2000 and 2005, eight countries reported a CFR of >5%, and three countries in 2009 exceeded 10% [31, 78]. CFR can exceed unfathomable numbers as occurred in Angola, when a *Vibrio cholera* O1 El Tor outbreak caused greater than 30% mortality in some provinces in a rapid outbreak affecting 46,758 [35]. With these exceptionally high CFRs, a disproportionate 99% of fatalities occurred in Africa since 2000 [42]. The CFR is reportedly below 1% in Asia [31]. The ICDDR-B in Bangladesh has shown that CFR can be as low as 0.2% [79]. In Africa, such low rates have been achieved only by relatively wealthy countries (Fig. 5.2) [77].

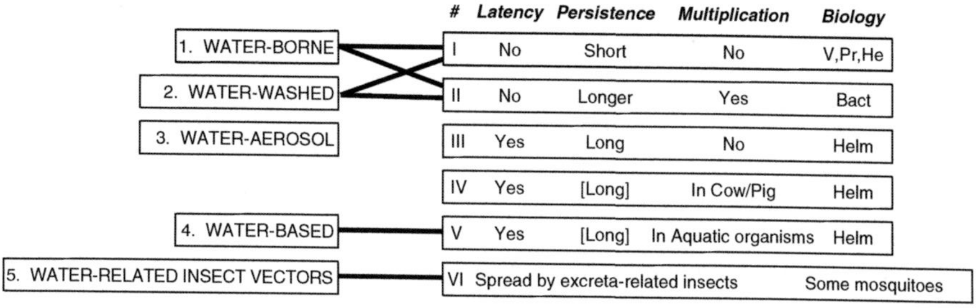

Fig. 5.3 Relation of water- and excreta-related transmission categories V=virus, Pr=protozoa, He=helminth [83]. Reprinted with permission from WHO

Mortality rates are highest among refugees of sociopolitical and natural disasters. The CFR following the October 2010 outbreak in Haiti was 13% on the first day but dropped rapidly to 2% once recognized [7, 77]. The experience in Haiti runs parallel to most outbreaks of the past decade. During the 2008–2009 outbreak in Zimbabwe, CFR was 4.3% [77]. During the Goma, Zaire outbreak in 1994, the CFR for the first month was between 19.5 and 31.2 per 10,000 per day, strikingly higher than the prewar CFR in Rwanda of only 0.6 per 10,000 per day. The most densely populated refugee camp, Muganga, at one point reported a CFR of 48% [80].

5.2.2 *Transmission*

5.2.2.1 Microbiology and Environment

Bradley first described the current public health paradigm of water-related illnesses in 1972 [81]. A recent modification of these principles categorizes diseases into the following: waterborne (ingestion of contaminated water such as typhoid, *Giardia*, *Cryptosporidium* in low-income settings, and hepatitis A); water-carried (accidental ingestion or aerosol exposure to contaminated recreational sources such as *Cryptosporidium* in high-income settings, *Pseudomonas* dermatitis, and trachoma); water-washed (person-person transmission through inadequate quantity of water and hygienic supplies such as hepatitis A and *Shigella*); water-based (water obligatory in pathogen life cycle; *Schistosomiasis*, *Dracunculiasis*, *Legionella*); and water-vectored (water-connected insects such as malaria, dengue, yellow fever, and Onchocerciasis) [81, 82]. Environmental survivability is another important factor for potential latent and persistent transmission of some excreta-transmitted organisms (Fig. 5.3) [83]. By this schema, *V. cholerae* is classified as both a waterborne and water-washed pathogen [33]. Additionally, food-borne outbreaks have been reported from contaminated vegetables and shellfish [84].

After Robert Koch first identified the curved gram-negative rod, *Vibrio cholerae*, as the "causative agent of cholera" in 1884, the organism was believed to be a human-specific parasite like typhoid, incapable of surviving permanently outside of the human host. In the 1990s, however, other vibrios were recognized as autochthonous inhabitants of brackish waters [85]. Current understandings are that the natural reservoir for cholera is marine and estuarine aquatic environments. Both *Vibrio cholerae* O1 and O139 can survive indefinitely by forming symbiotic relationships with aquatic zooplankton, plants, and crustaceans [26, 86]. Outbreaks typically follow a pattern of primary environmental exposure through breaches in water-sanitation systems, propagated secondarily by person-person spread [73]. Optimal growth conditions for vibrios include a salinity of 5–25%, temperatures near 35 °C, sunlight, alkaline pH, and iron-rich conditions. In addition to growth, increased sunlight, salinity of 2–2.5%, and moderate iron concentrations augment toxin production [74, 87–91]. When exposed to relatively nutrient-poor aquatic environments, however, *V. cholerae* O1 has a predilection for quickly entering a viable but non-culturable (VBNC) nonpathogenic state [74, 85]. Dramatic climate changes such as El Niño may trigger repopulation of vibrios previously in a predominately VBNC state [85]. Other enterics have been found to have long environmental persistence. *Campylobacter* displays a very long decay rate in aquatic environments [92]. Despite injury from copper, toxigenic *E. coli* retains the capacity to produce heat-stable toxin but is not detectable on selective culture media [87, 93]. Bacterial motility factors likely play an important survival role [94]. Norovirus is capable of persisting in food and fomites, even after disinfection with non-bleach detergents [95]. Parasitic pathogens such as *Giardia* [96], *Cryptosporidium* [97], and *E. histolytica* employ cystic forms allowing for survival times up to several months, even under extremely harsh conditions. The protection provided by the cysts and oocysts is so effective that these protozoa even show resistance to standard chlorination techniques.

When growing conditions are ideal, *V. cholerae* becomes even more toxigenic. The typical infectious dose of *V. cholerae* O1 is more than 10,000 organisms. Toxigenic *V. cholerae* shed in human stool, however, show increased expression of nutrient acquisition, motility, and acid-tolerance response genes, rendering it up to 50–700 times more capable of colonizing a naive host [98, 99]. This "hyperinfectious state" can be maintained for approximately 18 h outside of the gut, allowing ample time for transmission and the potential propagation of outbreaks through human hosts. Though the specific mechanisms are not yet clear, environmental lysogenic and lytic bacteriophages (vibriophages) possibly influence the extinction of cholera outbreaks [73, 100, 101]. Leading theories suggest that vibriophages counteract the hyperinfectious phenomenon, likely through phenotypic alterations in vibrio virulence factors such as motility [102]. The artificial introduction of these vibriophages into human stool leads to a tenfold increase in the infectious dose of *V. cholerae* [21]. Under natural conditions, vibriophage-positive index cases are less likely to secondarily transmit infection to household contacts than patients who were not phage positive [21, 103]. Eventual amelioration of outbreaks when phage predation outnumbers pathogenic bacteria has been demonstrated [104]. The complex interactions of these multiple environment factors are depicted in Fig. 5.4 [74].

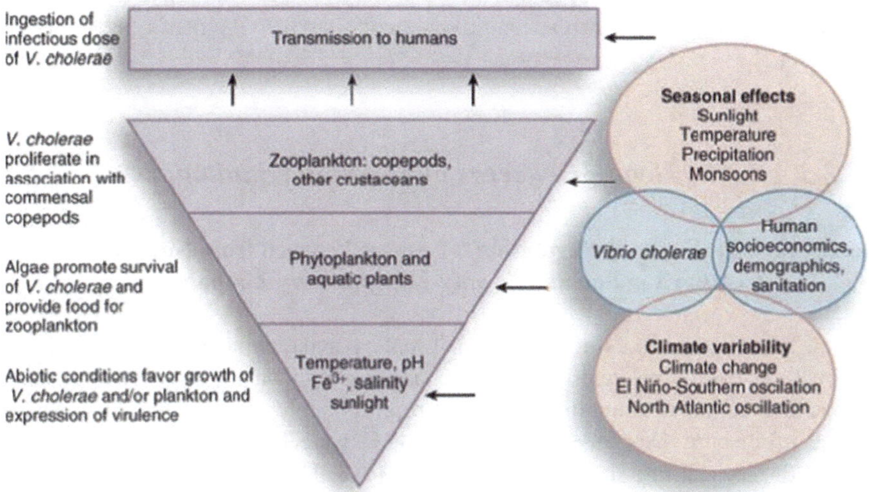

Fig. 5.4 Hierarchical environmental model for cholera transmission [74]. Reprinted with permission from WHO

5.2.2.2 Host Susceptibility

Host susceptibility factors also play an important role in severity of disease and the burden of organisms shed into stool. Among healthy volunteers, the reduction of stomach acid with bicarbonate solution just prior to inoculation has been shown to yield infectious rates of 90% with 10^4–10^8 bacteria compared with 10^8–10^{11} bacteria under normal conditions [21]. Associations between concomitant *Helicobacter pylori* and epidemic *Vibrio cholerae* in Bangladesh and Peru and an outbreak of cholera in achlorhydric patients in Italy have confirmed cholera susceptibility in states of hypochlorhydria [105, 106]. In the case of enteric infections, young age, malnutrition, impaired host defenses, inborn and acquired immunodeficiencies, and increasingly recognized genetic aberrations predispose to more severe infection. Micronutrient deficiencies such as those of vitamin A and zinc also increase morbidity due to diarrheal illnesses [107]. Humoral immunity is an important protectant against all enterics, as is common following infant breast milk weaning [108, 109]. Certain parasitic infections such as *Giardia* cause worse disease in individuals lacking adequate levels of IgA [110, 111]. Acquired cell-mediated immune defects increase severity of disease caused by *Strongyloides stercoralis, Cryptosporidium, Isospora*, *Salmonella*, and other enterics [112].

Host genetics are increasingly recognized risk factors for development of enteric disease [113]. Individuals of the O blood group type, for example, are at increased risk of *V. cholerae* O1 infection [114]. The APOE polymorphisms are a recently recognized variable in the cognitive effects subsequent to early childhood diarrhea. In particular, APOE2 frequency is higher among children with the heaviest diarrheal burden, whereas APOE4 appears to have a protective role in cognitive development despite its association with cognitive decline and Alzheimer's later in life [115–117].

5.2.3 *Public Health Concerns of Water and Sanitation*

5.2.3.1 "The Sanitary Revolution": Lessons Learned from Nineteenth-Century London and Twenty-First-Century Zimbabwe

In the late nineteenth century, diarrhea, dysentery, and typhoid accounted for almost 1 in 10 deaths in the United States, compared to less than 1% today [10]. Densely populated urban communities were disproportionately affected. Infant mortality rates in Pittsburg, Detroit, and Washington D.C. were 180/1,000 live births, nearly twice the present rate in sub-Saharan Africa [118, 119]. Between 1900 and 1929, however, there was a dramatic 20% drop in overall mortality and a concomitant 88% decrease in diarrheal illnesses [118]. Life expectancy in Britain climbed by 10 years during the same time span [10]. Parallel to these dramatic improvements in longevity were the near extinction of typhoid, cholera, and other severe enteric illnesses (Fig. 5.5) [27].

Three historical events in the nineteenth-century industrializing countries led to these rapid public health improvements: social dissatisfaction with poor living conditions and associated diseases, recognition of the route of cholera transmission, and municipalization of water and sanitation systems. "Asiatic" cholera was first seen in Britain in 1831. Epidemics of cholera (1832) and typhoid (1838) followed. The disproportionate affliction among the poor working class eventually led to "cholera riots" and widespread public fears [120, 121]. Commissioned by the government, Edwin Chadwick provided a quantitative linkage between poor living conditions and disease and life expectancy in his "Report on the Sanitary Condition of Laboring Population of Great Britain" [4]. Subsequently, The Public Health Act of 1848 was passed, affording London with provisions for public watering and sanitation services. Despite the new laws, in 1854, 23,000 people died in Ireland and Great Britain during one of the worst outbreaks of the third cholera pandemic [122]. Popular theory then posited that cholera was transmitted through vapors, or "miasmas", arising from fetid water [123, 124]. A London epidemiologist, John Snow, challenged the *miasma* theory in 1855. He argued that water, rather than *miasmas*, was the vehicle for cholera transmission. Snow carefully crafted a Voronoi diagram (Fig. 5.6) that demonstrated that 73 of 83 deaths occurred among residents closest to the Broad Street pump near the outbreak's epicenter. Mortality rates were lower at the adjacent Newcastle Arms pub, which used its own deep well. Snow's data led to removal of the pump handle, and deaths from cholera declined within days [125, 126].

In 1880, municipalities in Britain replaced private providers for clean water, leading to a decreased incidence of typhoid and cholera. Typhoid in the United States

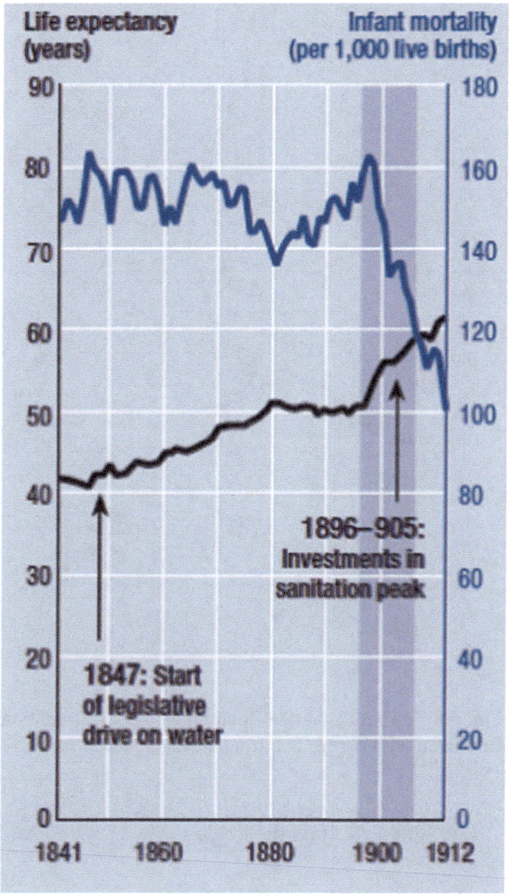

Fig. 5.5 Infant death rates and life expectancy in England and Wales, 1841–1912 [10]. Reprinted with permission from WHO

similarly declined after widespread use of water filters (Figs. 5.7 and 5.8) [10]. Unmanaged sewage, however, continued to contaminate surface and public water sources, and infant mortality due to diarrheal illness in Britain remained unchanged at 160/1,000 in 1890 [10]. Toward the close of the nineteenth century, Joseph Bazalgette discovered the technological means of providing municipal sanitation [27]. Social pressures and improved voting power for lower economic classes led to increased expenditures for sanitation services over the next two decades. This "sanitary revolution" led to increased life expectancy in London (Fig. 5.8). The United States experienced a drop in diarrhea-related mortality from over 120/100,000 people to less than 20/100,000, an unprecedented public health initiative [10].

The benefits of municipal water and sanitation systems, however, have failed to reach impoverished populations. The WHO defines access to water as 20 l a day of clean water per person from a source less than 1 km from home [10]. Currently, 1.1 billion people – 17% of the world's population – have no source of safe drinking

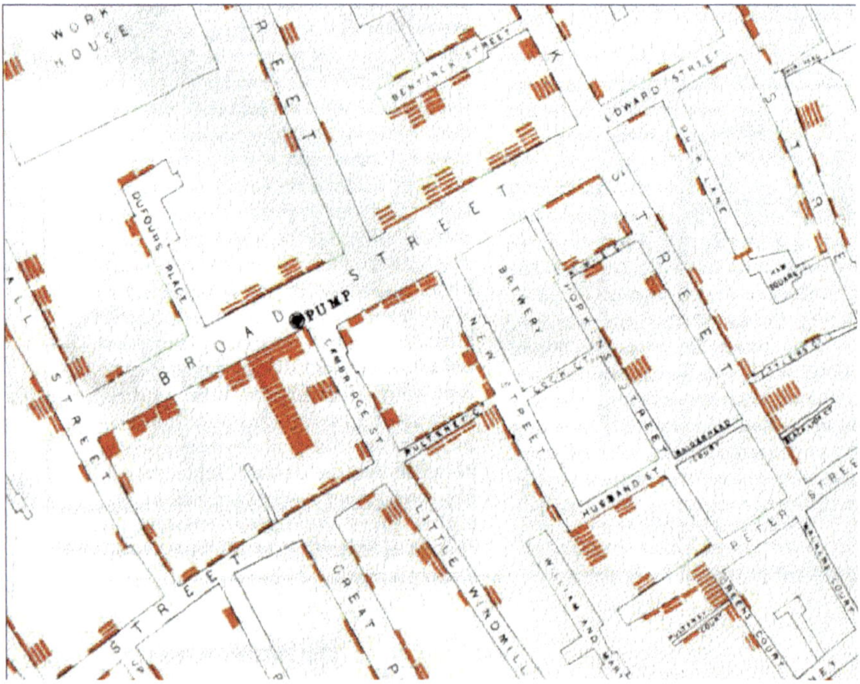

Fig. 5.6 Voronoi Diagram, John Snow, Broad Street Pump, Golden Square, London, 1855 [125]. Reprinted with permission from WHO

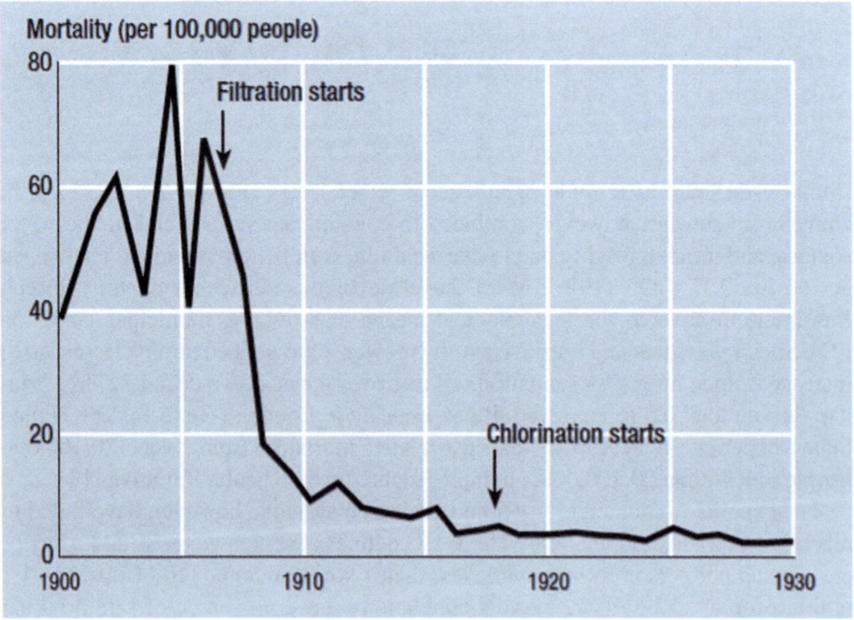

Fig. 5.7 Typhoid mortality in Cincinnati, Ohio, 1900–1930 [10]. Reprinted with permission from WHO

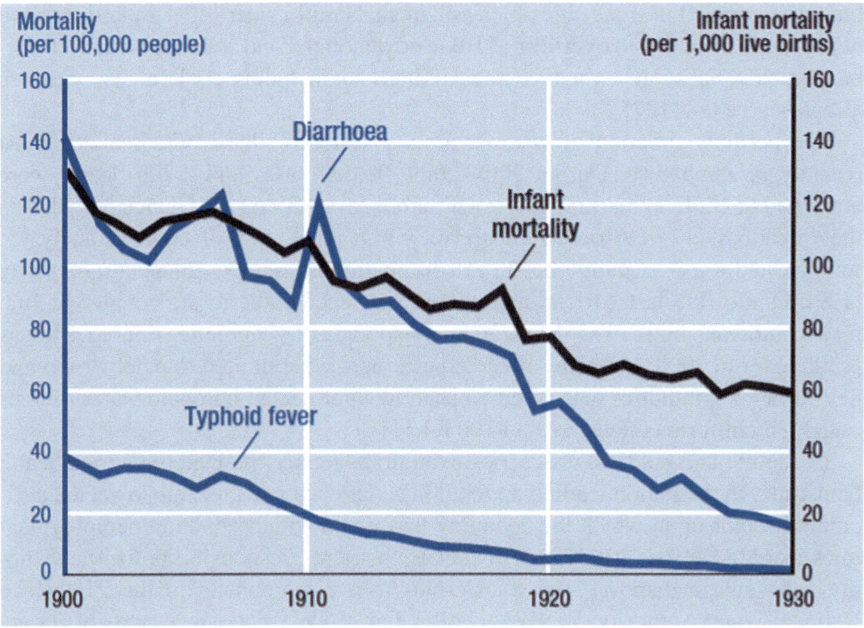

Fig. 5.8 Death rates from waterborne diseases in the United States, 1900–1930 [10]. Reprinted with permission from WHO

water [4]. Two-thirds of those without access to clean water live in Asia, and 42% of those living in sub-Saharan Africa have no safe water source. In pre-earthquake Haiti, the average water coverage was about 15 l/person/day, compared with the United States at >570 l/person/day [10]. Bangladesh, Kenya, Ghana, Nigeria, Burkina Faso, Niger, Angola, Ethiopia, Rwanda, Uganda, and Mozambique also fall below the "water-poverty" threshold. Basic sanitation coverage, defined as access to a pit latrine, is even worse; 2.6 billion people (42%) fall short. The number would increase to four billion if defined in terms of a "flush toilet" [4, 10]. In sub-Saharan Africa, 64% of all people lack basic sanitation [4]. This profound water-sanitation gap is the primary reason why cholera, typhoid, and other enteric infections are so prevalent in some communities but absent in others.

General country statistics fail to capture the dire state of water and hygiene access for the poorest of poor communities. While many cities such as Mumbai report improved coverage rates that include 90% of the population, the 18 million residents dwelling in peri-urban slums do not figure into the municipal data. These residents live in an environment with an estimated 1 toilet for every 1,440 people. For some households in Manila and Dar es Salaam, municipal waterworks connection fees may cost up to 3 months income, dramatically reducing utilization [10]. Similarly, while pit latrines may be in place, the removal of waste is often hindered by lack of a municipal sewage system. This has led to "flying toilets" of human excrement in some cities such as Kibera, Nairobi where 13% of latrines have become unusable due to overfilling [10]. And although hand washing with triclocarban antibacterial soap can reduce rates of diarrhea, including cholera, resources are all too scarce [64, 127].

The perilous situation of water-sanitation system collapse was realized most recently in Zimbabwe. During 2008–2009, 98,000 cases and 4,200 deaths were attributed to cholera, marking the worst outbreak in Africa [128]. Once heralded as the "breadbasket" of Africa, Zimbabwe, with a population of approximately ten million, had a model public health infrastructure and relative financial prosperity [129]. One of the last African nations to experience cholera, the country had no major outbreaks until 1992–1993, and only sporadically thereafter in border towns [130]. Prior to 2008, low rates of endemic cholera were limited to patchy rural and peri-urban communities that relied on shallow unprotected borehole water sources with high coliform counts (>1,800/100 mL) [131].

Economic and political crises, however, dramatically changed the public health landscape. In the period leading up to 2008 economic crisis in Zimbabwe, the agricultural sector upon which the economy was based collapsed, and unemployment rates soared to 94% [130]. Due to financial constraints, responsibility for water supply and sewage disposal was transferred from city councils to the Zimbabwe National Water Authority (ZINWA). Following ZINWA's takeover, parts of Harare and Chitungwiza were without running water for 2 years, forcing dependence on shallow wells, contaminated due to lack of sewage disposal [130]. Private domestic means of water purification, such as boiling water, was erratic due to widespread electrical outages [132]. These disruptions in water sanitation have been closely linked to subsequent disease outbreaks. Cases of acute diarrheal illness began being reported in Chitungwiza in August of 2008. A total of 118 cases were identified in the large urban center on the outskirts of Harare. *Vibrio cholerae* O1 was isolated in 18 (30%) of 59 specimens sent for analysis. Although this initial outbreak appeared to be contained, a second wave struck a few months later, infecting 600 people (CFR 15%) [130]. Within 4 months of onset, 11,735 cases were reported, and high mortality rates forced the nation to declare a state of emergency and a call for international aid [132, 133]. Densely populated urban centers, such as Budirio, quickly became the focal point of the outbreak [133]. All of Zimbabwe's ten provinces have since reported cases of cholera [134]. Extension into neighboring Mozambique, Botswana, Zambia, and South Africa via contamination of the Limpopo River occurred within months [128, 130, 135]. The health-care system, abandoned by professionals fleeing the squalor, was inadequately equipped for transfer and treatment. Consequently, the CFR was 5% in health-care facilities and surpassed 40% in some treated at home [136].

Poor living conditions, such as those in Zimbabwe, lead to characteristic secondary transmission patterns of cholera. During these outbreaks, spread of disease within households or via street vendors likely accounts for the majority of cases [137, 138]. Narrow-mouthed containers which prohibit the dipping of hands into storage water decrease intra-familial transmission by 74.6% [139]. Chlorination at water sources and directly in individual containers has been shown to reduce interfamilial transmission of cholera by 57.8% [139]. Boiling water or filtration with cloth, charcoal, and chemical coagulation can also reduce rates of secondary transmission [140]. An examination of water collection practices during outbreaks in Malawi refugee camps showed that contaminated water storage containers in houses usually show rising coliform counts between 30 and 60 min of collection and plateau around 2–6 h. Whether this reflected contamination at the time of collection or redistribution of organisms through agitation, a dramatic reduction in coliform counts was seen when containers with lids were introduced. This translated into a 31% reduction in episodes of diarrhea among children <5 years old [141].

With a well-functioning water-sanitation infrastructure, however, secondary transmission vanishes. The largest modern cholera outbreak in the United States occurred on February 14, 1992, when 75 of 336 Aerolineas Argentinas flight passengers from Lima landed in Los Angeles with cholera acquired after consuming cold seafood salad en route. Although ten patients were later hospitalized with severe cholera, there were no secondary cases [142, 143]. The most recent and nearest cholera epidemic in post-earthquake Haiti lead to only a handful of cases in the southern United States, all of which were returning relief workers [8]. Even when devastating natural disasters strike, as Hurricanes Katrina and Rita did in Louisiana in 2005, the environmental potential for crisis through disrupted water and sanitation systems is averted if there is adequate mobilization of public health resources and infrastructural support [144]. Unfortunately, in low-income settings, these disasters propagate channels for increased spread of enteric infections through disruption of already fragile water-sanitation infrastructures.

5.2.3.2 Disruptions in Water and Sanitation Due to Natural and Complex Disasters

Natural and sociopolitical (complex) disasters profoundly disrupt water-sanitation systems and hygiene. Natural disasters are rapid onset and rapidly abating events that have historically low epidemic potential [145–147]. Although a recent review of over 600 geophysical disasters showed that the risk of immediate post-disaster epidemics was negligible [148], historical accounts of diarrheal and dysentery outbreaks following flooding and hurricanes in particular are common [62, 149–151]. Contamination of water supplies by brackish flood water has been shown to raise coliform counts [152]. Following extensive flooding in Leningrad in 1924, infectious rates of typhoid fever rose from 9.9 to 53.3% and scarlet fever from 12 to 50.4% for several months. After a 1952 earthquake-tsunami in Kamchatka, Russia, local hospitals saw a 159% increase in infectious disease-related mortalities, many related to diarrheal illnesses, over the next year [149]. In the wake of torrential rains and flooding in Ethiopia in 2006, 150 of 600 deaths were attributed to diarrheal illness [62].

The influx of massive populations of natural disaster survivors and/or sociopolitical refugees into internally displaced population (IDP) camps has clearly become a common risk factor for enteric outbreaks [145–149, 153–155]. In refugee camps in eastern Sudan, Somalia, Malawi, Ethiopia, and Kenya in the 1980s, diarrhea was attributed to 25–50% of all deaths [150]. Outbreaks often occur several months after natural disasters and are more directly reflective of displaced living conditions than the catastrophe itself. When the 7.6 Richter-scale Kashmir earthquake shook northern Pakistan and India in 2005, international aid focused on rescue missions for missing persons. Less attention was placed on water, sanitary, and hygiene provisions [156]. Throughout the following year, 65% of all illnesses were due to infections, with a high percentage having acute watery diarrhea [28]. Confirmed cholera outbreaks among refugees have been reported in Sudan [157], Ethiopia [158, 159], Thailand [160], Turkey [161], Malawi [162, 163], Somalia [150], Ghana, Congo, Dominican Republic [29, 164], Tanzania [165], Nigeria [64], Uganda, Kenya [138], and most recently in Haiti [7].

Exposure to enteropathogens in IDP camps occurs through polluted water, unsanitary water transportation and storage, scarcity of soap and hygienic products, improper food preparation, and a contaminated food supply [28, 138, 146, 147, 166, 167]. One case-control study during a cholera outbreak among Mozambican refugees in Malawi in 1993 identified several sanitary risk factors: drinking river water within 1 week of illness onset (OR = 3.0, not statistically significant), submersing hands in household drinking water (OR = 6.0), and eating leftover cooked peas (OR = 8.0) [163]. Lack of soap, cooking pots, water containers, and latrines, no contact with oral rehydration solution (ORS), and contaminated dry fish are other risk factors [150, 163]. Recent arrival in a camp with ongoing cholera transmission (OR = 3.66) and sharing a latrine with three or more households (OR = 4.66) were risk factors during an outbreak among Sudanese and Somali refugees in Kenya in 1991. Storing water in sealed or covered containers was partially protective (OR = 0.55) [138].

Most enteric illnesses following natural disasters are caused by prevalent endemic pathogens: toxigenic *E. coli*, *Campylobacter*, non-typhoidal *Salmonella*, and *Norovirus* [149]. However, abrupt environmental changes, such as increased salinity of estuarine waters following flooding and hurricanes, may promote toxigenic shifts among otherwise nonpathogenic states. Fifty-five percent of tap, tube/bore well, and pond water samples collected after a cyclone in West Bengal, India in 2009, were positive for *V. cholerae* O1, including both Ogawa and Inaba serotypes [152]. Concentrations of both *V. cholerae* O1 and *V. cholerae* non-O1 were higher than prior to the cyclone. Prior to the disaster, all *V. cholerae* O1 isolates were nontoxigenic; however, 36% of isolates post-disasters produced *ctxB*. Water salinity at these sources had increased from 0.04 to 0.12% [152]. A similar phenomenon may have occurred following Hurricanes Katrina and Rita in Louisiana in October 2005, when 22 cases of vibrio (*V. vulnificus, V. parahaemolyticus,* and nontoxigenic *V. cholerae*) and rare sporadic cases of toxigenic *V. cholerae* were reported [142, 168].

The first appearance of the seventh pandemic in Haiti 7 months after a devastating 7.0 Richter-scale earthquake demolished the city of Port-au-Prince, causing the evacuation of more than 1.3 million IDPs, exemplifies how susceptible these populations can be in the setting of extreme poverty [7, 169]. Haiti is commonly cited as the poorest country in the western hemisphere; prior to the earthquake, 47% of the population lacked access to basic health care and 67% survived on less than

$2 US per day [170]. The threat of diarrheal illness after the earthquake was high. While national surveillance data was unavailable, individual studies prior to the earthquake suggest that acute diarrhea was the number one health problem among children 0–4 years of age [171]. Estimates approximated 4–6 episodes of diarrhea per child per year, and diarrhea accounted for 16% of all deaths under age five [172]. Waterborne enterics, such as norovirus, rotavirus, enterotoxigenic *Escherichia coli*, *Shigella*, *Campylobacter*, *Salmonella*, *Yersinia*, *Giardia*, *Cryptosporidium*, and *Entamoeba histolytica,* were common [171, 173]. Subsequent to the earthquake, all plumbing in the capital city of Port-au-Prince was destroyed [174], and early water quality testing performed by an independent German NGO, Technisches Hilfswerk, found unacceptably high coliform counts in preserved private wells around the Port-au-Prince area [70].

Combined efforts between WHO/PAHO, the UN, Haiti's MSPP, and other governmental and nongovernmental organizations initially succeeded in delivering 4.2 million liters of clean water daily and completing early installation of 11,000 latrines within weeks [174]. Infectious diarrheal rates were initially low [175]. Allocation for waste disposal, however, was lacking, and anecdotal accounts of inappropriate dumping of human waste into water sources had circulated. The risk for water contamination progressively increased. Once established, secondary transmission of cholera was inevitable. Many camps exceeded safe population density thresholds, with some in the Artibonite region where the outbreak began exceeding 30,000 people per camp. Exacerbated by inadequate hygienic supplies, by December 29, reported cases of cholera had risen to 148,787, including 83,166 hospitalized patients and 3,333 deaths [176].

Given that cholera had not been reported in Haiti since 1961, its appearance raised alarms among global humanitarian relief groups of the possible inadvertent introduction from international aid volunteers. An alternative explanation would be the reemergence from a previous VBNC state as likely occurred in South America in 1991. Based on single-nucleotide variations, the *V. cholerae* O1 El Tor strains in Haiti (H1/H2 Haiti 2010) are phylogenetically similar to the M4 (MDC126 Bangladesh 2008) strain and distinct from prior South American strains and circulating East African strains. Neither the C6 strain (C6706 Peru 1992) nor the circulating US Gulf Coast strain (2740–80) were phylogenetically similar (Fig. 5.9) [177]. Moreover, the SXT element of both M4 and H1/H2 strains is identical, and it is entirely absent from the C6 strain [177]. Ongoing epidemiological work is needed to determine the exact route of the introduction of a South Asian strain.

Overcrowded refugee camps require hypervigilant hygienic practices. Hurricane Katrina's devastation of southeastern gulf-coast communities of the United States in 2005 caused 1,800 immediate casualties and forced approximately 240,000 evacuees to Houston, Texas [166, 178–181]. Within three days of relocating to the large "megashelters" in Houston's Reliant Park Complex, more than 1,000 (17%) of the displaced population, including a disproportionate 75% of children, were afflicted. The acute gastrointestinal illness was later confirmed as norovirus [168, 181–183]. The short half-life of norovirus coupled with a substantial number of affected health-care providers despite abundant access to water and sanitation implicated

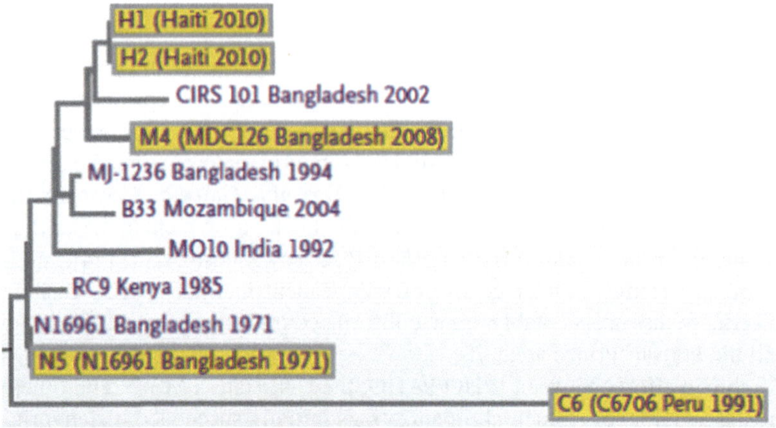

Fig. 5.9 The phylogenetic relationships among pandemic *V. cholerae* strains in the seventh pandemic, including H1, H2, M4, C6, and N5 on the basis of single-nucleotide variations [177]. Reprinted with permission from WHO

improper hygienic practices [181]. Educational awareness, together with increased provisions of alcohol-based gel hand sanitizers and portable sinks, eventually curbed the outbreak after 1 week [182]. Food preparation practices also strongly influence transmission [141, 163]. For example, among Mozambican refugees in Malawi, peas that had been cooked the previous night, but not re-cooked due to lack of firewood, contributed to transmission of cholera [163].

Outbreaks among refugees fleeing sociopolitical emergencies are notorious for high rates of infectivity and exceptionally high CFRs [150]. Inadequate outbreak preparation, geographic access barriers, and disorganized relocation efforts causing mass unexpected population displacement all contribute to dangerous situations with high risks of fatality [29, 163, 184]. Mortality rates of internally displaced populations and refugees may be 5–60 times the baseline for any given country [146, 147, 185]. Collectively, up to 40% of deaths in the initial phase of population relocation in complex emergencies are due to diarrheal illness, with over 80% occurring in children less than 2 years of age [147]. The post-conflict living conditions associated with outdoor taps; water sources less than 5 m from latrines; self-built, shallow, and unprotected wells; and open-air self-built latrines have been shown to lead to heavy fecal contamination [186]. Victims of complex sociopolitical disasters have often suffered with chronic illness and malnutrition for years secondary to economic and political turmoil [147]. Malnutrition strongly correlates with CFRs in refugee populations. When protein energy malnutrition (PEM) is less than 5%, the mean CFR is approximately 0.9/1,000/month, whereas CFR can climb to 4/1,000/month up to 177/1,000/month when PEM prevalence increases to 40% [150].

Failure to appreciate the risk of enteric outbreaks in IDPs leads to public health crises. One of the worst refugee outbreaks of *V. cholerae* on record occurred following the influx of 800,000 Rwandan refugees into North Kivu, Democratic Republic of the Congo, in 1994. From July 14–17, nearly 1.2 million Hutu refugees fleeing genocide sought security in the nearby North Kivu region. The overrun town of Goma, near Lake Kivu, was a common entry point, and four main camps were established to accommodate the massive influx: Munigi, Katale, Kibumba, and Mugunga [29]. During the first week of the crises, clean water availability was restricted to 200–1,000 ml per person daily [147, 187]. Consequently, Lake Kivu, used for bathing and washing, was the only reliable source for drinking water. Acute PEM was estimated in 18–23% of children aged 6–59 months [29]. By August 12, more than 62,000 cases of acute watery diarrhea were reported to health facilities, and within a few weeks of arrival, more than 50,000 refugees died [188–190]. Diarrheal illness accounted for 85–90% of deaths recorded in the first month alone. Final estimates of the total number affected likely exceeded 200,000 [190].

Vibrio cholerae O1, biotype El Tor, serotype Ogawa was isolated as early as July 20 and reached a single day peak of 6,000 cases on July 26. Cholera attributed to 35,500 (57%) documented cases and approximately 58,000–80,000 total cases (attack rate: 7.3–16%), excluding asymptomatic infection [29]. Between July 31 and August 4, cases of bloody diarrhea surpassed watery diarrhea. Multidrug-resistant (including resistance to tetracycline and nalidixic acid) *Shigella dysenteriae* type 1 was isolated [190]. Cases of dysentery represented approximately 40% of all deaths in the Mugunga camp during the first month, and 15,543 cases occurred between August 8 and 14 [29]. The combined cholera and shigellosis CFR for the first month was between 19.5 and 31.2 per 10,000 per day, strikingly greater than the baseline 0.6 per 10,000 per day CFR in prewar Rwanda. The largest population of refugees in the Muganga camp experienced the highest reported CFR of 48% on a single day [29]. More than 10,000 of fatalities were among unaccompanied children. Unaccompanied infant CFR was 100–800 per 10,000 per day. Acute malnutrition was present in 36% of children with dysentery, compared with 12% of children without dysentery [29]. Survival during the outbreak was entirely dependent on adequate fluid resuscitation. At an Israeli Army field hospital medical center, recovery rates of 94–96% were achieved through vigorous fluid administration and, in the case of presumed *Shigella* infection, through antibiotics [188]. Yet even after international agencies responded, the CFR still exceeded 3–5%. One challenge was reaching patients in the community who did not seek medical care. Deaths occurring in the community represented 47% and were directly due to lack of fluid resuscitation [29, 188]. Institution of simple life-sustaining oral rehydration solutions and isotonic intravenous fluids for severe cases would have saved thousands of lives [79, 190].

Restoring disrupted water sanitations is necessary to prevent years of ongoing *V. cholerae* O1 transmission after massive outbreaks. During November 16–24, 1996, an unexpected repatriation was announced. Nearly 500,000 returnees from five camps north of Goma reentered Rwanda through Gisenyi. Health facilities equipped with ORS, IV hydration centers, high-energy protein biscuits, water stations, and latrines were established every 6 km. Médecins Sans Frontières (MSF) estimated that 15,675 returnees sought medical consultation along the journey. Of these individuals, 8,916 (57%) had watery diarrhea, almost half (49%) of whom were children under 5 years old. That attack rate was 25.4/1,000, and 47 deaths were recorded. Stool sampling showed a high percentage of *V. cholerae* O1, biotype El Tor, Inaba serotype [184].

Rehydration centers prevented a high CFR. Another outbreak struck 90,000 remaining refugees in April 1997, causing 1,521 deaths in three temporary camps between Kisangani and Ubundu, in the Congo Democratic Republic [164]. Stool specimens were positive for *V. cholerae* O1, biotype El Tor, serotypes Inaba and Ogawa [39, 164, 191].

In response to persistently high CFRs in the post-disaster IDPs, new recommendations have been made to increase the provision of water in outbreak settings to 50 l/person/day. A protected well per every 200 people and latrines built no less than 30 m from water sources with one latrine per every 20 people are minimal standards [140].

5.2.3.3 Migrating Populations

Global urbanization contributes to increased demands on municipal water supplies and sewage containment. Historically, the rapid influx of rural migrants into urban slums established the social stimulus for the sanitary revolution. Presently, poor rural migrants are entering overcrowded slums and peri-urban communities lacking basic water and sanitation infrastructure at increasing rates worldwide. By 2015, the proportion of the developing world's population living in cities will likely change from 42 to 48%, representing an increase of 675 million [10]. In 1940 in Peru, 25% of the population was urban and 65% was rural and agricultural; in 1990, 1 year prior to the cholera outbreak, this ratio was reversed to 70% urban and 30% rural. By the time of the outbreak, more than 50% of the urban population lived in shantytowns and lacked basic services [10]. Unfortunately, for cities such as Lima in 1990 and other megacities worldwide today, the voices of unmet water needs are less audible than in the North American and European cities of the late 1800s.

The burden of diarrheal illness among international travelers is also great [192]. One-quarter to one-half of travelers to low-income countries experience an episode of diarrhea while abroad [193]. With 935 million people crossing international borders every year, there is potential for infected travelers to spread enteric disease [194]. During outbreaks, asymptomatic individuals have a high likelihood of travel outside of the outbreak region [74]. Cruise lines are notorious for outbreaks of Norwalk virus [195]. The largest enteric airline outbreak was the aforementioned cholera outbreak on the 1992 Aerolineas Argentinas flight from Lima, Peru to Los Angeles [143]. Just months following the outbreak in Haiti, news media reported cholera in Caracas, Venezuela, presumptively introduced from travelers to a large wedding in the Dominican Republic serving contaminated lobster.

Large transient international migrations of human populations add further stress to water sanitation systems. In Touba, Sengal, approximately 200 km from Dakar, population growths have led to high risks of enteric outbreaks. The city has grown from 5,000 to around 700,000 since 1960. The area is widely popular due to the provision of free land and water in the sacred area. Consequently, many have settled without establishing water or sewage systems that are unaffordable for most. Private septic tanks that do exist are often situated dangerously close to water lines. For the majority of the year, the population manages to remain free of epidemics, but matters become much more complicated every year when the population swells to two million during the Magal pilgrimage. A severe diarrheal outbreak occurred in 2005 causing 1,500 cases and 16 deaths. *V. cholerae* was identified in shared open-air basins that were being used for religious purposes. Although controversial, given the religious importance of the basins, outbreaks have not recurred after implementing plastic water bottles and sachets for the mass influx [195]. Similar threats exist in the annual Saudi Arabia Hajj.

5.2.4 New Understandings in Cholera Dynamics

5.2.4.1 Environmental Factors: Lessons Learned from South America

V. cholerae shares an environmental niche with phytoplankton and crustaceans. This association has led some to explicate geographic and temporal patterns of cholera outbreaks. Phytoplankton and vibrios share ideal growth conditions: namely, increased sunlight and temperature. Several biological processes ensue. Decomposing algal plumes provide nutrient content for the bacteria, and concomitantly, the increased CO_2 content as a by-product of algal metabolism reduces the aquatic pH, thus facilitating growth. Additionally, increased toxin expression is found in association with algae over time [74]. This relationship has led to the possibility that ponds are the primary reservoir for human infections in Bangladesh [196]. In East Africa, communities living near lakes with high colonization of water hyacinth (*Eichornia crassipes*) have been identified as having increased risk for cholera outbreaks. *V. cholerae* has been grown from water hyacinth in freshwater sources in India and Bangladesh [197], and experimental introduction of hyacinth into water leads to a 300-fold increase in concentration of *V. cholerae* adherent to the hyacinth compared with the surrounding water free-form bacteria [198]. The Nyanza Province in Kenya reported 38% [24, 309] of cholera cases in Kenya between 1994 and 2008. The peak years of the epidemic, 1997–1999, were also associated with the greatest hyacinth coverage in the nearby Winam Gulf ($r=0.83$; $P=0.0010$). Also, no hyacinth was observed from early 2002 to 2005 which correlated with no cases of cholera [198]. Confounders such as mean temperatures in the region showed only minimal fluctuations, and neither annual cumulative rainfall nor annual mean daily rainfall were associated [198].

V. cholerae is commensally associated with copepods and is found concentrated on carapaces and in zooplankton alimentary tracts [73]. Copepods, which flourish when phytoplankton populations are dense, may be another explanation for the apparent relationship between cholera and hyacinth. *V. cholerae* contain chitinase, an enzyme necessary to breakdown chitin, the protective outer coating of copepods [73]. The abundance of these aquatic organisms is so great that chitin is second most abundant organic compound in the world. *V. cholerae* cells attach and detach from chitin based upon its concentration and have a predilection for the oral region of copepods and egg cases. In both laboratory microcosms and field studies, copepods and crustaceans enhance *V. cholerae* survival, including VBNC forms adherent to chitin particles [74]. The crustaceans may benefit from the osmoregulation due to CTX, suggesting an essential symbiotic relationship. This may explain the apparent decrease in cholera cases during the monsoon season in India between June and July. During this time, zooplankton populations decrease as the heavy rains dilute nutrients, and a decrease in cases of cholera follows. Phytoplankton and subsequent zooplankton blooms occur in August and September with a peak in copepod egg levels during this time, correlating well with the peak incidence of diarrhea in the region. In Matlab, Bangladesh, seasonal outbreaks can be predicted by increases in water temperature (lagged 4–8 weeks) and in copepod and cyanobacterial concentrations in local water bodies [75]. Copepod concentrations occur simultaneously with seasonal peaks [75]. Further evidence is suggested by the 50% reduction in cholera infections by filtering water through a sari cloth, which catches chitin particles greater than 20 μm and 99% of chitin-bound cholera but which is much too porous to remove free-living cholera bacteria [198].

Another important factor includes the wide climate variation in the past several decades, with resurgence in interest in the relationship between weather patterns and infections. Use of satellite imaging has demonstrated climate factors correlating with cholera outbreaks [199]. Satellite imaging of coastal Bangladesh in 1992, 1994, and 1995 showed a consistent bimodal cycle of sea surface temperature (SST) that had statistical correlation with cholera outbreaks. Sea surface height (SSH), with resultant encroachment of tidal waters to inland water river systems, appears to modulate the influence of SST. Anomalies with low SSH in 1993 were associated with an uncharacteristically low rate of cholera, despite typical SST fluctuations. The pattern is not always consistent, however. Temperature and rainfall also heavily influence availability of water. During the dry season of semiarid regions of Nigeria, there is an increased proportion of households collecting water from a source more than 1 km away (4–23%). The average household water consumption during that time falls from 38 to 18 l per day [199]. An associated doubling of diarrheal illnesses occurred during the dry season [10].

Global temperature fluctuations may also play an important role. Wide temperature shifts and increasing overall mean temperatures could shift the distribution of plankton species and subsequently, of cholera. Increased SSH could bring plankton blooms into more estuarine locations, increasing population of halophilic bacteria [74]. One unifying theory of the reemergence of cholera in Latin America in 1991 incorporates the El Niño Southern Oscillation (ENSO) and North Atlantic Oscillation (NAO). Oceanographic studies over the past several decades show circulation of ocean water occurs back and forth between Pacific and Indian Oceans [200]. The ENSO phenomenon originates every few years in December–January, offshore from Peru in the eastern equatorial Pacific. During this time, a layer of warm water suppresses otherwise cool waters, triggering changes in global weather patterns [74]. The phenomenon is reversed during La Niña, following resultant cooling in the same region. El Niño events and cholera outbreaks have been increasing since the

1970s, and in Peru and the Bay of Bengal, ENSO-driven anomalies appear to affect cholera dynamics [200, 201]. In 1991, an extreme ENSO event preceded the Peruvian outbreak, raising the possibility of oceanic spread of vibrio organisms over time, which may explain the genetic variability between the Latin American and Asiatic strains. The spread of warm Pacific coastal current northward from South America has been shown to transport organisms to the Gulf of California and even as far north as Oregon. Interconnected sea waters through avenues such as the Amazon basin are thought to have been the portal by which the Latin American strain was detected on north Atlantic shores and in the Gulf of Mexico [200].

Providing further support for theories that link the emergence of cholera to the environment rather than human migration in Latin America was the pattern of several simultaneous foci at the outset of the epidemic. Cases appeared almost simultaneously in three separate costal Peruvian communities: Chimbote, Lima, and Chancay. Within 6 weeks, Chancay had reported 65,198 cases of suspected cholera and 363 deaths [200]. Initially, massive contamination of sea water from excreta of cholera patients on ships from Asia was incriminated [202]. However, port logs from Chimbote, the first city attacked, revealed that only two ships arrived from places outside of Latin America in the days preceding the outbreak. Both had come from Hong Kong, and no cholera-like illness was reported on either ship, nor were any antitoxin antibodies found in blood samples from the crew [200]. Retrospective clinical chart reviews also suggested that illnesses compatible with the WHO definition of cholera may have first surfaced in Trujillo 15 months prior to the 1991 outbreak [202]. Supporting the presence of sporadic cholera cases prior to 1991, public health officials isolated *V. cholerae* O1 El Tor and non-O1 vibrios from the environment for over a decade prior to the outbreak. DNA probes between 1993 and 1995 in different environmental sites including sewer systems also demonstrated the presence of increasing *V. cholerae* populations prior to outbreaks and with a seasonal pattern [203]. From 1991 to 2000, cholera outbreaks continued to occur seasonally, with the largest occurring in the summer months (January–March). During the summer of 1998, outbreaks were strongly associated with rises in SST temporally associated with an El Niño event and concomitant increases in planktonic blooms [204]. An El Niño event prior to the 1991 epidemic could have similarly led to the substantial increases in *V. cholerae* populations in coastal Peru. Such an occurrence, rather than intercity spread, could explain the phenomenon of simultaneous outbreaks in multiple cities [202]. High unemployment rates and inflation likely also contributed to conditions favorable for secondary cholera transmission. Untreated contaminated water, inadequate hygiene, and poor sanitary handling of contaminated food were all risk factors for acquiring cholera [205].

The paradigm of cholera-climate interactions leading to the Latin American outbreak has implications for future outbreaks in otherwise non-endemic regions [201]. Both non-O1 and O1 strains exist ubiquitously all over the world, including North American Pacific, Atlantic, and Gulf Coasts; Australia; South East Asia; South Pacific islands; Africa; Asia; and throughout Europe [74]. *V. cholerae* is endemic along the US Gulf Coast and in Australia but rarely causes infection, except through rare incidents of ingestion of undercooked or raw shellfish [74]. In these regions,

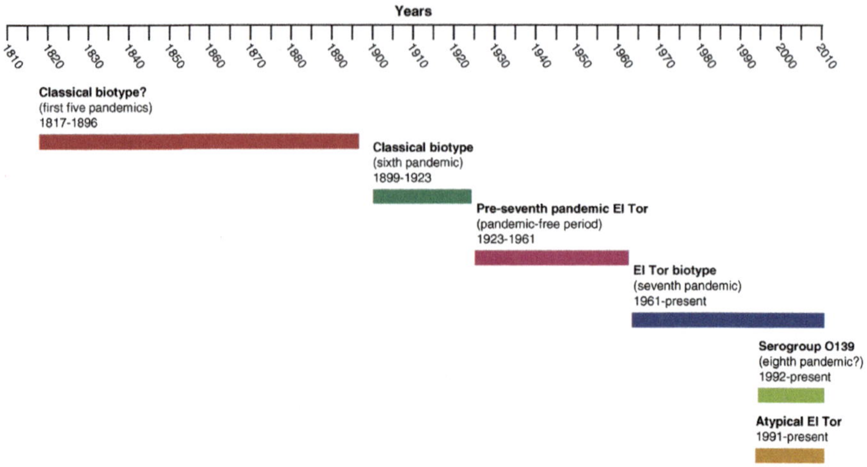

Fig. 5.10 Key evolutionary events in cholera epidemiology since 1817. The first five pandemics were caused by the classical biotype, whereas the classical strains appear to have caused the sixth pandemic. Between the sixth and seventh pandemics, there was an intervening period of 38 years during which cholera only occurred as local outbreaks caused by El Tor strains [20]. Reprinted with permission from WHO

planktonic associations are also recognized. In such cases, it is adequate water and sanitation systems, rather than the absence of pathogen in the environment, which mitigates secondary spread and thus prevents endemic patterns. The recognition of these environmental influences suggests that satellite imaging for SST and SSH could be potential future tools to predict when and where a cholera outbreak will occur [199, 206, 207].

5.2.4.2 Evolutionary Factors: Recent Trends in *V. cholera* O1 and O139 Molecular Epidemiology

The appearance of toxigenic potential in previously non-infectious strains (i.e., O139) and enhanced virulence of El Tor in the past two decades suggest that *V. cholerae* strains undergo more complicated environmental interactions than previously recognized (Fig.5.10). *V. cholera* species are differentiated serologically on the basis of the O antigen component of lipopolysaccharide (LPS). Of more than 200 serotypes, only the O1 and O139 serogroups cause major outbreaks [21]. Conversely, all other serogroups (non-O1/non-O139) are rarely toxigenic (<1%) and have almost negligible epidemic potential [20]. The O1 serogroup is further subdivided into two phenotypically different biotypes: classical, the cause of the first six pandemics; and El Tor, the cause of the current seventh pandemic [32]. Both biotypes may exist as one of three serotypes based on their nontoxigenic ABC antigens, Inaba (AC), Ogawa (AB), and Hikojima (ABC) [208]. Phenotypically, the classical biotype is more pathogenic, whereas the El Tor biotype is better suited for environmental survival [32]. Historically, the El Tor biotype has a lower symptomatic to asymptomatic ratio (1:30–1:101) and produces milder illness as compared with the classical biotype [138, 209]. There are several genotypic differences between the two biotypes contributing to their different clinical manifestations. Classical biotype has a more virulent toxin-producing *ctxB* gene. The *tcpA* (toxin-coregulated pilus) of the classical biotype confers enhanced colonization potential. Genetic sequencing of both the classical and El Tor strain has shown clustering of these and other essential virulence genes on a CTXϕ-encoded Vibrio pathogenicity island (VPI) [210].

Recently, the El Tor biotype has undergone unexpected changes in clinical disease pattern. Beginning in Matlab in the 1990s, rates of severe dehydration among hospitalized patients in Bangladesh with *V. cholera* O1 El Tor began increasing [211]. Ribotyping showed three new variants, Matlab I, II, and III, which later showed El Tor biotype profiles with acquisition of *tcpA* of the classical biotype in addition to other variations [211]. A comparison of an outbreak in southern Bangladesh occurring in 2006, however, showed severe dehydration, 78.8%, was significantly higher ($P<0.01$) than previous years (33.3% in 1998, 46.6% in 1999, 40% in 2000, and 41% in 2001) [212]. The El Tor biotype was confirmed in all biotypes, but ELISA demonstrated acquired ability to synthesize CTX of the classical biotype [212]. Subsequently, hybrid and altered El Tor strains (containing either both El Tor and classical *ctxB* or only classical *ctxB* subunits) have become increasingly common in Asia: Thailand in 2007, Orissa in 2007, and Malaysia in 2009 [38, 208, 213–216]. Variant El Tor strains have now entirely replaced prototypal El Tor in South Asia, and altered strains have also been documented in Mozambique [208, 214].

After appearing in Bangladesh in 1968, the El Tor biotype had almost completely replaced the classical biotype by 1973 [211]. In 1992, a non-O1 outbreak occurred, later that year identified as the O139 (Bengal) strain. Horizontal gene transfer of new LPS-biosynthesis encoding genes from a nontoxigenic vibrio into the El Tor biotype occurred in the environment [73, 100, 217–219]. This type of environmental serotype switching is likely common, given that under experimental conditions, the physiological state of cells, temperature, and salinity have been shown to induce conversion of *V. cholerae* non-O1 to O1 serotypes [87]. Though other isolated examples of non-O1 outbreaks had occurred previously, such as an O37 outbreak in Sudan in 1968, none had developed recurrent epidemic potential [211]. The O139 strain has continued to circulate, however, causing sporadic outbreaks in South Asia [220–222].

Similar to theories explaining the emergence of *V. cholerae* O139, horizontal gene transfer, in either environmental or human reservoirs, may explain the emergence of atypical El Tor variants. Whether El Tor biotypes acquired these changes from undetectable dormant classical biotypes in the VBNC state, free CTXϕ, or de novo mutations remains uncertain [20]. Multilocus gene analyses of *V. cholerae* O1 causing minor outbreaks, including the US Gulf Coast, Fijii, and Australia, show similarities with pre-seventh pandemic strains not present in the predominant El Tor [20, 223, 224]. Additionally, sequencing of the Peruvian *V. cholerae* O1 El Tor showed distinct VPI regions differentiating it from the prototypic strain [223].

This genetic diversity among El Tor biotypes, greater than previously appreciated, raises important questions regarding the potential for increasing virulence through acquisition of mobile genetic elements. One urgent threat would be the replacement of the 1990s South American strain, still present in the environment, with the newly introduced Haiti strain which has greater virulence and antimicrobial resistance determinants [177].

5.2.5 Therapeutic and Preventive Concerns

5.2.5.1 Therapy: Lessons Regarding Rehydration and Coordination

The ability of oral rehydration therapy (ORT), a simple salt-sugar-water cocktail, to counteract the morbidity and mortality of cholera and other diarrheal diseases is one of the greatest triumphs of the twentieth century [225]. Despite widespread diarrheal illness in the nineteenth-century industrializing world, it was not until the 1960s and 1970s that the lifesaving benefits of ORT and IV hydration were realized. The use of ORT and further nutritional modifications to rehydration therapy in low- and middle-income countries has led to dramatic declines in childhood mortality from diarrheal disease, especially in the first year of life [2]. Although simple to administer, ORT requires trained personnel, and the simple requirements of salt-sugar-water solution are not readily accessible.

The development of ORT is one of the first examples of orchestrated traditional practice, clinical observations, and scientific investigation. Documentation of rice water, coconut juice, and carrot soup for treatment can be found up to 3,000 years ago prescribed by the Indian physician Sushruta [226]. Thus, while cathartic purging and bloodletting were common treatment modalities during the first cholera pandemics in Europe, they were contentious when implemented in cholera outbreaks in India [227]. That profound losses of water and salt in cholera diarrhea led to dehydration, and eventual death was only first recognized in the mid-nineteenth century. Oral replacement of salt and water was considered to be insufficient, and O'Shaughnessy and Latta both proposed the use of intravenous water and salt replacement in 1831 and 1832, respectively [225, 228, 229]. When hypertonic intravenous fluids became common practice in 1906 [230], the CFR declined from 70 to 40%. Presently, isotonic intravenous fluids are preferred in severe cases, and either lactated Ringer's or normal saline may be used. No controlled studies of various IV solutions have been performed, but in the setting of potential critical hypokalemia, a saline-glucose-potassium regimen may have less consequences than lactated Ringer's since the bicarbonate component of the latter may cause further worsening of hypokalemia through intracellular shifts [188]. A change from lactated Ringer's to saline-glucose-potassium solution at an Israeli Army field hospital during the Goma outbreak seemed to decrease the rate of sudden death among patients receiving intravenous fluids [231]. Although intravenous fluids can rapidly restore circulating volume, the need to perform venipuncture is not without risk to patient and provider.

Additionally, the effect is rapidly lost when the fluids are not maintained. It was, therefore, not until an alternative more sustained rehydration therapy was implemented that significant mortality reductions were realized.

Physiologic research in the 1950s and 1960s first recognized the coupled intestinal transport of sodium with glucose in rodent models [232–234]. In 1960, demonstration of intact intestinal structure by histology and isotope studies dispelled beliefs that cholera was destructive to the mucosa [235]. During a cholera outbreak in Manila in 1961, Phillips and Wallace demonstrated that patients with cholera did not absorb orally administered sodium chloride, but when given with glucose, fluids were fully absorbed and sodium absorption was enhanced [236]. Concurrent studies in India confirmed the effectiveness of orogastrically administered glucose solutions [237]. Other studies later demonstrated the ability of ORT to reduce intravenous fluid requirements [238–240]. The effective oral administration of ORT without the need for an orogastric tube was important in demonstrating the feasibility of ORT in resource-limited rural settings [241]. When intravenous fluid supplies were exhausted in a Bangladeshi refugee camp of more than 350,000 people in 1972, Dr. Mahalanabis used ORT to treat more than 3,000 patients, dropping the CFR from 30 to 3.6%, thus definitively establishing the lifesaving role of ORT in outbreak settings [242]. Since official WHO endorsement of this solution in 1978 (WHO-ORS), an estimated 40 million deaths have been prevented worldwide [27, 122].

Despite its dramatic lifesaving capabilities, WHO-ORS does not dramatically reduce stool output, and, therefore, inexperienced practitioners, patients, and mothers of infected children may doubt its effectiveness, raising concerns for adequate treatment adherence [113]. Polyglucose (i.e., starch or rice)-based ORT have clinical benefits of reduced stool volumes, shorter duration of diarrhea, and lower ORS intake when compared with the standard WHO-ORS in adults and children with cholera [243]. Children and infants with acute non-cholera diarrhea also show a reduced rate of stool loss when compared with WHO-ORS [244]. Replacing the typical 20 g of glucose per liter solution with 50–80 g of rice has also shown reductions in potentially dangerous sodium concentrations due to the additional water requirements [245]. The rice-based solution may enhance sodium resorption by providing more glucose delivery through actions of brush-border disaccharidases without the high osmotic load of glucose monomer-based solutions. Moreover, mothers preferred rice-based ORS in one study [245]. For children with non-cholera diarrhea, early reintroduction of rice-based food can also reduce stool volume and duration of diarrhea when combined with traditional ORS [246].

The physiological basis for WHO-ORS in the treatment of cholera later paved the way for the discovery of its utility in other forms of childhood diarrhea. Molecular pathogenic differences between cholera toxin (which causes diarrhea with a fecal Na^+ concentration of ~90 mM) and rotavirus, one of the most common causes of acute watery diarrhea (which causes diarrhea with a fecal Na^+ concentration of ~40 mM), led to concerns that WHO-ORS could result in dangerous hypernatremia in children [227]. A meta-analysis examining treatment of non-cholera diarrhea in children showed equivalent efficacy between WHO-ORS (>310 mOsm/L) and a reduced-osmolar ORS (RO-ORS; 224 mOsm/L) with decreased stool volume and duration of diarrhea in the latter [227]. RO-ORS, therefore, has become the new preferred solution for the WHO and the Indian government [113]. There are concerns, however, of inducing hyponatremia in adults with cholera with RO-ORS, as most studies were underpowered to properly evaluate this risk [247]. A low-sodium rice-based ORS may be even more effective in reducing stool output than traditional ORS or RO-ORS [248].

Attempts to better utilize the colon's absorptive capacity to increase overall fluid resorption and consequently reduce stool output have included incorporation of amylase-resistant starches (RS) to ORS. Unlike rice and similar starches that are readily digested by amylase in the upper small intestine, when RS reaches the colon, it is metabolized by colonic bacteria into short-chain fatty acids (SCFA), which stimulate fluid and sodium absorption in the colon in a manner that is not inhibited by cAMP. Amylase-resistant maize starch enhances ORS efficacy for both cholera in adults and non-cholera diarrhea in children in the first 48 h of therapy but may necessitate delay in administering antibiotics [16, 249]. Similarly, green banana starch and pectin also showed more rapid resolution of diarrhea compared with rice-based ORS alone [250, 251]. Green bananas were also shown to increase percentage of clinical cure (from 67 to 85%) at day 5 when used as an adjunct against shigellosis [252]. RS-containing RO-ORS may become the next gold standard therapy for acute diarrhea if supported by more extensive efficacy studies [253].

While diarrhea mortality decreased dramatically after the implementation of ORS, the global diarrhea morbidity remains significant, with a stable or even increasing median number of diarrheal episodes per child per year [2]. While ORS saves lives lost to acute dehydration, it fails to remove the etiologic factors contributing to diarrheal illnesses or their long-term consequences. Thus, until water and sanitation are reality for all, interventions other than ORS are needed to fully address the ongoing enteric threats in low-income settings. Exclusive breast-feeding is beneficial for episodes of both acute watery diarrhea and early childhood diarrhea [108]. The protective benefits of calorie and antibody-rich breast milk are well known. In addition, antimicrobial breast milk proteins (i.e., lactoferrin and lysozyme), when added to rice-based ORS, reduced the duration of acute watery diarrhea and led to a greater percentage of formed stools in the first 48 h among Peruvian children [254]. A randomized clinical trial demonstrated improved growth in children receiving bovine lactoferrin supplementation [255]. This may be due in part to experimentally documented lactoferrin-induced decreased pathogenicity of a variety of enteric pathogens, including rotavirus, enterotoxigenic *E. coli, Shigella, Salmonella, Giaridia,* and *E. histolytica* [109].

Glutamine, a crucial source of enterocyte energy, has been demonstrated to regulate important processes of epithelial repair and barrier function [256, 257]. Experimental models of cholera, rotavirus, and cryptosporidiosis have demonstrated glutamine's capability to generate electrogenic sodium absorption [225]. A glutamine-containing ORS was well tolerated and equally effective as standard WHO-ORS in infants [258]. Unfortunately, clinical trials of glutamine [259], as well as other amino acids such as glycine [260, 261] and alanine, have failed to show significant additional benefit over ORS alone [262]. The heat-stable glutamine derivative, alanyl-glutamine, may hold more future potential promise. Lima AA et al.

demonstrated the potency of alanyl-glutamine to enhance intestinal water and electrolyte absorption compared with glutamine or glucose-only containing regimens [263]. Arginine, often deficient in malnourished patients, may also have intestinal reparative properties and has been shown to reduce the incidence of necrotizing enterocolitis in premature infants [113]. Recently, *ApoE4* was demonstrated to upregulate arginine-selective cationic amino acid transport, a phenomenon which may explain why this allele has cognitive protective effects in chronic diarrhea and malnutrition [117, 264]. Additionally, ongoing studies in Brazil suggest that APOE4 may potentially raise cholesterol among non-exclusively breastfed children receiving poor-fat diets, thus aiding recovery from early childhood infection and malnutrition [115].

Micronutrient deficiency is widespread in low-income countries, and adjunctive use offers several benefits [265]. Zinc supplementation in conjunction with ORS reduces acute diarrhea by 15–25% [266] and decreases the rate of prolonged diarrhea by 38–47% in various studies [267–269]. The particular mechanisms of zinc benefits remain uncertain, although it appears to enhance cellular immunity and maintain gut mucosal cell function [113]. Zinc supplementation also decreases duration of persistent diarrhea in children greater than 6 months of age [270, 271]. Zinc improves growth in malnourished children, though detrimental overdoses have occurred in the severely malnourished [265]. While having no effect on the duration of acute watery diarrhea, vitamin A supplementation in a pooled analysis of trials in Asia showed a reduction in persistent diarrhea of 55% [265]. Micronutrients, therefore, may play a role in cases of acute diarrhea, especially those that are "ORS-resistant" and more importantly, may help to reverse the vicious cycle of persistent diarrhea and malnutrition by reducing the risk of chronic diarrhea [225]. Currently, the WHO recommends zinc supplementation for children with acute or persistent diarrhea, though it is not yet integrated into any particular ORT [272].

ORT is most beneficial when given in appropriate amounts and before severe dehydration occurs, thus raising the importance of rapid detection of dehydrating diarrhea and rapid fluid administration. Analysis of deaths during the Zimbabwe outbreak showed not only high overall CFR but particularly worse conditions for people outside of health clinics [129]. An estimated CFR of 22–48% occurred among individuals treated outside of health clinics, representing 40% of all deaths. Many deaths occurred for want of simple ORT which, despite the government's efforts to encourage its use, remained unaffordable for most Zimbabweans [122]. In contrast, CFRs were just over 5% at health clinics, where rehydrating solutions were more accessible [136]. Following an increased response from the WHO, foreign governmental agencies, and nongovernmental organizations, a Cholera Command and Control Center was eventually established in Harare, and CFR began to fall to 0.8% by July 2009 [136].

Increased mortality with inadequate resuscitation, either due to lack of supplies or lack of understanding; withholding of treatment until laboratory confirmation of disease; and inadequately sized intravenous catheters are a recurring problem in many outbreaks [78, 142]. The benefit of a highly coordinated rehydration response was exemplified during the Goma outbreak. At one temporary treatment center in

Katindo, initial CFRs exceeded 14%, with 115 deaths among 790 cases. When international relief arrived, the CFR decreased dramatically in two days from 12 deaths in 399 cases (3.0%) to 3 deaths among 536 cases (CFR=0.6%) [190]. This dramatic change was possible when ICDDR-B relief workers implemented greater emphasis on rehydration with a screening section within the treatment center, intensive care, and most importantly, on rehydration maintenance centers where ORS was available [80]. In light of this dramatic example, the WHO now recommends quick identification of cholera treatment units (CTU) for severe dehydration and ORS stations with 24-h access in the community for mild to moderate dehydration [273].

Antibiotics may be helpful in severe cases of cholera and for dysentery [21]. Increasingly, cholera outbreaks in Africa demonstrate antibiotic-resistant strains [274] but resistance patterns vary between regions. Tetracycline sensitivity varies from 100% in Tanzania and Rwanda, 80–100% in Kenya and South Sudan, 65–90% in Somalia, to as low as 44% in Mogadishu [275]. Also, sensitivity to particular antibiotics can fluctuate rapidly. In Kenya and Somalia, sensitivity to chloramphenicol and co-trimoxazole decreased dramatically from 85% in 1994 to less than 10% in 1996 [275]. Antibiotic resistance testing at the onset and periodically throughout an outbreak is necessary. During the Goma outbreak, four million nalidixic acid tablets were distributed for intensive treatment of dysentery [80]. Mutant forms of both *S. dysenteriae* type 1 and *V. cholerae* resistant to nalidixic acid rapidly emerged. Due to the presence of preexisting tetracycline, trimethoprim-sulfamethoxazole, and aminopenicillin resistance among both species, the only effective agents were fluoroquinolones which were cost-restricted in Africa at that time [80, 276].

Despite their ability to improve severe cases and likely decrease shedding and epidemic propagation, the future role of antibiotics may become increasingly limited. Neither reactive nor preemptive mass chemoprophylaxis is a proven effective strategy. The time required for distribution of drug exceeds the rapidity of transmission, and the short-lived effect of the antibiotic is too short for the typical duration of pathogens persisting in the environment. While adjuvant antibiotic use as part of a campaign to decrease disease burden has been proposed, increasing reports of antibiotic resistance with decreasing fluoroquinolone activity are very concerning [71, 277]. Other preventive strategies such as vaccines have historically been discouraged by the WHO. This has been readdressed in light of frequent outbreaks during the past 5 years. In 2010, the WHO modified its recommendations that vaccines in the appropriate setting may be considered adjuvant options (Table 5.1) [37]. The challenges of vaccine implementation, including practical, pathogen, and biotechnology considerations, are explored in the next section.

5.2.5.2 Vaccination Strategies

Though the sanitary revolution had nearly negated the risk of autochthonous cholera and typhoid in industrializing nations, the ongoing threat of introduced pandemics, the need to protect travelers and military personnel, and the threat of ongoing epidemics stimulated interest in vaccine development. Only after advancements

Table 5.1 WHO cholera vaccination recommendations [37]

Situation	Target population	Delivery
Epidemic[a]	*Preemptive*: • May be considered by local health authorities to prevent potential outbreaks or spread of a current outbreak to new areas • Predictive risk-assessment tools need to be developed to determine when to use vaccine • Field test risk-assessment tools if available *Reactive*: • May be considered by local health authorities as an additional control • Conduct a thorough investigation of current and historical epidemiological situation • Identify clear geographic areas • Document and disseminate feasibility and impact of vaccination if used	*Administration*: • Conduct as quickly as possible • As many as possible, all eligible people (≥ 1 year (Schancholl®) and mORCVAX) or ≥2 years(Dukoral®), depending on the vaccine available) • Two doses
Endemic[b]	*High risk areas and populations*: • Preschool-aged and school-aged children • Other susceptible conditions such as pregnancy and HIV-infection • Older age groups if funding permits	*Administration*: Ages ≥6 years old: Dukoral®, two initial doses ≥7 days apart booster every second year if continued risk Children 2–5 years: Dukoral®, three initial doses ≥7 days apart followed by a 1 booster dose every 6 months • If any interval between doses exceeds recommended booster interval, revaccination with initial dose is recommended *Periodic mass vaccination campaigns*: • Schools, health-care facilities, religious institutions, other community settings • Incorporating cholera vaccination into routine vaccination schedules is an alternative or complementary strategy to mass vaccination

Information obtained from WHO Cholera Vaccine Recommendations, updated 2009 (WHO Publication 2010 [37])

[a]The mainstay of control measures should remain (1) providing appropriate treatment to people with cholera, (2) implementing interventions to improve water and sanitation, and (3) mobilizing communities

[b]Endemic is defined as the occurrence of fecal culture-confirmed cholera diarrhea in a population at least 3 of the past 5 years

were made in wealthier populations, however, did attention divert to include vaccination for highly endemic and impoverished regions. The struggles experienced in the development of an effective cholera vaccine and the ability to implement it in both endemic and epidemic settings exemplify the feasibility challenges of all enteric vaccines. The lengthy and expensive process of vaccine development often requires hundreds of millions of dollars and several decades to deliver a candidate vaccine from conception to use as a public health tool [113]. The inherent challenges encompass expert understandings of host-immune interactions, biotechnological feasibility, epidemiological behavior of the pathogen, public perception, and eventual marketing. Thus, there are only a few commercially available enteric vaccines: rotavirus, *V. cholerae* O1, and *S. typhi* [113].

The first-generation parental vaccines against cholera had limited efficacy and safety profiles [40]. Although an early trial of parenteral vaccine in Indonesia showed 88% efficacy among 1–4-year-old children for 6 months, protection rapidly declined to only 50% between 11 and 14 months postvaccination [278]. Older adults were even less protected, with immediate protection rates of 50–60%. The WHO did not recommend vaccines against cholera until a more sustained response could be achieved. Also during the 1970s, Jan Holmgren and colleagues at the University of Gothenburg in Sweden began early work on an oral vaccine, proposing the benefits of easier administration and more sustained immunity. Their product, Dukoral® (SBL Vaccines) was first licensed in 1991. The vaccine consisted of a formalin-killed whole-cell (WC) *V. cholerae* O1, plus cholera toxin B subunit (BS). Newer generations have substituted recombinant cholera toxin B (rBS-WC) for the native toxin [30]. Currently, Dukoral® includes heat-inactivated Inaba classic strain, formalin-inactivated Inaba El Tor, both heat- and formalin-inactivated Ogawa classic strain, and recombinant toxin B subunit [279]. It has a shelf life of 3 years at 2–8 °C and is stable at 37 °C for 1 month [37]. Field trials in Bangladesh and among Peruvian military personnel demonstrated efficacy at 6 months near 85% with WC-BS formulations and near 60% with the WC component alone [40, 280]. A 3-year follow-up in Bangladesh showed a persistent protective efficacy of 50% for BS-WC and 52% for WC alone. The rate of protection was similar for severe and non-severe cases. Adults had significantly more protection, 65%, compared with children aged 2–5, 25% [281]. Efficacy has been demonstrated in areas with high HIV prevalence. In Beira, Mozambique, Dukoral® showed 78% protection in short-term intention-to-vaccinate analysis, with 57% of participants completing two doses and 72% at least one dose. Among HIV-positive individuals, protection rates were 72% [282]. Though not a single case of cholera was confirmed, preemptive mass vaccination was shown to be feasible in Aceh, Indonesia, following the 2004 tsunami [283]. Reactive mass vaccination was successful in Mozambican refugee camps with endemic cholera [284] and during cholera epidemics in Uganda [285]. The WHO's current recommendations are outlined in Table 5.1 [37].

The second licensed vaccine, Shanchol® (Shantha Biotechnics Ltd., Hyderabad, AP, India), is a bivalent inactivated whole-cell vaccine licensed in India following clinical trials in Vietnam and Kolkata [38, 286]. Both *V. cholerae* O1 (modified immunizing strains from ORC-Vax (VABIOTECH, Hanoi, Vietnam) with increased

LPS content) and O139 are included, with documented stronger immunogenicity to O1 than O139 [287]. A double-blind, randomized, placebo-controlled trial demonstrated safety and immunogenicity among vaccinated individuals in Kolkata [288]. Among adults, 53% showed immunogenicity, and 80% of children vaccinated showed a greater than fourfold rise in serum *V. cholerae* O1 antibody titers. An interim analysis demonstrated 65% protection against clinically significant cholera for children at least 2 years after vaccination in an intention-to-vaccinate analysis [289].

CVD 103-HgR, Orochol®, was a single-dose, oral live attenuated vaccine derived from the classical Inaba 569B strain, which has a unique deletion of 94% of enzymatically active A-subunit with a residual B subunit [40]. It was proven safe and immunogenic in North America, Switzerland, Peru, Indonesia, and in HIV-positive individuals in Mali [40]. Efficacy, however, was poor among 67,000 subjects in Indonesia [40]. The vaccine has had a limited market due to concerns of its monovalent nature hindering protection against Ogawa-strain infection. Consequently, the oral formulation of this vaccine is no longer produced, and while still available, the injectable form is not widely recommended given its limited efficacy and short duration of protection [37].

Current approaches to improve efficacy involve not only strain diversity but also improvements in vaccine delivery. Epithelial cell adhesion and engulfment are necessary for an effective oral vaccine. Encasing the vaccine into lipid particles called outer membrane vesicles may facilitate greater uptake of antigen and improve immunogenicity. Use of this strategy for *Salmonella typhi* and *N. meningitidis* serogroup B (not present in the current parenteral *N. meningitidis* vaccine) has shown immunogenicity of innate and adaptive immune response in mice and safety with immunogenicity in humans [30]. Vaccine efficacy may also be improved with zinc supplementation [290]. Maternal immunoglobulin in breast milk may neutralize the vaccine rendering it immunologically inert, and, therefore, withholding breastfeeding for 3 h prior to vaccination of young children may improve efficacy [290]. Finally, various oral polio, rotavirus, and cholera vaccines have been less immunogenic when given to disadvantaged populations in low-income countries than in more affluent test populations. It is likely that a combination of factors, including environmental enteropathy, malnutrition, helminthic infestation, and bacterial overgrowth, play a role in reducing vaccine immunogenicity in endemic populations [113].

The biotechnological challenges of immunogenicity and serotype variability are only one component in actualizing a successful enteric vaccination strategy [27]. Despite the dramatic improvements of the oral vaccines over first-generation parenteral vaccines, proper adherence to the full vaccination series is necessary to confer adequate immunogenicity, and this remains a barrier to implementation in public health programs. The oral vaccines require a two-dose regimen, administered greater than 10 days apart for adults, and three doses for children 2–6 years old [40]. Two other oral vaccines with potentially easier administration are undergoing Phase II–III development: Peru-15 (CholeraGarde) [291] and *V. cholerae* 638 [292]. Peru-15, developed at Harvard University, is a live attenuated Inaba strain with deletions of ctx A and rtx A genes rendering it nontoxigenic, nonmotile, and non-recombinational [293, 294]. It is given as a single dose with safety proven both among healthy volunteers in the United States [295, 296] as well as adults and children from Bangladesh [292]. *V. cholerae* 638 is derived from an Ogawa strain with results showing immunogenicity in Cuban volunteers [297, 298]. Other vaccines, CVD 11 (Ogawa), VA1.3 (Inaba/Ogawa), IEM 108 (Ogawa), CVD 112 (O139), and Bengal-15 (O139) are in early development stages [40, 299].

A cost-benefit ratio analysis of vaccine global implementation is difficult to gauge given that millions of at-risk populations have ongoing exposure and the half-life of protection from available vaccines is relatively poor. Mass production and distribution costs are also prohibitive, especially considering that targeted at-risk populations are among the world's poorest. Also, some argue competing markets, such as the use of Dukoral® for traveler's diarrhea [300], limit vaccine availability for less privileged populations. In Vietnam, an attempt to circumvent dependence on international suppliers was made by instituting a mass vaccination campaign with a locally produced vaccine. Since the mid-1980s, the Company for Vaccine and Biological Production No. 1 in Hanoi (VABIOTECH) has produced several versions of the vaccine at a cost of US$ 0.10–0.40 per dose [300, 301]. An open-labeled, non-randomized trial of a two-dose regimen of an oral whole-cell vaccine against *V. cholerae* O1 without placebo control in Hue conferred 66% protective efficacy during an outbreak of El Tor Ogawa in the early 1990s [302]. At that time, cholera was endemic in 35 of the country's 45 provinces. During the outbreak and for 8–10 months thereafter, protection against hospitalization for cholera was 60% (95% CI=40–73, $P<0.001$), which increased slightly to 66% for those who completed both doses across all vaccinated age groups [302]. After the emergence of the O139 serotype, killed O139 was safely added to the vaccine [303]. A large-scale efficacy trial of mass vaccination campaign between 1998 and 2000 reached 75–80% of the targeted population and costs US $0.91 per fully vaccinated person. Vaccine costs represented 75% of the total immunization campaign costs [301, 304]. Passive surveillance from 1998 to 2000 showed no substantial amount of cholera, and intensive surveillance was stopped [301]. Over the next 5 years, approximately 77% of the city's 286,639 eligible population was fully immunized [301]. Unexpectedly, an outbreak of 323 cases of severe diarrhea due to *V. cholerae* O1, El Tor, Inaba occurred in 2003. A small case-control study showed vaccination in 1998 or 2000 afforded a 50% protection rate (95% CI=9–63%; $P=0.0235$) [301]. There was no demonstrable protection against non-cholera diarrhea. The most significant finding was that, of patients with cholera, only 43% had appropriate sanitation [301]. In 2007–2008, an outbreak caused by an altered *V. cholerae* O1 El Tor producing classical cholera toxin B occurred in northern Vietnam, causing 3,271 cases [305].

Controversy exists regarding the appropriate utilization of cholera vaccines in other endemic regions. A mathematical model based on oral cholera vaccine efficacy rates and transmission patterns in Matlab, Bangladesh, suggested that if biennial vaccine coverage rates exceeded 50–70%, cholera could be reduced to an annual incidence rate of less than 1 per 1,000 in endemic areas [306]. Some argue, however, that to implement a costly vaccine may not have sustained compliance or benefit if basic measures such as improved water and hand hygiene practices are not met [307]. Currently available cholera vaccines have practical limitations as well, prohibiting incorporation into immunization campaigns [40]. The coordination of vaccine administration following complex emergencies is especially challenging. Infection, especially during secondary transmission of hyperinfective vibrios, is extremely rapid. In Malawi, for example, 52% of Mozambican refugees admitted for intravenous treatment presented within 16 days of arrival to camp [163]. Additionally, while cost-benefit analyses in endemic settings suggest a low cost for mass vaccine campaigns, following the 2004 earthquake-tsunami in Aceh, Indonesia, the cost of vaccine distribution alone was 8 USD per person.

Long-term efficacy of enteric vaccines efficacy is limited given that neither vaccine-derived immunogenicity nor natural infection confers complete serotype crossover protection for *V. cholerae* O1, *Shigella spp.*, or toxigenic *E. coli* [113, 306]. Despite the exposure of the majority of Rwandan refugees to *V. cholerae* O1 Ogawa serotype in the Goma disaster, for example, a second outbreak (this time an Inaba strain) occurred only 2 years later [308]. Concomitant circulating vibrio strains led to an Ogawa cholera outbreak just 6 months after an Inaba outbreak in Orissa [101, 309]. Novel serotypes, genetic variants, and serotype switching from the previously predominant strain has been concurrent during non-cholera enteric epidemics as well [252]. During an outbreak of *S. flexneri* (serotype X variant isolate, 200217) in China, a new variant rapidly expanded in eight of eleven provinces and underwent multiple serotype switching events [310]. Contrarily, the heat-labile toxin of ETEC shares approximately 80% homology with CTX [279], and Dukoral® has shown 67% efficacy in patients known to have had infection with ETEC [311].

Given that Dukoral® has a modest benefit against even non-cholera acute watery diarrhea, some argue that more widespread vaccination could also reduce inappropriate antibiotic use by a total reduction in the attack rates of outbreaks. Proponents of this argument cite the widespread misuse of antibiotics and emerging resistance among Enterobacteriaceae. In Africa, cholera epidemics are frequently initiated by antibiotic-resistant strains, and inappropriate use of prophylactic antibiotics is widespread [274]. Antibiotic resistance patterns of *V. cholerae* in eastern Africa are varied between countries [275]. Other enteric outbreaks in Africa also show high rates of antibiotic resistance. During the multi-enteric outbreak among the Ethiopian refugee population fleeing drought in 1984, there was a high rate (53%) of multidrug resistance among many tested Enterobacteriaceae. Among *E. coli* strains, 53% were resistant to ampicillin, 47% to chloramphenicol, 30% to co-trimoxazole, and 67% to tetracycline. Of 7 *Shigella* strains, three were resistant to chloramphenicol and four were resistant to tetracycline [312]. *S. dysenteriae* type 1 and *V. cholerae* isolates from the Goma outbreak showed multidrug resistance to tetracyclines, aminopenicillins, and trimethoprim-sulfamethoxazole [79, 276].

The legacy of *V. cholerae* vaccines is only a glimpse of the obstacles facing global vaccine coverage for enteric infections. Since the early 1990s, the WHO has prioritized vaccine development for rotavirus, ETEC, *Shigella* (*S. dysenteriae* 1), *V. cholerae* O1, and *S. typhi* [313]. While rotavirus vaccines RotaTeq (Merck) and Rotarix (GlaxoSmithKline) have dramatically reduced infant rotaviral infections in high- and middle-income countries, field trials in resource-limited areas of Asia and Africa are only now under way [113]. Typhoid vaccine (Ty21a attenuated live oral vaccine and purified Vi capsular polysaccharide parenteral vaccine) efficacy in resource-poor settings is less than in the case of its more common use among travelers [314]. One exception has been the typhoid Vi conjugate vaccine (Vi-rEPA) which has been shown to give effective protection, even in young children as was demonstrated in Vietnam [315]. Yet despite advocacy for use of typhoid during epidemics or as an adjunct to improved sanitation, the waning protection provided over time and the emergence of *S. paratyphi* (not covered by the current vaccines) have unmasked significant holes in typhoid vaccine coverage for endemic populations [316, 317]. Global coverage for *Shigella* spp. would need to protect against 16 (of 50) epidemiologically important serotypes [16]. Current *Shigella* vaccines, at best, incorporate a pentavalent mix of five serotypes: *S. dysenteriae* 1, *S. sonnei*, *S. flexneri* 2a, *S. flexneri* 3a, and *S. flexneri* 6 [16, 113]. Vaccines against ETEC must aim to induce immunity to a variety of common ETEC fimbrial colonization factor antigens (CFA) together as well as neutralization of LT-toxin [113]. Other enterics receiving attention for vaccine development include pathogenic noroviruses, *C. jejuni*, *Clostridium difficile*, EPEC, *E. histolytica*, *Cryptosporidium* spp., EAEC, and *Salmonella* Paratyphi A and B [113]. While promising when effective, vaccines alone cannot overcome the vast array of organisms transmissible when basic water and sanitation are lacking.

5.3 In the Wake of Cholera: Enteric Infections and Malnutrition and Childhood Cognitive Development

Through the lens of publicly feared epidemics such as cholera, we begin to appreciate the hazardous conditions faced by the majority of the world's population living in conditions of inadequate water and sanitation (Fig. 5.11) [10]. The rapid demise of some of these afflicted persons and the extensive epidemics following disasters periodically headline newspapers and media sites worldwide. While resources from high-income benefactors flow in response to media pleas, a more silent scourge looms. Cholera represents but the "tip of the iceberg" of the huge, largely underappreciated personal and societal costs of repeated enteric infections in early childhood and their long-term effects on growth stunting and impaired cognitive development [11]. These, too, are the direct result of inadequate water and sanitation that still plague billions of people around the world. Although oral rehydration therapy is lifesaving for acute watery diarrhea and dehydration, since the sanitary revolution has yet to reach 42% of the world's population [4], prolonged or persistent intestinal infections and their staggering morbidity continue unabated [2]. In low-income countries, children under 5 years of age experience a median of 3.2 episodes of diarrhea per child-year [2]. Disease-adjusted life years (DALYs) due to diarrheal disease rank second among global burden of disease after respiratory illnesses. In addition to nearly 1.8 million child deaths each year (4,500 deaths per day) as a result of diarrhea [4], the burden of infectious diarrhea is a staggering 72 million (4.8%) DALYs [1]. Moreover, this burden does not fully account for the

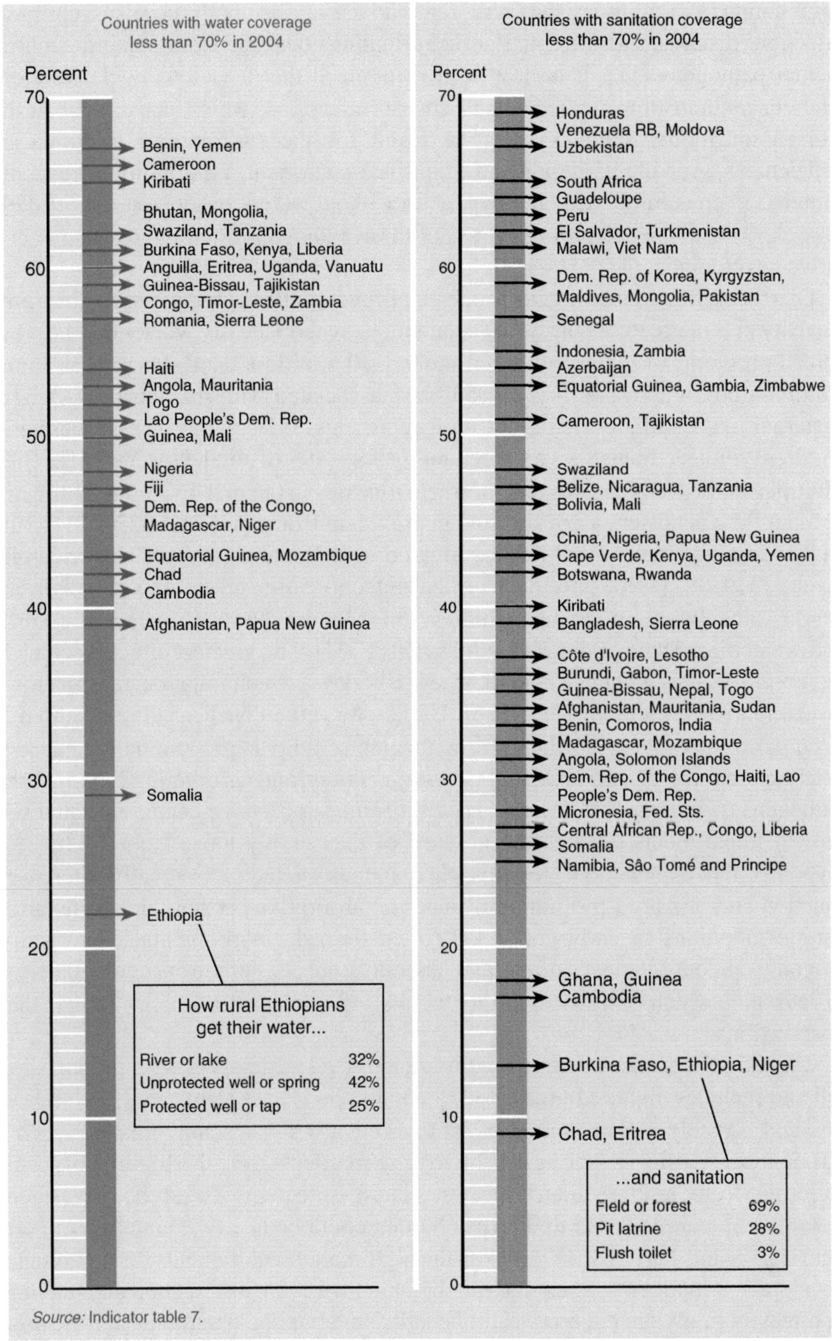

Fig. 5.11 Countries with water and sanitation coverage less than 70% [10]. Reprinted with permission from WHO

large numbers of malnourished children who are at once both more susceptible to infectious diseases and suffer the further crippling consequences of enteric environmental pathogens [11]. It is now well recognized that a vicious cycle develops, wherein malnutrition predisposes to enteric infections, which conversely further worsen nutritional status [318]. The result for the survivors is micronutrient deficiencies, growth retardation and cognitive impairment, a morbidity infrequently captured in epidemiological surveys. Even without watery or loose stools, children may experience the deleterious effects of these pathogens on both growth and cognitive development [11, 319–329].

Diarrheal illness impairs gastrointestinal function through decreased absorptive capacity and ineffective nutritional acquisition, synergistically worsening the widespread problems of malnutrition. Of the 9.7–10.6 million deaths each year among children under the age of 5 years, 53% are associated with malnutrition [2, 318]. Maternal and childhood undernutrition represents 35% of the disease burden in children younger than 5 years, accounting for 11% of total DALYs [318, 330]. Multiple studies have shown that diarrheal illnesses in the first 1–2 years of life may account for a persistent 4-cm shortfall in growth in Brazil [11, 318, 323–325]. Other studies in Guatemala, West Africa, Mexico, and Bangladesh have shown similar results [319–322]. Not only do diarrheal infections impair childhood weight and height gains, but malnourished children suffer longer duration, increased severity, and greater incidence of diarrheal illness [318, 331]. The greatest effect is seen with recurrent illnesses and persistent diarrhea (>14 days) which impair catch-up growth in malnourished children [113, 326]. Unlike the acute diarrheal illness caused by *V. cholerae*, persistent diarrhea in low-income settings is predominately cause by enteroaggregative *E. coli* (EAEC), *Cryptosporidium*, and *Giardia* [332–335]. These pathogens (primarily EAEC and *Cryptosporidium spp.*) have been associated with growth impairments even in the absence of measurably loose stools [336–338]. Hypothesized explanations for this phenomenon include chronically altered gut function and impaired restoration of mucosal absorptive capacity due to recurring enteric infections in early childhood (often termed environmental enteropathy). Ongoing epidemiological surveys and laboratory corollaries are currently underway to determine which host susceptibility factors and mechanistic biology explain these observations.

The range of consequences from this vicious cycle extends beyond growth shortfall and includes impaired fitness [327], cognition [11, 328], fluency [329], schooling, and possibly malabsorption of drugs necessary for systemic diseases such as AIDS, tuberculosis, and malaria. The long-term effects over the lifetime of a child suffering from both malnutrition and enteric infections could be devastating. Cognitive impairment due to diarrhea burden could be nearly 10 intelligence quotient (IQ) points [11, 318, 339]. Given the high energy requirements for neurological development in the first 5 years of life, breaking the cycle of infection and malnutrition may not only have direct health benefits but could be paramount for the populace of low-income countries struggling to compete in a global economy. Indeed, the differences between national IQs may correlate best with the intensity of infectious diseases [340]. A working model of the vicious cycle of poverty and poor sanitation,

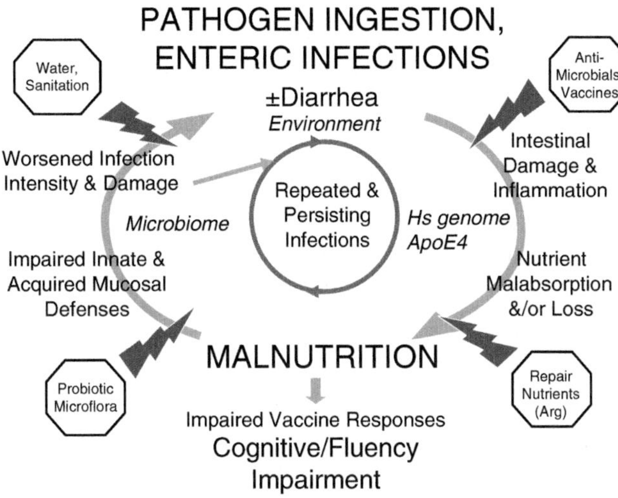

Fig. 5.12 The vicious cycle between malnutrition and diarrhea [RL Guerrant, LA Bartelt]. Reprinted with permission from WHO

leading to enteric infections, intestinal damage, malnutrition, and ultimately, cognitive and fitness impairment, is depicted in Fig. 5.12 [318].

Enteric outbreaks, therefore, test not only our ability to aggressively halt rapidly spreading disease and its horrific potential for loss of lives. When they occur, these epidemics also challenge us to recognize the underlying structural inequalities that render populations increasingly vulnerable to affliction. Careful observations have highlighted that epidemics such as cholera are just one of the many consequences of ongoing enteropathogen transmission that will continue to plague at-risk communities until sustainable water-sanitation-hygiene infrastructures are secured.

References

1. Mathers C, Boerma T, Ma Fat D (2008) The global burden of disease: 2004 update. World Health Organization, Geneva
2. Kosek M, Bern C, Guerrant RL (2003) The global burden of diarrhoeal disease, as estimated from studies published between 1992 and 2000. Bull World Health Organ 81:197–206
3. Prüss A, Kay D, Fewtrell L, Bartram J (2002) Estimating the burden of disease from water, sanitation, and hygiene at a global level. Environ Health Perspect 110:537–542
4. Mara DD (2003) Water, sanitation and hygiene for the health of developing nations. Public Health 117:452–456
5. Yoder JS, Hlavsa MC, Craun GF, Hill V, Roberts V, Yu PA et al (2008) Surveillance for waterborne disease and outbreaks associated with recreational water use and other aquatic facility-associated health events–United States, 2005–2006. MMWR Surveill Summ 57:1–29
6. Yoder J, Roberts V, Craun GF, Hill V, Hicks LA, Alexander NT et al (2008) Surveillance for waterborne disease and outbreaks associated with drinking water and water not intended for drinking–United States, 2005–2006. MMWR Surveill Summ 57:39

7. Centers for Disease Control and Prevention (CDC) (2010) Cholera outbreak – Haiti, October 2010. MMWR Morb Mortal Wkly Rep 59:1411
8. Centers for Disease Control and Prevention (CDC) (2010) Update on cholera – Haiti, Dominican Republic, and Florida, 2010. MMWR Morb Mortal Wkly Rep 59:1637–1641
9. Bhattacharya SK (1994) History of development of oral rehydration therapy. Indian J Public Health 38:39–43
10. Watkins K (2006) Human Development Report 2006. Beyond scarcity: power, poverty and the global water crisis. United Nations Development Project, New York
11. Guerrant R, Kosek M, Lima A, Lorntz B, Guyatt H (2002) Updating the DALYs for diarrhoeal disease. Trends Parasitol 18:191–193
12. Pawlowski S, Warren C, Guerrant R (2009) Diagnosis and treatment of acute or persistent diarrhea. Gastroenterology 136:1874–1886
13. Leclerc H, Schwartzbrod L, Dei-Cas E (2002) Microbial agents associated with waterborne diseases. Crit Rev Microbiol 28:371–409
14. Pegues M (2009) Salmonella species, including *Salmonella typhi.* In: Mandell GL (ed) Mandell, Douglas, and Bennett's principles and practice of infectious diseases, 7th edn. Elsevier, Churchill Livingstone, Orlando
15. Seas C, Gotuzzo G (2009) *Vibrio cholerae.* In: Mandell GL (ed) Mandell, Douglas, and Bennett's principles and practice of infectious diseases, 7th edn. Elsevier, Churchill Livingstone, Orlando
16. Guerrant R, Steiner T, Lima A, Bobak D (1999) How intestinal bacteria cause disease. J Infect Dis 179(Suppl 2):S331–S337
17. Debellis L, Diana A, Arcidiacono D, Fiorotto R, Portincasa P, Altomare DF et al (2009) The *Vibrio cholerae* cytolysin promotes chloride secretion from intact human intestinal mucosa. PLoS One 4:e5074
18. Sack DA, Sack RB, Nair GB, Siddique AK (2004) Cholera. Lancet 363(9404):223–233
19. Shinoda S, Nakagawa T, Hirakawa N, Miyoshi S, Arakawa E, Ramamurthy T et al (2008) Molecular epidemiological studies of *Vibrio cholerae* in Bengal region. Biocontrol Sci 13:1–8
20. Safa A, Nair GB, Kong RY (2010) Evolution of new variants of *Vibrio cholerae* O1. Trends Microbiol 18:46–54
21. Nelson EJ, Harris JB, Morris JG, Calderwood SB, Camilli A (2009) Cholera transmission: the host, pathogen and bacteriophage dynamic. Nat Rev Microbiol 7:693–702
22. Childers B, Klose K (2007) Regulation of virulence in *Vibrio cholerae*: The *toxr* regulon. Future Microbiol 2:335–344
23. Levine M, Gotuzzo E, Sow S (2005) Cholera infections. In: Guerrant RL, Walker DH, Weller PF (eds) Tropical infectious diseases, 2nd edn. Elsevier, Churchill Livingstone, Philadelphia, pp 273–282
24. Pan American Health Organization (1992) The economic impact of the cholera epidemic, Peru, 1991. Epidemiol Bull 13:9–11
25. Sack RB, Siddique AK, Longini IM, Nizam A, Yunus M, Islam MS et al (2003) A 4-year study of the epidemiology of *Vibrio cholerae* in four rural areas of Bangladesh. J Infect Dis 187:96–102
26. Gaffga NH, Tauxe RV, Mintz ED (2007) Cholera: a new homeland in Africa? Am J Trop Med Hyg 77:705–713
27. Mintz ED, Guerrant RL (2009) A lion in our village–the unconscionable tragedy of cholera in Africa. N Engl J Med 360:1060–1063
28. Chan EY, Kim JJ (2010) Characteristics and health outcomes of internally displaced population in unofficial rural self-settled camps after the 2005 Kashmir, Pakistan earthquake. Eur J Emerg Med 17:136–141
29. Public health impact of Rwandan refugee crisis (1995) What happened in Goma, Zaire, in July, 1994? Goma epidemiology group. Lancet 345:339–344
30. Ryan ET (2011) The cholera pandemic, still with us after half a century: time to rethink. PLoS Negl Trop Dis 5:e1003

31. World Health Organization (2010) Cholera, 2009. Wkly Epidemiol Rec 85:293–310
32. Goel AK, Jiang SC (2010) Genetic determinants of virulence, antibiogram and altered biotype among the *Vibrio cholerae* O1 isolates from different cholera outbreaks in India. Infect Genet Evol 10:815–819
33. Morris JG (2003) Cholera and other types of vibriosis: a story of human pandemics and oysters on the half shell. Clin Infect Dis 37:272–280
34. Zuckerman JN, Rombo L, Fisch A (2007) The true burden and risk of cholera: implications for prevention and control. Lancet Infect Dis 7:521–530
35. Sack DA, Sack RB, Chaignat CL (2006) Getting serious about cholera. N Engl J Med 355:649–651
36. Sur D, Deen JL, Manna B, Niyogi SK, Deb AK, Kanungo S et al (2005) The burden of cholera in the slums of Kolkata, India: data from a prospective, community based study. Arch Dis Child 90:1175–1181
37. World Health Organization (2010) Cholera vaccines: WHO position paper. Wkly Epidemiol Rec 85:117–128
38. Kanungo S, Sah BK, Lopez AL, Sung JS, Paisley AM, Sur D et al (2010) Cholera in India: an analysis of reports, 1997–2006. Bull World Health Organ 88:185–191
39. Griffith DC, Kelly-Hope LA, Miller MA (2006) Review of reported cholera outbreaks worldwide, 1995–2005. Am J Trop Med Hyg 75:973–977
40. Lopez AL, Clemens JD, Deen J, Jodar L (2008) Cholera vaccines for the developing world. Hum Vaccin 4:165–169
41. Lanata CF, Mendoza W, Black RE (2002) Improving diarrhoea estimates. World Health Organization, Geneva
42. Schaetti C, Hutubessy R, Ali SM, Pach A, Weiss MG, Chaignat CL, Khatib AM (2009) Oral cholera vaccine use in Zanzibar: socioeconomic and behavioural features affecting demand and acceptance. BMC Public Health 9:100
43. Mukherjee P, Ghosh S, Ramamurthy T, Bhattacharya MK, Nandy RK, Takeda Y et al (2010) Evaluation of a rapid immunochromatographic dipstick kit for diagnosis of cholera emphasizes its outbreak utility. Jpn J Infect Dis 63:234–238
44. Lam C, Octavia S, Reeves P, Wang L, Lan R (2010) Evolution of seventh cholera pandemic and origin of 1991 epidemic, Latin America. Emerg Infect Dis 16:1130–1132
45. Scrascia M, Pugliese N, Maimone F, Mohamud KA, Grimont PA, Materu SF, Pazzani C (2009) Clonal relationship among *Vibrio cholerae* O1 El Tor strains isolated in Somalia. Int J Med Microbiol 299:203–207
46. Moszynski P (2006) Angolan cholera epidemic could have been prevented says, MSF. BMJ 332:1235
47. Dao S, Konaté I, Oumar AA, Sacko M, Maiga I, Toure K et al (2009) Cholera epidemics in Mali between 1995 and 2004. Sante Publique 21:263–269
48. Luque Fernández MA, Bauernfeind A, Jiménez JD, Gil CL, El Omeiri N, Guibert DH (2009) Influence of temperature and rainfall on the evolution of cholera epidemics in Lusaka, Zambia, 2003–2006: analysis of a time series. Trans R Soc Trop Med Hyg 103:137–143
49. Sasaki S, Suzuki H, Igarashi K, Tambatamba B, Mulenga P (2008) Spatial analysis of risk factor of cholera outbreak for 2003–2004 in a peri-urban area of Lusaka, Zambia. Am J Trop Med Hyg 79:414–421
50. Harris JR, Cavallaro EC, de Nóbrega AA, Dos S, Barrado JC, Bopp C, Parsons MB et al (2009) Field evaluation of crystal VC rapid dipstick test for cholera during a cholera outbreak in Guinea-Bissau. Trop Med Int Health 14:1117–1121
51. Zarocostas J (2005) Cholera outbreaks in West Africa kill more than 700. BMJ 331:800
52. Gunnlaugsson G, Angulo FJ, Einarsdóttir J, Passa A, Tauxe RV (2000) Epidemic cholera in Guinea-Bissthe challenge of preventing deaths in rural west Africa. Int J Infect Dis 4:8–13
53. Mugoya I, Kariuki S, Galgalo T, Njuguna C, Omollo J, Njoroge J et al (2008) Rapid spread of *Vibrio cholerae* O1 throughout Kenya, 2005. Am J Trop Med Hyg 78:527–533
54. Scrascia M, Maimone F, Mohamud KA, Materu SF, Grimont F, Grimont PA, Pazzani C (2006) Clonal relationship among *Vibrio cholerae* O1 El Tor strains causing the largest cholera epidemic in Kenya in the late 1990s. J Clin Microbiol 44:3401–3404

55. Urassa WK, Mhando YB, Mhalu FS, Mjonga SJ (2000) Antimicrobial susceptibility pattern of *Vibrio cholerae* O1 strains during two cholera outbreaks in Dar es Salaam, Tanzania. East Afr Med J 77:350–353
56. Smith AM, Keddy KH, De Wee L (2008) Characterization of cholera outbreak isolates from Namibia, December 2006 to February 2007. Epidemiol Infect 136:1207–1209
57. Osei FB, Duker AA (2008) Spatial and demographic patterns of cholera in Ashanti region – Ghana. Int J Health Geogr 7:44
58. Sidley P (2001) Cholera sweeps through South African province. BMJ 322:71
59. Mendelsohn J, Dawson T (2008) Climate and cholera in Kwazulu-Natal, South Africa: the role of environmental factors and implications for epidemic preparedness. Int J Hyg Environ Health 211:156–162
60. Manga NM, Ndour CT, Diop SA, Dia NM, Ka-Sall R, Diop BM et al (2008) Cholera in Senegal from 2004 to 2006: lessons learned from successive outbreaks. Med Trop (Mars) 68:589–592
61. Moszynski P (2006) Cholera outbreak in Darfur is made worse by advent of rains. BMJ 332:1472
62. Moszynski P (2006) Floods wreak havoc in East Africa. BMJ 333:464
63. Noeske J, Guévart E, Kuaban C, Solle J, Fonkoua MC, Mouangue A, Fouda AB (2006) Routine use of antimicrobial drugs during the 2004 cholera epidemic in Douala, Cameroon. East Afr Med J 83:596–601
64. Hutin Y, Luby S, Paquet C (2003) A large cholera outbreak in Kano City, Nigeria: the importance of hand washing with soap and the danger of street-vended water. J Water Health 1:45–52
65. Wendo C (2003) Cholera spreads in Liberia. Lancet 362:966
66. Centers for Disease Control and Prevention (2003) Cholera epidemic after increased civil conflict–Monrovia, Liberia, June–September 2003. MMWR Morb Mortal Wkly Rep 52:1093–1095
67. Kondo H, Seo N, Yasuda T, Hasizume M, Koido Y, Ninomiya N, Yamamoto Y (2002) Post-flood–infectious diseases in Mozambique. Prehosp Disaster Med 17:126–133
68. Naidoo A, Patric K (2002) Cholera: a continuous epidemic in Africa. J R Soc Promot Health 122:89–94
69. Legros D, McCormick M, Mugero C, Skinnider M, Bek'Obita DD, Okware SI (2000) Epidemiology of cholera outbreak in Kampala, Uganda. East Afr Med J 77:347–349
70. World Health Organization (2010) Water and sanitation in health emergencies: the role of WHO in the response to the earthquake in Haiti, 12 January 2010. Wkly Epidemiol Rec 85:349–354
71. Andrews JR, Basu S (2011) Transmission dynamics and control of cholera in Haiti: an epidemic model. Lancet 377:1248–1255
72. Ali A, Chen Y, Johnson JA, Redden E, Mayette Y et al (2011) Recent clonal origin of cholera in Haiti. Emerg Infect Dis 17:699–701
73. Ruiz-Moreno D, Pascual M, Emch M, Yunus M (2010) Spatial clustering in the spatiotemporal dynamics of endemic cholera. BMC Infect Dis 10:51
74. Lipp EK, Huq A, Colwell RR (2002) Effects of global climate on infectious disease: the cholera model. Clin Microbiol Rev 15:757–770
75. Longini IM, Yunus M, Zaman K, Siddique AK, Sack RB, Nizam A (2002) Epidemic and endemic cholera trends over a 33-year period in Bangladesh. J Infect Dis 186:246–251
76. Sasaki S, Suzuki H, Fujino Y, Kimura Y, Cheelo M (2009) Impact of drainage networks on cholera outbreaks in Lusaka, Zambia. Am J Public Health 99:1982–1987
77. Harris JB, Larocque RC, Charles RC, Mazumder RN, Khan AI, Bardhan PK (2010) Cholera's western front. Lancet 376:1961–1965
78. Shikanga OT, Mutonga D, Abade M, Amwayi S, Ope M, Limo H et al (2009) High mortality in a cholera outbreak in western Kenya after post-election violence in 2008. Am J Trop Med Hyg 81:1085–1090
79. Ryan ET, Dhar U, Khan WA, Salam MA, Faruque AS, Fuchs GJ et al (2000) Mortality, morbidity, and microbiology of endemic cholera among hospitalized patients in Dhaka, Bangladesh. Am J Trop Med Hyg 63:12–20

80. Siddique AK, Salam A, Islam MS, Akram K, Majumdar RN, Zaman K et al (1995) Why treatment centres failed to prevent cholera deaths among Rwandan refugees in Goma, Zaire. Lancet 345:359–361
81. Steiner TS, Thielman NM, Guerrant RL (1997) Protozoal agents: what are the dangers for the public water supply? Annu Rev Med 48:329–340
82. Schneider RE, Shiffman M, Faigenblum J (1978) The potential effect of water on gastrointestinal infections prevalent in developing countries. Am J Clin Nutr 31:2089–2100
83. Choffnes ER, Mack A (2009) Global issues in water, sanitation, and health: workshop summary, Forum on Global Threats, Institute of Medicine
84. Centers for Disease Control and Prevention (2004) Cholera epidemic associated with raw vegetables–Lusaka, Zambia, 2003–2004. MMWR Morb Mortal Wkly Rep 53:783–786
85. Colwell RR, Huq A (1994) Environmental reservoir of *Vibrio cholerae*. The causative agent of cholera. Ann N Y Acad Sci 740:44–54
86. Tamplin ML, Gauzens AL, Huq A, Sack DA, Colwell RR (1990) Attachment of *Vibrio cholerae* serogroup O1 to zooplankton and phytoplankton of Bangladesh waters. Appl Environ Microbiol 56:1977–1980
87. Montilla R, Chowdhury MA, Huq A, Xu B, Colwell RR (1996) Serogroup conversion of *Vibrio cholerae* non-O1 to *Vibrio cholerae* O1: effect of growth state of cells, temperature, and salinity. Can J Microbiol 42:87–93
88. Tamplin ML, Colwell RR (1986) Effects of microcosm salinity and organic substrate concentration on production of *Vibrio cholerae* enterotoxin. Appl Environ Microbiol 52:297–301
89. Kay BA, Bopp CA, Wells JG (1994) Isolation and identification of *Vibrio cholerae* O1 from fecal specimens in *Vibrio cholerae* and cholera. In: Wachsmuth K, Wachsmuth IK, Blake PA, Olsvik Ø (eds) *Vibrio cholerae* and cholera: molecular to global perspectives. American Society for Microbiology, Washington, DC
90. Singleton FL, Attwell R, Jangi S, Colwell RR (1982) Effects of temperature and salinity on *Vibrio cholerae* growth. Appl Environ Microbiol 44:1047–1058
91. Singleton FL, Attwell RW, Jangi MS, Colwell RR (1982) Influence of salinity and organic nutrient concentration on survival and growth of *Vibrio cholerae* in aquatic microcosms. Appl Environ Microbiol 43:1080–1085
92. Rollins DM, Colwell RR (1986) Viable but nonculturable stage of *Campylobacter jejuni* and its role in survival in the natural aquatic environment. Appl Environ Microbiol 52:531–538
93. Singh A, McFeters GA (1986) Recovery, growth, and production of heat-stable enterotoxin by *Escherichia coli* after copper-induced injury. Appl Environ Microbiol 51:738–742
94. Austin B (2010) Vibrios as causal agents of zoonoses. Vet Microbiol 140:310–317
95. Barker J, Vipond IB, Bloomfield SF (2004) Effects of cleaning and disinfection in reducing the spread of norovirus contamination via environmental surfaces. J Hosp Infect 58:42–49
96. Flanagan PA (1992) Giardia–diagnosis, clinical course and epidemiology. A review. Epidemiol Infect 109:1–22
97. Robertson LJ, Campbell AT, Smith HV (1992) Survival of *Cryptosporidium parvum* oocysts under various environmental pressures. Appl Environ Microbiol 58:3494–3500
98. Codeço CT, Coelho FC (2006) Trends in cholera epidemiology. PLoS Med 3:e42
99. Merrell DS, Butler SM, Qadri F, Dolganov NA, Alam A, Cohen MB et al (2002) Host-induced epidemic spread of the cholera bacterium. Nature 417:642–645
100. Hartley DM, Morris JG, Smith DL (2006) Hyperinfectivity: a critical element in the ability of *V. cholerae* to cause epidemics? PLoS Med 3:e7
101. Kendall EA, Chowdhury F, Begum Y, Khan AI, Li S, Thierer JH et al (2010) Relatedness of *Vibrio cholerae* O1/O139 isolates from patients and their household contacts, determined by multilocus variable-number tandem-repeat analysis. J Bacteriol 192:4367–4376
102. Faruque SM, Islam MJ, Ahmad QS, Faruque AS, Sack DA, Nair GB, Mekalanos JJ (2005) Self-limiting nature of seasonal cholera epidemics: role of host-mediated amplification of phage. Proc Natl Acad Sci U S A 102:6119–6124
103. Nelson EJ, Chowdhury A, Harris JB, Begum YA, Chowdhury F, Khan AI et al (2007) Complexity of rice-water stool from patients with *Vibrio cholerae* plays a role in the transmission of infectious diarrhea. Proc Natl Acad Sci U S A 104:19091–19096

104. Jensen MA, Faruque SM, Mekalanos JJ, Levin BR (2006) Modeling the role of bacteriophage in the control of cholera outbreaks. Proc Natl Acad Sci U S A 103:4652–4657
105. Shahinian ML, Passaro DJ, Swerdlow DL, Mintz ED, Rodriguez M, Parsonnel J (2000) *Helicobacter pylori* and epidemic *Vibrio cholerae* O1 infection in Peru. Lancet 355:377–378
106. Schiraldi O, Benvestito V, Di Bari C, Moschetta R, Pastore G (1974) Gastric abnormalities in cholera: epidemiological and clinical considerations. Bull World Health Organ 51:349–352
107. Qadri F, Svennerholm AM, Faruque AS, Sack RB (2005) Enterotoxigenic *Escherichia coli* in developing countries: epidemiology, microbiology, clinical features, treatment, and prevention. Clin Microbiol Rev 18:465–483
108. Qureshi K, Mølbak K, Sandström A, Kofoed PE, Rodrigues A, Dias F et al (2006) Breast milk reduces the risk of illness in children of mothers with cholera: observations from an epidemic of cholera in Guinea-Bissau. Pediatr Infect Dis J 25:1163–1166
109. Ochoa TJ, Cleary TG (2009) Effect of lactoferrin on enteric pathogens. Biochimie 91:30–34
110. Gillin FD, Reiner DS, Wang CS (1983) Killing of *Giardia lamblia* trophozoites by normal human milk. J Cell Biochem 23:47–56
111. Perlmutter DH, Leichtner AM, Goldman H, Winter HS (1985) Chronic diarrhea associated with hypogammaglobulinemia and enteropathy in infants and children. Dig Dis Sci 30:1149–1155
112. Marcos LA, Terashima A, Dupont HL, Gotuzzo E (2008) Strongyloides hyperinfection syndrome: an emerging global infectious disease. Trans R Soc Trop Med Hyg 102:314–318
113. Petri WA, Miller M, Binder HJ, Levine MM, Dillingham R, Guerrant RL (2008) Enteric infections, diarrhea, and their impact on function and development. J Clin Invest 118:1277–1290
114. Glass RI, Holmgren J, Haley CE, Khan MR, Svennerholm A, Stoll BJ et al (1985) Predisposition for cholera of individuals with O blood group. Possible evolutionary significance. Am J Epidemiol 121:791–796
115. Oriá RB, Patrick PD, Oriá MO, Lorntz B, Thompson MR, Azevedo OG et al (2010) APOE polymorphisms and diarrheal outcomes in Brazilian shanty town children. Braz J Med Biol Res 43:249–256
116. Oriá RB, Patrick PD, Blackman JA, Lima AA, Guerrant RL (2007) Role of apolipoprotein E4 in protecting children against early childhood diarrhea outcomes and implications for later development. Med Hypotheses 68:1099–1109
117. Oriá RB, Patrick PD, Zhang H, Lorntz B, de Castro Costa CM, Brito GA et al (2005) APOE4 protects the cognitive development in children with heavy diarrhea burdens in Northeast Brazil. Pediatr Res 57:310–316
118. Cain L, Rotella E (2001) Death and spending: urban mortality and municipal expenditure on sanitation. Annales de démographie historique 101:139–154
119. Hains MR (2001) The urban mortality transition in the United States, 1800–1940. Annales de démographie historique 101:33–64
120. Burrell S, Gill G (2005) The Liverpool cholera epidemic of 1832 and anatomical dissection–medical mistrust and civil unrest. J Hist Med Allied Sci 60:478–498
121. Gill G, Burrell S, Brown J (2001) Fear and frustration – the Liverpool cholera riots of 1832. Lancet 358:233–237
122. Cumberland S (2009) An old enemy returns. Bull World Health Organ 87:85–86
123. Halliday S (2001) Death and miasma in Victorian London: an obstinate belief. BMJ 323:1469–1471
124. Paz S, Broza M (2007) Wind direction and its linkage with *Vibrio cholerae* dissemination. Environ Health Perspect 115:195–202
125. Snow J (1855) On the mode of communication of cholera, 2nd edn. Churchill, London
126. Brody H, Rip MR, Vinten-Johansen P, Paneth N, Rachman S (2000) Map-making and myth-making in Broad Street: the London cholera epidemic, 1854. Lancet 356:64–68
127. Luby SP, Agboatwalla M, Feikin DR, Painter J, Billhimer W, Altaf A, Hoekstra RM (2005) Effect of handwashing on child health: a randomised controlled trial. Lancet 366:225–233
128. Fisher D (2009) Cholera in Zimbabwe. Ann Acad Med Singapore 38:82

129. Koenig R (2009) Public health. International groups battle cholera in Zimbabwe. Science 323:860–861
130. Mason PR (2009) Zimbabwe experiences the worst epidemic of cholera in Africa. J Infect Dev Ctries 3:148–151
131. Nyati H (2004) Evaluation of the microbial quality of water supplies to municipal, mining and squatter communities in the Bindura urban area of Zimbabwe. Water Sci Technol 50:99–104
132. Editorial team (2008) Concerted international response to control ongoing cholera epidemic in Zimbabwe. Euro Surveill 13:19064
133. World Health Organization (2008) Outbreak news. Cholera, Zimbabwe. Wkly Epidemiol Rec 83:449–450
134. Hug A (2009) Inside Zimbabwe's cholera epidemic. Can Med Assoc J 180:285–286
135. Truscott R (2008) Zimbabwe appeals for medical aid as it declares state of emergency over cholera epidemic. BMJ 337:a2942
136. World Health Organization (2009) Cholera outbreak, Zimbabwe. Wkly Epidemiol Rec 84:50–52
137. Scapoli C, Guidi E, Angelini L, Stefanati A, Gregorio P (2003) Sociomedical indicators in the cholera epidemic in Ferrara of 1855. Eur J Epidemiol 18:617–621
138. Shultz A, Omollo JO, Burke H, Qassim M, Ochieng JB, Weinberg M et al (2009) Cholera outbreak in Kenyan refugee camp: risk factors for illness and importance of sanitation. Am J Trop Med Hyg 80:640–645
139. Deb BC, Sircar BK, Sengupta PG, De SP, Mondal SK, Gupta DN et al (1986) Studies on interventions to prevent El Tor cholera transmission in urban slums. Bull World Health Organ 64:127–131
140. World Health Organization Global Task Force on Cholera Control (2010) Cholera outbreak: assessing the outbreak response and improving preparedness. World Health Organization, Geneva
141. Roberts L, Chartier Y, Chartier O, Malenga G, Toole M, Rodka H (2001) Keeping clean water clean in a Malawi refugee camp: a randomized intervention trial. Bull World Health Organ 79:280–287
142. Besser RE, Feikin DR, Eberhart-Phillips JE, Mascola L, Griffin PM (1994) Diagnosis and treatment of cholera in the United States. Are we prepared? JAMA 272:1203–1205
143. Eberhart-Phillips J, Besser RE, Tormey MP, Koo D, Feikin D, Araneta MR et al (1996) An outbreak of cholera from food served on an international aircraft. Epidemiol Infect 116:9–13
144. Centers for Disease Control and Prevention (2006) Two cases of toxigenic *Vibrio cholerae* O1 infection after hurricanes Katrina and Rita–Louisiana, October 2005. MMWR Morb Mortal Wkly Rep 55:31–32
145. Toole MJ (1997) Communicable diseases and disease control. In: Noji EK (ed) The public health consequences of disasters. Oxford University Press, New York, pp 79–100
146. Wilder-Smith A (2005) Tsunami in South Asia: what is the risk of post-disaster infectious disease outbreaks? Ann Acad Med Singapore 34:625–631
147. Connolly MA, Gayer M, Ryan MJ, Salama P, Spiegel P, Heymann DL (2004) Communicable diseases in complex emergencies: impact and challenges. Lancet 364:1974–1983
148. Floret N, Viel JF, Mauny F, Hoen B, Piarroux R (2006) Negligible risk for epidemics after geophysical disasters. Emerg Infect Dis 12:543–548
149. Beinin L (1985) Medical consequences of natural disasters. Springer, Berlin
150. Centers for Disease Control (1992) Famine-affected, refugee, and displaced populations: recommendations for public health issues. MMWR Recomm Rep 41:1–76
151. Christenson B (2006) Oscar Costa-Mandry and post hurricane bacillary dysentery. Clin Infect Dis 42:1650–1651
152. Palit A, Batabyal P (2010) Toxigenic *Vibrio cholerae* from environmental sources associated with the cholera outbreak after 'AILA' cyclone in west Bengal, India. Lett Appl Microbiol 51:241–243

153. Qadri F, Khan AI, Faruque AS, Begum YA, Chowdhury F, Nair GB et al (2005) Enterotoxigenic *Escherichia coli* and *Vibrio cholerae* diarrhea, Bangladesh, 2004. Emerg Infect Dis 11:1104–1107
154. Waring SC, Brown BJ (2005) The threat of communicable diseases following natural disasters: a public health response. Disaster Manag Response 3:41–47
155. de Ville de Goyet C (2000) Stop propagating disaster myths. Lancet 356:762–764
156. Brennan RJ, Waldman RJ (2006) The South Asian earthquake six months later–an ongoing crisis. N Engl J Med 354:1769–1771
157. Malholland K (1985) Cholera in Sudan: an account of an epidemic in a refugee camp in eastern Sudan, May-June 1985. Disasters 9:247–258
158. Otten M (1986) Nutritional and mortality aspects of the 1985 famine in north-central Ethiopia. Presented as a report to the save the Children Federation, Westport, CT
159. Seaman J (1992) Famine mortality in Ethiopia and Sudan. In: Mortality and society in sub-Saharan Africa. Oxford University Press, New York, pp 349–366
160. Toole MJ, Waldman RJ (1988) An analysis of mortality trends among refugee populations in Somalia, Sudan, and Thailand. Bull World Health Organ 66:237–247
161. Centers for Disease Control (1991) Public health consequences of acute displacement of Iraqi citizens–March-May 1991. MMWR Morb Mortal Wkly Rep 40:443–447
162. Moren A, Stefanaggi S, Antona D, Bitar D, Etchegorry MG, Tchatchioka M, Lungu G (1991) Practical field epidemiology to investigate a cholera outbreak in a Mozambican refugee camp in Malawi, 1988. J Trop Med Hyg 94:1–7
163. Swerdlow DL, Malenga G, Begkoyian G, Nyangulu D, Toole M, Waldman RJ et al (1997) Epidemic cholera among refugees in Malawi, Africa: treatment and transmission. Epidemiol Infect 118:207–214
164. Centers for Disease Control and Prevention (1998) Cholera outbreak among Rwandan refugees–Democratic Republic of Congo, April 1997. MMWR Morb Mortal Wkly Rep 47:389–391
165. Birmingham ME, Lee LA, Ndayimirije N, Nkurikiye S, Hersh BS, Wells JG, Deming MS (1997) Epidemic cholera in Burundi: patterns of transmission in the Great Rift Valley Lake region. Lancet 349:981–985
166. Sur D, Dutta P, Nair GB, Bhattacharya SK (2000) Severe cholera outbreak following floods in a northern district of west Bengal. Indian J Med Res 112:178–182
167. Bissell RA (1983) Delayed-impact infectious disease after a natural disaster. J Emerg Med 1:59–66
168. Centers for Disease Control and Prevention (2005) Vibrio illnesses after Hurricane Katrina–multiple states, August-September 2005. MMWR Morb Mortal Wkly Rep 54:928–931
169. Broach JP, McNamara M, Harrison K (2010) Ambulatory care by disaster responders in the tent camps of Port-au-Prince, Haiti, January 2010. Disaster Med Public Health Prep 4:116–121
170. Pan American Health Organization (2011) Basic health indicator data base Haiti. PAHO, Washington, DC. Available from: http://www.paho.org/english/dd/ais/cp_332.htm. Accessed 20 Feb 2011
171. Centers for Disease Control and Prevention (2010) Haiti pre-decision briefs for public health action. CDC, Atlanta. Available from: http://www.bt.cdc.gov/disasters/earthquakes/Haiti/pre-decision_briefs.asp
172. Pan American Health Organization (2010) Basic health indicator data base Haiti, Country Profile. PAHO, Washington, DC
173. Pape JW, Levine E, Beaulieu ME, Marshall F, Verdier R, Johnson WD (1987) Cryptosporidiosis in Haitian children. Am J Trop Med Hyg 36:333–337
174. Pan American Health Organization (2010) Earthquake in Haiti PAHO/WHO situation report on health activities post earthquake. Pan American Health Organization, Washington, DC
175. Centers for Disease Control and Prevention (2010) Launching a national surveillance system after an earthquake – Haiti, 2010. MMWR Morb Mortal Wkly Rep 59:933–938

176. World Health Organization (2010) Outbreak news. Cholera, Haiti – update. Wkly Epidemiol Rec 85:489–490
177. Chin CS, Sorenson J, Harris JB, Robins WP, Charles RC, Jean-Charles RR et al (2011) The origin of the Haitian cholera outbreak strain. N Engl J Med 364:33–42
178. Centers for Disease Control and Prevention (CDC) (2006) Morbidity surveillance after Hurricane Katrina – Arkansas, Louisiana, Mississippi, and Texas, September 2005. MMWR Morb Mortal Wkly Rep 55:727–731
179. Cavey AM, Spector JM, Ehrhardt D, Kittle T, McNeill M, Greenough PG, Kirsch TD (2009) Mississippi's infectious disease hotline: a surveillance and education model for future disasters. Prehosp Disaster Med 24:11–17
180. Cookson ST, Soetebier K, Murray EL, Fajardo GC, Hanzlick R, Cowell A, Drenzek C (2008) Internet-based morbidity and mortality surveillance among Hurricane Katrina evacuees in Georgia. Prev Chronic Dis 5:1–7
181. Yee EL, Palacio H, Atmar RL, Shah U, Kilborn C, Faul M et al (2007) Widespread outbreak of norovirus gastroenteritis among evacuees of Hurricane Katrina residing in a large "megashelter" in Houston, Texas: lessons learned for prevention. Clin Infect Dis 44:1032–1039
182. Murray KO, Kilborn C, DesVignes-Kendrick M, Koers E, Page V, Selwyn BJ et al (2009) Emerging disease syndromic surveillance for Hurricane Katrina evacuees seeking shelter in Houston's Astrodome and Reliant Park Complex. Public Health Rep 124:364–371
183. Todd B (2006) Infection control and Hurricane Katrina. What nurses can learn in the aftermath of the disaster. Am J Nurs 106:29–31
184. Brown V, Reilley B, Ferrir MC, Gabaldon J, Manoncourt S (1997) Cholera outbreak during massive influx of Rwandan returnees in November, 1996. Lancet 349:214
185. Toole MJ, Waldman RJ (1993) Refugees and displaced persons. War, hunger, and public health. JAMA 270:600–605
186. Colombatti R, Vieira CS, Bassani F, Cristofoli R, Coin A, Bertinato L, Riccardi F (2009) Contamination of drinking water sources during the rainy season in an urban post-conflict community in Guinea Bissimplications for sanitation priority. Afr J Med Med Sci 38:155–161
187. Salama P, Buzard N, Spiegel P (2001) Improving standards in international humanitarian response: the Sphere Project and beyond. JAMA 286:531–532
188. Heyman SN, Ginosar Y, Shapiro M, Kluger Y, Marx N, Maayan S (1997) Diarrheal epidemics among Rwandan refugees in 1994. Management and outcome in a field hospital. J Clin Gastroenterol 25:595–601
189. World Health Organization (1994) Cholera. Outbreak among Rwandan refugees. Wkly Epidemiol Rec 69:223
190. Siddique AK (1994) Cholera epidemic among Rwandan refugees: experience of ICDDR, B in Goma, Zaire. Glimpse 16:3–4
191. Bhattacharya S, Black R, Bourgeois L, Clemens J, Cravioto A, Deen JL et al (2009) Public health. The cholera crisis in Africa. Science 324:885
192. Powell B, Ford C (2010) Risks of travel, benefits of a specialist consult. Cleve Clin J Med 77:246–254
193. World Tourism Organization. International tourism 2010: multi-speed recovery. UNWTO; 11. Available from: http://unwto.org/en. Accessed 16 April 2011
194. Centers for Disease Control and Prevention (2002) Outbreaks of gastroenteritis associated with noroviruses on cruise ships–United States, 2002. MMWR Morb Mortal Wkly Rep 51:1112–1115
195. Thompson F (2010) Water woes in Senegal's Holy City. Bull World Health Organ 88:7–8
196. Cockburn TA, Cassanos JG (1960) Epidemiology of endemic cholera. Public Health Rep 75:791–803
197. Feikin DR, Tabu CW, Gichuki J (2010) Does water hyacinth on East African lakes promote cholera outbreaks? Am J Trop Med Hyg 83:370–373

198. Colwell RR, Huq A, Islam MS, Aziz KM, Yunus M, Khan NH et al (2003) Reduction of cholera in Bangladeshi villages by simple filtration. Proc Natl Acad Sci U S A 100:1051–1055
199. Lobitz B, Beck L, Huq A, Wood B, Fuchs G, Faruque AS, Colwell R (2000) Climate and infectious disease: use of remote sensing for detection of *Vibrio cholerae* by indirect measurement. Proc Natl Acad Sci U S A 97:1438–1443
200. Mourino-Perez RR (1998) Oceanography and the 7th cholera pandemic. Epidemiology 9(3):355–357
201. Colwell RR (1996) Global climate and infectious disease: the cholera paradigm. Science 274:2025–2031
202. Seas C, Miranda J, Gil AI, Leon-Barua R, Patz J, Huq A et al (2000) New insights on the emergence of cholera in Latin America during 1991: the Peruvian experience. Am J Trop Med Hyg 62:513–517
203. Franco AA, Fix AD, Prada A, Paredes E, Palomino JC, Wright AC et al (1997) Cholera in Lima, Peru, correlates with prior isolation of *Vibrio cholerae* from the environment. Am J Epidemiol 146:1067–1075
204. Gil AI, Louis VR, Rivera IN, Lipp E, Huq A, Lanata CF et al (2004) Occurrence and distribution of *Vibrio cholerae* in the coastal environment of Peru. Environ Microbiol 6:699–706
205. Swerdlow DL, Mintz ED, Rodriguez M, Tejada E, Ocampo C, Espejo L et al (1992) Waterborne transmission of epidemic cholera in Trujillo, Peru: lessons for a continent at risk. Lancet 340:28–33
206. Ford TE, Colwell RR, Rose JB, Morse SS, Rogers DJ, Yates TL (2009) Using satellite images of environmental changes to predict infectious disease outbreaks. Emerg Infect Dis 15:1341–1346
207. Constantin de Magny G, Murtugudde R, Sapiano MR, Nizam A, Brown CW, Busalacchi AJ et al (2008) Environmental signatures associated with cholera epidemics. Proc Natl Acad Sci U S A 105:17676–17681
208. Choi SY, Lee JH, Jeon YS, Lee HR, Kim EJ, Ansaruzzaman M et al (2010) Multilocus variable-number tandem repeat analysis of *Vibrio cholerae* O1 El Tor strains harbouring classical toxin B. J Med Microbiol 59:763–769
209. Woodward WE, Mosley WH (1972) The spectrum of cholera in rural Bangladesh. II. Comparison of El Tor Ogawa and classical Inaba infection. Am J Epidemiol 96:342–351
210. Karaolis DK, Lan R, Kaper JB, Reeves PR (2001) Comparison of *Vibrio cholerae* pathogenicity islands in sixth and seventh pandemic strains. Infect Immun 69:1947–1952
211. Nair GB, Faruque SM, Bhuiyan NA, Kamruzzaman M, Siddique AK, Sack DA (2002) New variants of *Vibrio cholerae* O1 biotype El Tor with attributes of the classical biotype from hospitalized patients with acute diarrhea in Bangladesh. J Clin Microbiol 40: 3296–3299
212. Siddique AK, Nair GB, Alam M, Sack DA, Huq A, Nizam A et al (2010) El Tor cholera with severe disease: a new threat to Asia and beyond. Epidemiol Infect 138:347–352
213. Okada K, Chantaroj S, Roobthaisong A, Hamada S, Sawanpanyalert P (2010) A cholera outbreak of the *Vibrio cholerae* O1 El Tor variant carrying classical *ctxb* in Northeastern Thailand in 2007. Am J Trop Med Hyg 82:875–878
214. Pal BB, Khuntia HK, Samal SK, Kar SK, Patnaik B (2010) Epidemics of severe cholera caused by El Tor *Vibrio cholerae* O1 Ogawa possessing the *ctxb* gene of the classical biotype in Orissa, India. Int J Infect Dis 14:e384–e389
215. Ang GY, Yu CY, Balqis K, Elina HT, Azura H, Hani MH, Yean CY (2010) Molecular evidence of cholera outbreak caused by a toxigenic *Vibrio cholerae* O1 El Tor variant strain in Kelantan, Malaysia. J Clin Microbiol 48:3963–3969
216. Taneja N, Mishra A, Sangar G, Singh G, Sharma M (2009) Outbreaks caused by new variants of *Vibrio cholerae* O1 El Tor, India. Emerg Infect Dis 15:352–354
217. Talyzina NM, Ingvarsson PK, Zhu J, Wai SN, Andersson A (2009) Molecular diversification in the quorum-sensing system of *Vibrio cholerae*: Role of natural selection in the emergence of pandemic strains. Appl Environ Microbiol 75:3808–3812

218. Shimada T, Nair GB, Deb BC, Albert MJ, Sack RB, Takeda Y (1993) Outbreak of *Vibrio cholerae* non-O1 in India and Bangladesh. Lancet 341:1346–1347
219. Albert MJ, Ansaruzzaman M, Bardhan PK, Faruque ASG, Faruque SM, Islam MS et al (1993) Large epidemic of cholera-like disease in Bangladesh caused by *Vibrio cholerae* O139 synonym Bengal. Cholera working group, International Centre for Diarrhoeal Diseases Research, Bangladesh. Lancet 342:387–390
220. Siddiqui FJ, Bhutto NS, von Seidlein L, Khurram I, Rasool S, Ali M et al (2006) Consecutive outbreaks of *Vibrio cholerae* O139 and *V. Cholerae* O1 cholera in a fishing village near Karachi, Pakistan. Trans R Soc Trop Med Hyg 100:476–482
221. Qu M, Xu J, Ding Y, Wang R, Liu P, Kan B et al (2003) Molecular epidemiology of *Vibrio cholerae* O139 in China: polymorphism of ribotypes and CTX elements. J Clin Microbiol 41:2306–2310
222. Sinha S, Chakraborty R, De K, Khan A, Datta S, Ramamurthy T et al (2002) Escalating association of *Vibrio cholerae* O139 with cholera outbreaks in India. J Clin Microbiol 40:2635–2637
223. Nusrin S, Gil AI, Bhuiyan NA, Safa A, Asakura M, Lanata CF et al (2009) Peruvian *Vibrio cholerae* O1 El Tor strains possess a distinct region in the vibrio seventh pandemic island-ii that differentiates them from the prototype seventh pandemic El Tor strains. J Med Microbiol 58:342–354
224. Safa A, Bhuiyan NA, Murphy D, Bates J, Nusrin S, Kong RY et al (2009) Multilocus genetic analysis reveals that the Australian strains of *Vibrio cholerae* O1 are similar to the pre-seventh pandemic strains of the El Tor biotype. J Med Microbiol 58:105–111
225. Guerrant RL, Carneiro-Filho BA, Dillingham RA (2003) Cholera, diarrhea, and oral rehydration therapy: triumph and indictment. Clin Infect Dis 37:398–405
226. da Cunha FRM, Cash RA (1990) History of the development of oral rehydration therapy. Clin Ther 12(Suppl A):2–11
227. Rao MC (2004) Oral rehydration therapy: new explanations for an old remedy. Annu Rev Physiol 66:385–417
228. MacGillivray N (2006) Dr Latta of Leith: pioneer in the treatment of cholera by intravenous saline infusion. J R Coll Physicians Edinb 36:80–85
229. Foëx BA (2003) How the cholera epidemic of 1831 resulted in a new technique for fluid resuscitation. Emerg Med J 20:316–318
230. Carpenter CC (1990) The erratic evolution of cholera therapy: from folklore to science. Clin Ther 12(Suppl A):22–27
231. Heyman SN, Haim N, Horovitz J, Sofer S, Orbach J, Yaakov A (1994) Sudden death during fluid resuscitation: lesson from Rwanda. Lancet 344:1509–1510
232. Rikliss E, Quastel JH (1958) Effects of cations on sugar absorption by isolated surviving guinea pig intestine. Can J Biochem Physiol 36:347–362
233. Curran PF (1960) Sodium chloride and water transport by rat ileum *in vitro*. J Gen Physiol 43:1137–1148
234. Crane RK (1962) Hypothesis for mechanism of intestinal active transport of sugars. Fed Proc 21:891–895
235. Gangarosa EF, Beisel WR, Benyajati C, Sprinz H, Piyaratn P (1960) The nature of the gastrointestinal lesion in Asiatic cholera and its relation to pathogenesis: a biopsy study. Am J Trop Med Hyg 9:125–135
236. Phillips RA (1964) Water and electrolyte losses in cholera. Fed Proc 23:705–712
237. Pierce NF, Banwell JG, Rupak DM, Mitra RC, Caranasos GJ, Keimowitz RI et al (1968) Effect of intragastric glucose-electrolyte infusion upon water and electrolyte balance in Asiatic cholera. Gastroenterology 55:333–343
238. Nalin DR, Cash RA, Islam R, Molla M, Phillips RA (1968) Oral maintenance therapy for cholera in adults. Lancet 292:370–372
239. Nalin DR, Cash RA (1970) Oral or nasogastric maintenance therapy for diarrhoea of unknown aetiology resembling cholera. Trans R Soc Trop Med Hyg 64:769–771

240. Nalin DR, Cash RA, Rahman M (1970) Oral (or nasogastric) maintenance therapy for cholera patients in all age-groups. Bull World Health Organ 43:361–363
241. Cash RA, Nalin DR, Rochat R, Reller LB, Haque ZA, Rahman AS (1970) A clinical trial of oral therapy in a rural cholera-treatment center. Am J Trop Med Hyg 19:653–656
242. Mahalanabis D, Choudhuri AB, Bagchi NG, Bhattacharya AK, Simpson TW (2001) Oral fluid therapy of cholera among Bangladesh refugees. 1973. Bull World Health Organ 79:473–479
243. Thillainayagam AV, Hunt JB, Farthing MJ (1998) Enhancing clinical efficacy of oral rehydration therapy: is low osmolality the key? Gastroenterology 114:197–212
244. Gore SM, Fontaine O, Pierce NF (1992) Impact of rice based oral rehydration solution on stool output and duration of diarrhoea: meta-analysis of 13 clinical trials. BMJ 304:287–291
245. Molla AM, Bari A, Greenough WB, Molla AM, Budhiraja P, Sharma PN (2000) Bangladeshi rural mothers prepare safer rice oral rehydration solution. Acta Paediatr 89:791–794
246. Fayad IM, Hashem M, Duggan C, Refat M, Bakir M, Fontaine O, Santosham M (1993) Comparative efficacy of rice-based and glucose-based oral rehydration salts plus early reintroduction of food. Lancet 342:772–775
247. Pulungsih SP, Punjabi NH, Rafli K, Rifajati A, Kumala S, Simanjuntak CH et al (2006) Standard WHO-ORS versus reduced-osmolarity ORS in the management of cholera patients. J Health Popul Nutr 24:107–112
248. Dutta D, Bhattacharya MK, Deb AK, Sarkar D, Chatterjee A, Biswas AB et al (2000) Evaluation of oral hypo-osmolar glucose-based and rice-based oral rehydration solutions in the treatment of cholera in children. Acta Paediatr 89:787–790
249. Ramakrishna BS, Venkataraman S, Srinivasan P, Dash P, Young GP, Binder HJ (2000) Amylase-resistant starch plus oral rehydration solution for cholera. N Engl J Med 342:308–313
250. Rabbani GH, Teka T, Saha SK, Zaman B, Majid N, Khatun M et al (2004) Green banana and pectin improve small intestinal permeability and reduce fluid loss in Bangladeshi children with persistent diarrhea. Dig Dis Sci 49:475–484
251. Alam NH, Meier R, Schneider H, Sarker SA, Bardhan PK, Mahalanabis D et al (2000) Partially hydrolyzed guar gum-supplemented oral rehydration solution in the treatment of acute diarrhea in children. J Pediatr Gastroenterol Nutr 31:503–507
252. Kosek M, Yori PP, Olortegui MP (2010) Shigellosis update: advancing antibiotic resistance, investment empowered vaccine development, and green bananas. Curr Opin Infect Dis 23:475–480
253. Gregorio GV, Gonzales ML, Dans LF, Martinez EG (2009) Polymer-based oral rehydration solution for treating acute watery diarrhoea. Cochrane Database Syst Rev 2:CD006519
254. Zavaleta N, Figueroa D, Rivera J, Sánchez J, Alfaro S, Lönnerdal B (2007) Efficacy of rice-based oral rehydration solution containing recombinant human lactoferrin and lysozyme in Peruvian children with acute diarrhea. J Pediatr Gastroenterol Nutr 44:258–264
255. Ochoa TJ, Chea-Woo E, Campos M, Pecho I, Prada A, McMahon RJ, Cleary TG (2008) Impact of lactoferrin supplementation on growth and prevalence of *Giardia* colonization in children. Clin Infect Dis 46:1881–1883
256. Neu J, DeMarco V, Li N (2002) Glutamine: clinical applications and mechanisms of action. Curr Opin Clin Nutr Metab Care 5:69–75
257. Rhoads JM, Argenzio RA, Chen W, Rippe RA, Westwick JK, Cox AD et al (1997) L-Glutamine stimulates intestinal cell proliferation and activates mitogen-activated protein kinases. Am J Physiol 272:G943–G953
258. Ribeiro Júnior H, Ribeiro T, Mattos A, Palmeira C, Fernandez D, Sant'Ana I et al (1994) Treatment of acute diarrhea with oral rehydration solutions containing glutamine. J Am Coll Nutr 13:251–255
259. Gutiérrez C, Villa S, Mota FR, Calva JJ (2007) Does an l-glutamine-containing, glucose-free, oral rehydration solution reduce stool output and time to rehydrate in children with acute diarrhoea? A double-blind randomized clinical trial. J Health Popul Nutr 25:278–284
260. Nalin DR, Cash RA, Rahman M, Yunus M (1970) Effect of glycine and glucose on sodium and water adsorption in patients with cholera. Gut 11:768–772

261. World Health Organization (1991) Impact of glycine-containing ORS solutions on stool output and duration of diarrhoea: a meta-analysis of seven clinical trials. The international study group on improved ORS. Bull World Health Organ 69:541–548
262. Bhan MK, Mahalanabis D, Fontaine O, Pierce NF (1994) Clinical trials of improved oral rehydration salt formulations: a review. Bull World Health Organ 72:945–955
263. Lima AA, Carvalho GH, Figueiredo AA, Gifoni AR, Soares AM, Silva EA, Guerrant RL (2002) Effects of an alanyl-glutamine-based oral rehydration and nutrition therapy solution on electrolyte and water absorption in a rat model of secretory diarrhea induced by cholera toxin. Nutrition 18:458–462
264. Colton CA, Czapiga M, Snell-Callanan J, Chernyshev ON, Vitek MP (2001) Apolipoprotein E acts to increase nitric oxide production in macrophages by stimulating arginine transport. Biochim Biophys Acta 1535:134–144
265. Mahalanabis D, Bhan MK (2001) Micronutrients as adjunct therapy of acute illness in children: impact on the episode outcome and policy implications of current findings. Br J Nutr 85(Suppl 2):S151–S158
266. Sazawal S, Black RE, Bhan MK, Bhandari N, Sinha A, Jalla S (1995) Zinc supplementation in young children with acute diarrhea in India. N Engl J Med 333:839–844
267. Bhatnagar S, Bahl R, Sharma PK, Kumar GT, Saxena SK, Bhan MK (2004) Zinc with oral rehydration therapy reduces stool output and duration of diarrhea in hospitalized children: a randomized controlled trial. J Pediatr Gastroenterol Nutr 38:34–40
268. Black RE, Sazawal S (2001) Zinc and childhood infectious disease morbidity and mortality. Br J Nutr 85(Suppl 2):S125–S129
269. Strand TA, Chandyo RK, Bahl R, Sharma PR, Adhikari RK, Bhandari N et al (2002) Effectiveness and efficacy of zinc for the treatment of acute diarrhea in young children. Pediatrics 109:898–903
270. Lukacik M, Thomas RL, Aranda JV (2008) A meta-analysis of the effects of oral zinc in the treatment of acute and persistent diarrhea. Pediatrics 121:326–336
271. Lazzerini M, Ronfani L (2008) Oral zinc for treating diarrhoea in children. Cochrane Database Syst Rev 6:CD005436
272. Atia AN, Buchman AL (2009) Oral rehydration solutions in non-cholera diarrhea: a review. Am J Gastroenterol 104:2596–2604, quiz 2605
273. Curioso WH, Miranda JJ, Kimball AM (2004) Learning from low income countries: what are the lessons? Community oral rehydration units can contain cholera epidemics. BMJ 329:1183–1184
274. Okeke IN (2009) Cholera vaccine will reduce antibiotic use. Science 325:674
275. Materu SF, Lema OE, Mukunza HM, Adhiambo CG, Carter JY (1997) Antibiotic resistance pattern of *Vibrio cholerae* and *Shigella* causing diarrhoea outbreaks in the Eastern Africa region: 1994–1996. East Afr Med J 74:193–197
276. Cavallo JD, Niel L, Talarmin A, Dubrous P (1995) Antibiotic sensitivity to epidemic strains of *Vibrio cholerae* and *Shigella dysenteriae* 1 isolated in Rwandan refugee camps in Zaire. Med Trop (Mars) 55:351–353
277. Saha D, Karim MM, Khan WA, Ahmed S, Salam MA, Bennish ML (2006) Single-dose azithromycin for the treatment of cholera in adults. N Engl J Med 354:2452–2462
278. Saroso JS, Bahrawi W, Witjaksono H, Budiarso RL, Brotowasisto, Bencić Z et al (1978) A controlled field trial of plain and aluminium hydroxide-adsorbed cholera vaccines in Surabaya, Indonesia, during 1973–75. Bull World Health Organ 56:619–627
279. Wiedermann U, Kollaritsch H (2006) Vaccines against traveler's diarrhoea and rotavirus disease – a review. Wien Klin Wochenschr 118:2–8
280. Clemens JD, Harris JR, Khan MR, Kay BA, Yunus M, Svennerholm AM et al (1986) Field trial of oral cholera vaccines in Bangladesh. Lancet 328:124–127
281. Clemens JD, Sack DA, Harris JR, Van Loon F, Chakraborty J, Ahmed F et al (1990) Field trial of oral cholera vaccines in Bangladesh: results from three-year follow-up. Lancet 335:270–273
282. Lucas ME, Deen JL, von Seidlein L, Wang XY, Ampuero J, Puri M et al (2005) Effectiveness of mass oral cholera vaccination in Beira, Mozambique. N Engl J Med 352:757–767

283. Chaignat CL, Monti V, Soepardi J, Petersen G, Sorensen E, Narain J, Kieny MP (2008) Cholera in disasters: do vaccines prompt new hopes? Expert Rev Vac 7:431–435
284. Cavailler P, Lucas M, Perroud V, McChesney M, Ampuero S, Guérin PJ et al (2006) Feasibility of a mass vaccination campaign using a two-dose oral cholera vaccine in an urban cholera-endemic setting in Mozambique. Vaccine 24:4890–4895
285. Dorlencourt F, Legros D, Paquet C, Neira M, Ivanoff B, Le Saout E (1999) Effectiveness of mass vaccination with WC/rBS cholera vaccine during an epidemic in Adjumani District, Uganda. Bull World Health Organ 77:949–950
286. Shamsuzzaman S, Ahmed T, Mannoor K, Begum YA, Bardhan PK, Sack RB et al (2009) Robust gut associated vaccine-specific antibody-secreting cell responses are detected at the mucosal surface of Bangladeshi subjects after immunization with an oral killed bivalent *V. cholerae* O1/O139 whole cell cholera vaccine: comparison with other mucosal and systemic responses. Vaccine 27:1386–1392
287. Anh DD, Canh do G, Lopez AL, Thiem VD, Long PT, Son NH et al (2007) Safety and immunogenicity of a reformulated Vietnamese bivalent killed, whole-cell, oral cholera vaccine in adults. Vaccine 25:1149–1155
288. Mahalanabis D, Lopez AL, Sur D, Deen J, Manna B, Kanungo S et al (2008) A randomized, placebo-controlled trial of the bivalent killed, whole-cell, oral cholera vaccine in adults and children in a cholera endemic area in Kolkata, India. PLoS One 3:e2326
289. Sur D, Lopez AL, Kanungo S, Paisley A, Manna B, Ali M et al (2009) Efficacy and safety of a modified killed-whole-cell oral cholera vaccine in India: an interim analysis of a cluster-randomised, double-blind, placebo-controlled trial. Lancet 374:1694–1702
290. Ahmed T, Arifuzzaman M, Lebens M, Qadri F, Lundgren A (2009) CD4+ T-cell responses to an oral inactivated cholera vaccine in young children in a cholera endemic country and the enhancing effect of zinc supplementation. Vaccine 28:422–429
291. Chowdhury MI, Sheikh A, Qadri F (2009) Development of Peru-15 (choleragarde), a live-attenuated oral cholera vaccine: 1991–2009. Expert Rev Vac 8:1643–1652
292. García L, Jidy MD, García H, Rodríguez BL, Fernández R, Año G et al (2005) The vaccine candidate *Vibrio cholerae* 638 is protective against cholera in healthy volunteers. Infect Immun 73:3018–3024
293. Kenner JR, Coster TS, Taylor DN, Trofa AF, Barrera-Oro M, Hyman T et al (1995) Peru-15, an improved live attenuated oral vaccine candidate for *Vibrio cholerae* O1. J Infect Dis 172:1126–1129
294. Sack DA, Sack RB, Shimko J, Gomes G, O'Sullivan D, Metcalfe K, Spriggs D (1997) Evaluation of Peru-15, a new live oral vaccine for cholera, in volunteers. J Infect Dis 176:201–205
295. Cohen MB, Giannella RA, Bean J, Taylor DN, Parker S, Hoeper A et al (2002) Randomized, controlled human challenge study of the safety, immunogenicity, and protective efficacy of a single dose of Peru-15, a live attenuated oral cholera vaccine. Infect Immun 70: 1965–1970
296. Qadri F, Chowdhury MI, Faruque SM, Salam MA, Ahmed T, Begum YA et al (2005) Randomized, controlled study of the safety and immunogenicity of Peru-15, a live attenuated oral vaccine candidate for cholera, in adult volunteers in Bangladesh. J Infect Dis 192:573–579
297. Valera R, García HM, Jidy MD, Mirabal M, Armesto MI, Fando R et al (2009) Randomized, double-blind, placebo-controlled trial to evaluate the safety and immunogenicity of live oral cholera vaccine 638 in Cuban adults. Vaccine 27:6564–6569
298. Tacket CO, Losonsky G, Nataro JP, Comstock L, Michalski J, Edelman R et al (1995) Initial clinical studies of CVD 112 *Vibrio cholerae* O139 live oral vaccine: Safety and efficacy against experimental challenge. J Infect Dis 172:883–886
299. Vu DT, Hossain MM, Nguyen DS, Nguyen TH, Rao MR, Do GC et al (2003) Coverage and costs of mass immunization of an oral cholera vaccine in Vietnam. J Health Popul Nutr 21:304–308

300. López-Gigosos R, García-Fortea P, Reina-Doña E, Plaza-Martín E (2007) Effectiveness in prevention of travellers' diarrhea by an oral cholera vaccine WC/rBS. Travel Med Infect Dis 5:380–384
301. Thiem VD, Deen JL, von Seidlein L, Canh do G, Anh DD, Park JK et al (2006) Long-Term effectiveness against cholera of oral killed whole-cell vaccine produced in Vietnam. Vaccine 24:4297–4305
302. Trach DD, Clemens JD, Ke NT, Thuy HT, Son ND, Canh DG et al (1997) Field trial of a locally produced, killed, oral cholera vaccine in Vietnam. Lancet 349:231–235
303. Trach DD, Cam PD, Ke NT, Rao MR, Dinh D, Hang PV et al (2002) Investigations into the safety and immunogenicity of a killed oral cholera vaccine developed in Vietnam. Bull World Health Organ 80:2–8
304. Naficy AB, Trach DD, Ke NT, Chuc NT, Sorkin A, Rao MR et al (2001) Cost of immunization with a locally produced, oral cholera vaccine in Vietnam. Vaccine 19:3720–3725
305. Nguyen BM, Lee JH, Cuong NT, Choi SY, Hien NT, Anh DD et al (2009) Cholera outbreaks caused by an altered *Vibrio cholerae* O1 El Tor biotype strain producing classical cholera toxin B in Vietnam in 2007 to 2008. J Clin Microbiol 47:1568–1571
306. Longini IM, Nizam A, Ali M, Yunus M, Shenvi N, Clemens JD (2007) Controlling endemic cholera with oral vaccines. PLoS Med 4:e339
307. Arvelo W, Blum LS, Nahar N, VON Seidlein L, Nahar L, Pack RP et al (2011) Community perceptions of bloody diarrhoea in an urban slum in South Asia: implications for introduction of a Shigella vaccine. Epidemiol Infect 139(4):599–605
308. Preston NW (1997) Cholera vaccines: lessons from Rwanda and elsewhere. Lancet 349:957
309. Khuntia HK, Samal SK, Kar SK, Pal BB (2010) An Ogawa cholera outbreak 6 months after the Inaba cholera outbreaks in India, 2006. J Microbiol Immunol Infect 43:133–137
310. Ye C, Lan R, Xia S, Zhang J, Sun Q, Zhang S et al (2010) Emergence of a new multidrug-resistant serotype X variant in an epidemic clone of *Shigella flexneri*. J Clin Microbiol 48:419–426
311. Jelinek T, Kollaritsch H (2008) Vaccination with Dukoral against travelers' diarrhea (ETEC) and cholera. Expert Rev Vaccines 7:561–567
312. Desenclos JC, Zergabachew A, Desmoulins B, Chouteau L, Desve G, Admassu M (1988) Clinical, microbiological and antibiotic susceptibility patterns of diarrhoea in Korem, Ethiopia. J Trop Med Hyg 91:296–301
313. Levine MM (2006) Enteric infections and the vaccines to counter them: future directions. Vaccine 24:3865–3873
314. Levine MM (2006) Mass vaccination to control epidemic and endemic typhoid fever. Curr Top Microbiol Immunol 304:231–246
315. Lin FY, Ho VA, Khiem HB, Trach DD, Bay PV, Thanh TC et al (2001) The efficacy of a *Salmonella typhi* Vi conjugate vaccine in two-to-five-year-old children. N Engl J Med 344:1263–1269
316. Michel R, Garnotel E, Spiegel A, Morillon M, Saliou P, Boutin JP (2005) Outbreak of typhoid fever in vaccinated members of the French armed forces in the Ivory Coast. Eur J Epidemiol 20:635–642
317. Kanungo S, Dutta S, Sur D (2008) Epidemiology of typhoid and paratyphoid fever in India. J Infect Dev Ctries 2:454–460
318. Guerrant RL, Oriá RB, Moore SR, Oriá MO, Lima AA (2008) Malnutrition as an enteric infectious disease with long-term effects on child development. Nutr Rev 66:487–505
319. Mata LJ, Urrutia JJ, Lechtig A (1971) Infection and nutrition of children of a low socioeconomic rural community. Am J Clin Nutr 24:249–259
320. Martorell R, Habicht JP, Yarbrough C, Lechtig A, Klein RE, Western KA (1975) Acute morbidity and physical growth in rural Guatemalan children. Am J Dis Child 129:1296–1301
321. Rowland MG, Cole TJ, Whitehead RG (1977) A quantitative study into the role of infection in determining nutritional status in Gambian village children. Br J Nutr 37:441–450
322. Black RE, Brown KH, Becker S (1984) Effects of diarrhea associated with specific enteropathogens on the growth of children in rural Bangladesh. Pediatrics 73:799–805

323. Guerrant RL, Kirchhoff LV, Shields DS, Nations MK, Leslie J, de Sousa MA et al (1983) Prospective study of diarrheal illnesses in northeastern Brazil: patterns of disease, nutritional impact, etiologies, and risk factors. J Infect Dis 148:986–997
324. Moore SR, Lima AA, Conaway MR, Schorling JB, Soares AM, Guerrant RL (2001) Early childhood diarrhoea and helminthiases associate with long-term linear growth faltering. Int J Epidemiol 30:1457–1464
325. Rowland MG, Rowland SG, Cole TJ (1988) Impact of infection on the growth of children from 0 to 2 years in an urban west African community. Am J Clin Nutr 47:134–138
326. Schorling JB, Guerrant RL (1990) Diarrhoea and catch-up growth. Lancet 335:599–600
327. Guerrant DI, Moore SR, Lima AA, Patrick PD, Schorling JB, Guerrant RL (1999) Association of early childhood diarrhea and cryptosporidiosis with impaired physical fitness and cognitive function four-seven years later in a poor urban community in northeast Brazil. Am J Trop Med Hyg 61:707–713
328. Berkman DS, Lescano AG, Gilman RH, Lopez SL, Black MM (2002) Effects of stunting, diarrhoeal disease, and parasitic infection during infancy on cognition in late childhood: a follow-up study. Lancet 359:564–571
329. Patrick PD, Oriá RB, Madhavan V, Pinkerton RC, Lorntz B, Lima AA, Guerrant RL (2005) Limitations in verbal fluency following heavy burdens of early childhood diarrhea in Brazilian shantytown children. Child Neuropsychol 11:233–244
330. Black RE, Allen LH, Bhutta ZA, Caulfield LE, de Onis M, Ezzati M et al (2008) Maternal and child undernutrition: global and regional exposures and health consequences. Lancet 371:243–260
331. Guerrant RL, Schorling JB, McAuliffe JF, de Souza MA (1992) Diarrhea as a cause and an effect of malnutrition: diarrhea prevents catch-up growth and malnutrition increases diarrhea frequency and duration. Am J Trop Med Hyg 47:28–35
332. Bhan MK, Raj P, Levine MM, Kaper JB, Bhandari N, Srivastava R et al (1989) Enteroaggregative *Escherichia coli* associated with persistent diarrhea in a cohort of rural children in India. J Infect Dis 159:1061–1064
333. Lima AA, Guerrant RL (1992) Persistent diarrhea in children: epidemiology, risk factors, pathophysiology, nutritional impact, and management. Epidemiol Rev 14:222–242
334. Henry FJ, Udoy AS, Wanke CA, Aziz KM (1992) Epidemiology of persistent diarrhea and etiologic agents in Mirzapur, Bangladesh. Acta Paediatr Suppl 381:27–31
335. Bhan MK, Bhandari N, Sazawal S, Clemens J, Raj P, Levine MM, Kaper JB (1989) Descriptive epidemiology of persistent diarrhoea among young children in rural Northern India. Bull World Health Organ 67:281–288
336. Steiner TS, Lima AA, Nataro JP, Guerrant RL (1998) Enteroaggregative *Escherichia coli* produce intestinal inflammation and growth impairment and cause interleukin-8 release from intestinal epithelial cells. J Infect Dis 177:88–96
337. Checkley W, Epstein LD, Gilman RH, Black RE, Cabrera L, Sterling CR (1998) Effects of *Cryptosporidium parvum* infection in Peruvian children: growth faltering and subsequent catch-up growth. Am J Epidemiol 148:497–506
338. Checkley W, Gilman RH, Epstein LD, Suarez M, Diaz JF, Cabrera L et al (1997) Asymptomatic and symptomatic cryptosporidiosis: their acute effect on weight gain in Peruvian children. Am J Epidemiol 145:156–163
339. Niehaus MD, Moore SR, Patrick PD, Derr LL, Lorntz B, Lima AA, Guerrant RL (2002) Early childhood diarrhea is associated with diminished cognitive function 4 to 7 years later in children in a northeast Brazilian shantytown. Am J Trop Med Hyg 66:590–593
340. Eppig C, Fincher CL, Thornhill R (2010) Parasite prevalence and the worldwide distribution of cognitive ability. Proc R Soc Lond B Biol Sci 277:3801–3808

Chapter 6
Challenges in the Control and Eradication of Malaria

Ignatius W. Fong

6.1 Introduction

Malaria is still the most important parasitic disease in the world, and tropical developing countries or resource-poor areas face daunting challenges to control and eradicate this pervasive infection. Although progress has been made over the past century in shrinking the malaria map, more than 40% of the world's population are at risk of contracting malaria [1]. Most recent estimates on the annual burden of malaria worldwide are several hundred million cases with about 800,000 deaths per year [1]. Snow et al. [2] estimated that there were 515 million cases of clinical malaria caused by *Plasmodium falciparum* alone in 2002. However, in the past 150 years, about half of the countries in the world eliminated malaria [3]. Presently, there are 99 countries with endemic malaria, of which 67 are controlling malaria to a large degree and 32 are in the process of trying to eliminate this parasite [3].

Although we now associate malaria with tropical and subtropical areas of the world, it was previously worldwide even in temperate regions of the world including North America and Western Europe. The burden of malaria diminishes with distance from the equator, and it predominantly occurs in areas ideal for breeding mosquitoes, such as marshy areas, river deltas, swampy valleys, and alluvial regions. After the Second World War, 41.5% of the European countries were at risk for malaria, which was eliminated by the beginning of the 1970s, except Turkey (on the border of Europe and Asia Minor) which experienced 100,000 cases in 1977 [4]. In North America, malaria was eliminated between 1947 and 1951, through a campaign of spraying of the residual insecticide dichlorodiphenyltrichloroethane (DDT), industrialization, and urbanization [5].

I.W. Fong, M.B.B.S., F.R.C.P.C (✉)
Department of Medicine, University of Toronto, Toronto, ON, Canada

Division of Infectious Diseases, St. Michael's Hospital, Toronto, ON, Canada
e-mail: FONGI@smh.ca; fongi@smh.toronto.on.ca

I.W. Fong (ed.), *Challenges in Infectious Diseases*, Emerging Infectious Diseases of the 21st Century 502, DOI 10.1007/978-1-4614-4496-1_6,

6.2 Historical Aspects

Historical records indicate that malaria existed in the old world for several thousand years. It likely originated from nonhuman primates, gorillas, and chimpanzees and subsequently adapted to humans with estimates varying from 3,200 to 7,700 years or 25,000 to 50,000 years ago [6]. Medical writings of disease with periodic fever and splenic enlargement suggest malaria was described in China 2700 BC, Mesopotamia 2000 BC, and Egypt 1570 BC [7]. Moreover, Hippocrates' (460–370 BC) description of tertian and quartan fever indicate that malaria existed in Greece in ancient times, and malaria antigen have been detected in Egyptian mummies of more than 3,000 years old [7, 8]. The malaria parasite *Plasmodium* was first detected in the blood of malaria patients in Constantine by the French physician Charles Laveran in 1880 and subsequently confirmed by Ronald Ross in the Indian Medical Service, who concluded that mosquitoes inoculated humans with the disease when he reported in 1895 that the parasite was found in the stomach and blood of anophelines mosquito [4]. Both investigators were awarded the Nobel Prize in Medicine.

6.3 Microbiology

The genus *Plasmodium* belongs to the phylum Apicomplexa and consists of almost 200 species that are parasitic to reptiles, birds, and mammals [6]. Malaria in humans is caused mainly by four *Plasmodium* species: *P. falciparum*, *P. vivax*, *P. ovale*, and *P. malariae*. However, there are increased reports of a nonhuman primate parasite *Plasmodium knowlesi* transmission to humans in Asia (often misdiagnosed as *P. malariae*), widely distributed in Malaysian Borneo and extending to Peninsular Malaysia but also found in Thailand, Philippines, and other Asian countries [9, 10]. *P. falciparum* causes the most severe form of malaria (due to high parasitic burden) and the most morbidity and mortality in sub-Saharan Africa (nearly 85% of the total), but *P. vivax* is the most geographically widespread of human malarias, with 70–80 million clinical cases across Asia, Central and South America, the Middle East, and parts of Africa (North) [6]. Although *P. vivax* is traditionally considered a benign disease, there is evidence that severe disease is common with malaria caused by this parasite [11].

6.4 Progress in Control of Malaria

Attempts to control and eliminate malaria started in the nineteenth century soon after discovery of the parasite and mode of transmission but were hampered by the two great world wars. During the First World War, the English partly controlled malaria by draining swampy regions and treatment of water surfaces with paraffin to arrest development of the anophelines larvae. Around 1920, trioxymethylene was used to spray water surfaces, which was simpler and cheaper than paraffin [4]. However, in 1923, the USSR suffered a major malaria epidemic with five million cases and 60,000 deaths [4]. It was not until DDT was introduced by 1939 that malaria could be controlled and eliminated in developed Western nations. However, even after the Second World War, 41.5% of the European population lived in malaria-endemic areas, and by 1950, only 30% of the world population lived in malaria-free areas [12]. In 1955, the WHO initiated the Global Malaria Eradication Programme [13], built on accessible treatment and prevention with chloroquine and vector control with DDT. This campaign was partly successful in areas of low transmission rates, such as in regions of India and Sri Lanka, but was subsequently hampered by the development of chloroquine-resistant *P. falciparum* and DDT-resistant anophelines mosquito, lack of political will, and financial constraints in highly endemic areas. This initial global eradication program was officially terminated as a goal in 1972 [14]; but it was never implemented in most parts of Africa with the highest burden of malaria.

Since the termination of the Global Malaria Eradication Programme, some countries have seen substantial increase in the burden of malaria in some areas of the world, with epidemics in Sri Lanka in 1968–1969 and in Madagascar in 1987–1988 [15]. Although some countries continued to show decline in malaria through continuation of antivector measures, economic development, and improved health-care infrastructure (i.e., Thailand) [16]. Failure of the malaria eradication campaign had largely been attributed to development of chloroquine-resistant *P. falciparum* and subsequent multidrug-resistant strains. Effective chemotherapy is a key cornerstone in efforts to control malaria and reduce the burden of disease in endemic areas. Chloroquine resistance first emerged in Southeast Asia and South America in the late 1950s and made its appearance in Africa about the late 1970s [17]. The development of chloroquine resistance had resulted in four- to eightfold increase in mortality [18]. After termination of the global eradication program, there was an increase in malaria burden in the world especially in the 1970s and 1980s, but renewed efforts have resulted in shrinkage of the malaria global map. However, although the global population at risk decreased from 77% at the start of the twentieth century to a low of 46% in 1994, it increased to 48% in 2002 due to population growth in the same geographic distribution [12]. This translates to an increase of 0.9–3 billion people at risk.

Since the start of the twenty-first century, there have been renewed efforts to ramp up malaria control in endemic areas with the goal of eventual elimination. This has been due to increased finances from developed nations and charitable foundations (i.e., Bill and Melinda Gates Foundation), widespread use of residual insecticide-treated bednets, improved rapid diagnostic tests, and implementation of artemisinin-based combination therapy [3]. More than 70% of the global burden of malaria resides in Africa, and just over 10 years ago, the African heads of states signed a declaration in Nigeria to reduce the malaria mortality in half by 2010 [19].

This declaration was initiated by the UN in 1995 as a special initiative for Africa and adopted in 1998 by the WHO as part of the roll back malaria movement. The Global Fund to Fight AIDS, Tuberculosis and Malaria was established in 2002 to facilitate funding for large-scale health-related Millenium Development Goals (MDGs) [20]. Roll back malaria program's main focus was on countries with high burden of disease, and Africa was the primary target.

Worldwide spending on malaria control was about US$100 million in 1998 but by 2009, the Global Fund had approved $5.3 billion for 191 malaria grants in 82 countries [21]. The priority interventions supported across most African countries included insecticide-treated nets, selective indoor house spray of residual insecticide, reduction of maternal infection during pregnancy, widespread use of artemisinin combination therapy (ACT), and improvement of rapid diagnostic methods. By 2010, ACTs were first-line treatment in every African malaria-endemic country, and more countries were adopting indoor residual spraying and insecticide-treated nets [22]. These recent changes have resulted across different regions of Africa marked reductions in transmission and incidence of clinical malaria [22–25].

The incidence of severe malaria in coastal Kenya fell by more than 90% in 5 years, with a major impact on childhood illness and mortality [22, 25].

Similar success story have been seen in the island of Bioko, Equatorial Guinea which instituted an integrated malaria control program in 2003. In 4–5 years, there was a major reduction in transmission and rates of parasitemia and anemia and a two-thirds reduction in mortality of children under 5 years of age [24]. The effect of malaria reduction may not only have an effect on malaria-related morbidity and mortality but on invasive bacterial infection as well [22], which appears to be increased with severe malaria in children. Africa is considered the key continent in the fight against global malaria, and there have been major success in recent years. However, the countries that dramatically reduced malaria (about a dozen) are small and peaceful [26]. These include Zambia (population 1.1 million) and Rwanda (population 10 million) that have reduced malaria cases by more than 50%, and the two-island state of Sâo Tom and Principe has almost eliminated malaria [26]. However, Ethiopia is the only large country (population 81 million) through international funding that have introduced integrated control methods on a large scale (ACTs, bednets, indoor spraying), and the efficacy of these measures are still pending assessment as malaria in this country comes in waves with the last outbreak in 2003–2004.

The major bulk of the burden of malaria in Africa (>50%) resides in large countries where the challenges for control are greatest. These include Nigeria (population155 million) where bednet coverage is less than 10% and the Democratic Republic of the Congo (population 69 million) where war and poor infrastructure pose major barriers to malaria control (which is still the number 1 killer); Sudan, Tanzania, and Uganda have all shown little progress in controlling malaria [26].

Recent success in malaria control in some countries of Africa and hopes for global eradication has been dampened with recent emergence of artemisinin resistance in *P. falciparum* along the Thai-Cambodian border [27].

6.5 Drug Resistance

Drug resistance in malaria has been and continues to be a barrier to controlling and eradicating this persistent parasite over the past six decades. Widespread occurrence of artemisinin resistance, as occurred with chloroquine and others, will be a major obstacle and would jeopardize the plan for global control and eradication of malaria. Resistance has already developed to all the antimalarial drug classes, and widespread resistance to artemisinin would be a disaster. In vivo resistance to antimalarial drugs has been described for three of the four main species that infect humans, *P. falciparum*, *P. vivax*, and to a lesser degree *P. malariae* [28]. Clinically, the development of resistance to antimalarial drugs to a high degree requires the accumulation of multiple mutations. This has led to the recommendations for combination therapy – i.e., artemisinin combination. The appearance of clinically significant resistance to ACTs along the Thai-Cambodian border has been attributed to the availability of artemisinin monotherapy in Western Cambodia for more than 30 years. Despite the implementation of active malaria control and introduction of ACTs in 2001, 78% of artemisinin use in Western Cambodia consisted of monotherapy through the private sector [29]. *P. falciparum* has developed resistance to all antimalarials in current use, but the degree is widely variable depending on the geographic region of the world. Chloroquine-resistant *P. falciparum* is widespread in all regions with endemic malaria, except for Central America, the Caribbean (the island of Hispaniola), and parts of the Middle East. Antifolate drug combinations such as sulfadoxine-pyrimethamine (SP) resistance similar to chloroquine and artemisinin started on the Thai-Cambodian border and spread across Asia and Africa and also reported in South America [30–32]. Mefloquine resistance is frequent in several regions of Southeast Asia, Amazon region of South America, and areas of Africa [33–35]. Similarly, amodiaquine resistance has also appeared in South America, Southeast Asia, and Africa [33–35]. Quinine resistance has been limited to East/Southeast Asia and infrequently in South America [28], despite the fact that quinine has been used as an antimalarial for over a century. Multidrug-resistant malaria is now established in Southeast Asia, South America, and parts of Africa [36].

P. vivax resistance to chloroquine and/or primaquine has drawn less attention but has been expanding surreptitiously. In the past two decades, emergence and spread of drug- resistant strains of *P. vivax* has extended through Asia from Papua New Guinea and Indonesia to India, Vietnam, and Thailand to South America, the Horn of Africa (Ethiopia), and Madagascar [28, 37]. *P. vivax* resistance to mefloquine and SP has also been reported on the western border of Thailand and Indonesia [28].

6.6 Epidemiology of Drug-Resistant Malaria

The Thailand-Cambodia border is the hotbed of malaria drug resistance, and this region has been the forerunner and probable source of antimalarial drug resistance before spreading through Southeast Asia, then to Africa and other parts of the world.

Resistance along the Thai-Cambodia border started with chloroquine, followed by resistance to SP, mefloquine, and now artemisinin. Development of drug-resistant malaria is one of the most important factors and challenge that will be a barrier to global malaria control and eradication. Chloroquine resistance of *P. falciparum* was first documented in Asia (Thai-Cambodia border) and South America in 1959–1960, spread to Africa by 1978, and became widespread throughout sub-Saharan Africa during the 1980s [38] and is now worldwide except for isolated areas.

Resistance to the antifolate combination SP was first detected along the Thai-Cambodia border in the mid-1960s [39], and widespread resistance subsequently developed in large areas of Southeast Asia, Southern China, and the Amazon Basin after 1975 and by 1999 [40, 41]. In Africa, SP resistance appeared in the late 1980s and has spread through the continent to a variable degree, greater in the east than in the west. In vitro SP resistance was documented across sub-Saharan Africa (13–50%) even before widespread clinical use [40]. Despite increasing resistance in Africa, this combination drug is still used for intermittent preventive treatment (IPT) as a malaria control strategy in certain high- risk groups, pregnant women, and children [42].

Quinine has been in use for over two centuries and malaria resistance to monotherapy appeared in the mid-1960s primarily along the Thai-Cambodia border [43]. Clinical resistance to quinine monotherapy occurs sporadically in Southeast Asia and Western Oceania, and in vitro resistance is less frequent in South America and Africa [44, 45]. Mefloquine, chemically related to quinine, resistance was also first observed along the Thai-Cambodia border in the late 1980s [46, 47]. Resistant strains are now common in the neighboring countries, and migrant gem miners returning from Cambodia are believed to propagate the spread of mefloquine resistance to Bangladesh and India. Clinical resistance to mefloquine is present in the Amazon Basin and South America but to a lesser degree than in Asia. In vitro resistance to mefloquine has been reported from Africa, but clinical resistance is still sporadic [48].

Malarone, a combination tablet of atovaquone (250 mg) and proguanil (100 mg), has been marketed for malaria prophylaxis and treatment since 1997 for chloroquine- resistant *P. falciparum*. However, it is mainly used by tourists and returning travelers from developed nations visiting endemic regions because of its expense. Atovaquone as a single agent was first introduced in 1996 and resistance was first reported in the same year in Thailand [49]. Resistance to malarone has been reported in Africa since 2004 [50], and the presence of two-point mutations in the parasite cytochrome b gene (associated with malarone resistance) was detected at the initial treatment of naïve African patients in 5–10%, reported in 2006 [51].

Multidrug resistance (resistance to >2 operational antimalarial drugs of different chemical classes) is established in Southeast Asia, South America, and Africa and appears to be spreading rather than localized to focal areas in these regions. However, resistance to artemisinin isolated in China in the 1970s from the sweet wormwood plant (used for treating fever for centuries) is currently limited to the Thai-Cambodian border.

6.7 Factors in Drug-Resistant Malaria

It is unclear why the Thai-Cambodian border or the Thai-Myanmar border appears to be the cradle of malaria drug resistance. There are multiple complex issues that appear to be involved in the progressive evolution and selection of drug-resistant malaria. Thailand is almost malaria-free except for occurrence of disease along its borders. The factors that determine drug resistance are interrelated and overlapping (see Fig. 6.1) and may involve the interaction of host, parasite, operational and pharmacological factors.

The southeastern border of Thailand and Cambodia has long been considered the epicenter of malaria drug resistance. Mefloquine resistance has since heightened on the Thai-Cambodian border and the western Thai-Myanmar border from mid-1980s to mid-1990s [46, 52]. Subsequently, an area on the central part of the Thai-Myanmar border became a new focus of multidrug-resistant (MDR) problem. Since the mid-1990s, the number of falciparum malaria has declined along the Thai-Cambodian border and within Thailand territory, but in immigrants from Myanmar, a large number of cases occur annually [47].

Changes in the population dynamics along the Thai borders from 1988 are believed to have contributed to the malaria drug-resistant problem. Migration of gem miners to Western Cambodia near Bo Rai district and the town of Pailin began soon after opening of check points [49]. Pailin in Western Cambodia, where gem mining and logging occurred year-round, represented an epicenter of intense malaria transmission. Estimates of 3,000 gem miners from nonendemic malaria areas (mainly from Thailand but also from neighboring Myanmar, Bangladesh, and India) crossed the Bo Rai border daily. These predominantly nonimmune workers (migrants), in an area of high malaria transmission without protection and control program in place, easily became infected after 2–3 weeks stay, with an estimate of 50% infection of the first-trip returnees [47]. A large outbreak of malaria occurred in a region of high drug pressure, which predisposed to selection of resistant strains. Many patients reentered Thailand with severe malaria, and survivors often returned after treatment.

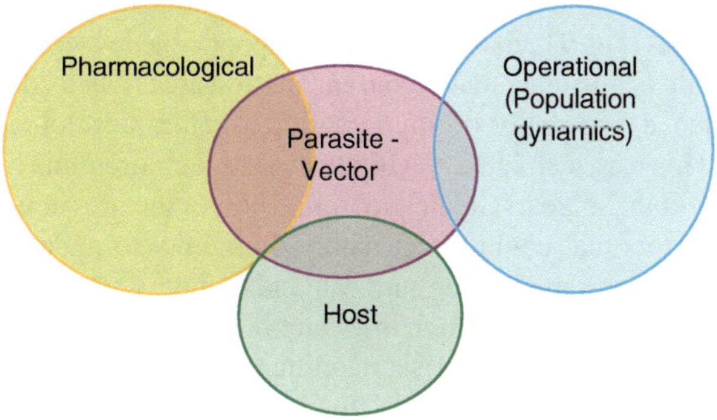

Fig. 6.1 Factors in malaria drug resistance

The spread of MDR strains from Bo Rai (Thai-Cambodia border) to the Mae Sot provide further fodder for this outbreak and allow MDR malaria to become established along the Thai-Myanmar border. The Thai malaria control program in 1995 instituted malaria clinics along these high-risk borders and provided mefloquine-artesunate combination drug therapy [41]. These measures initially led to control and stabilization within the Thai borders for 5 or more years. However, mefloquine resistance in Cambodia was associated with high failure rates with artesunate-mefloquine combination in recent years [53, 54].

Although Cambodia instituted artemisinin-based combination therapies in 2001, it appears that 78% of artemisinin use was monotherapy provided by the private sector [55]. This, combined with partial resistance to artesunate-mefloquine (providing one active drug), extended period of. suboptimal therapies, genetic background of parasites from an area of high resistance, and high transmission, all likely contributed to the emergence of artemisinin-resistant malaria in Cambodia [27].

6.7.1 Host Factors

Besides population dynamics or movement characteristics that may have contributed to the spread of MDR malaria in Asia, the host immunity may play a major role. It has been postulated that in areas of high or intense transmission, community immunity against malaria is significant, and symptomatic disease occurs in only a small proportion of about 1–2% of clinical attacks [55]. Since only a small fraction of the population receives treatment, development of resistance to new drugs is slow to develop, whereas in areas of lower transmission where substantial protective community immunity is lacking, infection is more likely to result in clinical disease and require more frequent drug therapies, which predispose to drug resistance [57]. In this model, the population with high endemic rates and significant herd immunity, usually when infected, have lower parasitic load (with one clone), whereas in low endemic areas without much herd immunity, infection usually results in higher parasitic load (with multiple clones); thus, there is greater risk of multiple mutations leading to resistance [56]. This would be applicable to immigrants from low-transmission malaria areas that migrate to the Thai-Cambodian or Thai-Myanmar borders. The general observation that resistance developed earlier in low-transmission areas (i.e., Thailand and Brazil) supports the low-transmission hypothesis. However, others postulate that high transmission areas can lead to increased risk of drug resistance, especially in young children before development of partial immunity [57]. This was seen in East Africa where full chloroquine resistance occurred and spread within 2.5 years, related to high chloroquine pressure [58]. Theoretically, other host factors that could affect natural immunity to malaria such as malnutrition, where epidemics may occur with war and famine, and the human immune deficiency virus (HIV) epidemic, which is greater in underdeveloped and areas endemic for malaria, could increase the risk of clinical disease and severity of malaria. Hence, the resulting greater parasitic load and high drug pressure could predispose to rapid malaria drug resistance. However, there have been no significant reports on these issues which should be investigated.

Other human factors that likely have some role in drug-resistance development include misuse of antimalarials. This may include overuse of drugs for febrile conditions without confirming the diagnosis (estimated to be a common practice in endemic areas) and underuse with premature discontinuation of active drugs before complete eradication of parasites; use of partially effective regimens or single agents intentionally or unintentionally (fake drugs) can also encourage drug resistance.

6.7.2 Pharmacological Factors

Pharmacological, host, and parasitic factors are closely intertwined. The pharmacokinetics and pharmacodynamic characteristics of the drugs used to treat malaria may affect the development of selecting resistant strains. It has been proposed that drugs with slow killing effect and long half-lives, with a long "selective window" (periods during which blood levels are 20–80% of the maximum inhibitory concentration) when drug concentration is adequate to suppress susceptible parasites but too low to prevent replication of drug-resistant parasites [59, 60], are prone to drug resistance soon after introduction. Drugs with long terminal half-life where pharmacokinetic factors have been postulated to contribute to rapid drug resistance and impaired efficacy include SP (pyrimethamine component) and mefloquine.

Artemisinin and its more potent derivatives (artemether, artesunate, and dihydroartemisinin) not only kill parasites effectively and rapidly but disappear from the blood within a day after administration. When used as monotherapy, artemisinins are associated with recurrent parasitemia unless the medication is administered for 5–7 days. Thus, artemisinins are coadministered with longer-acting agents to protect against recrudescent infections and theoretically prevent resistance. Artesunate plus mefloquine and fixed combination artemether-lumefantrine (Coartem) are examples of these artemisinin combination therapies (ACTs). In areas of intense transmission, reinfections are common, and this may occur during the selection window of the partner drug (with prolonged terminal half-life), and subtherapeutic levels may allow for rapid emergence of drug resistance [61]. Studies in Africa with the use of ACTs indicate that selection of resistant parasites to the long-acting partner drugs may be emerging [61, 62].

The pharmacokinetic characteristics of drugs have only recently been noted to play a role in malaria drug resistance. Previously, clinical failure of treatment was always attributed to inherent parasite resistance without assessing drug levels. Some drugs such as lumefantrine have highly variably drug absorption (determined by fat consumption and other factors), and low drug levels 7 days after treatment could lead to recurrent parasitemia [63]. Better knowledge and application of the principles of the drugs' pharmacokinetics may have slowed the spread of drug resistance. Premarketing dose-finding studies of most antimalarial drugs were performed before drug resistance was a problem or a consideration. Thus, the selected dose was usually the lowest dose to achieve a good performance with the least adverse effect [61]. The therapeutic levels are usually adequate to clear fully susceptible parasites but allow mildly resistant parasites to multiply and spread. It has been proposed, using a pharmacokinetic-pharmacodynamic model, that had mefloquine dosed at 24 mg/kg rather than 15 mg/kg, resistance to mefloquine could have been slower to develop [64]. In Guinea-Bissau, where chloroquine has been used at 2–3 times the dose administered by other countries (50–70 mg/kg vs. 25 mg/kg over 3 days), chloroquine resistance is more rare compared to neighboring countries [65, 66].

Most antimalarial drugs, except for artemisinins and quinine, are slowly eliminated and, in endemic areas, provide a gradient of drug concentrations to which new parasites (reinfection) are exposed and predisposed to development of resistant mutants. Stepniewska and White [60] used a mathematical model to examine pharmacokinetic-pharmacodynamic properties of antimalarial drugs and the selection window. The window of selection was determined mainly by the terminal half-life ($T_{½}$) of the drug, the degree of resistance, the blood concentration of the drug, and the slope of the concentration-effect relationship. The longer the $T_{½}$, the flatter the concentration-effect curve and the wider the selection window [60]. Artemisinin and quinine with $T_{½}$ of less than 24 h usually do not select for resistance during the elimination phase.

6.7.3 Parasitic Factors

The molecular basis of drug resistance in malaria has been established for the majority of antimalarials, but the mechanisms for initiation of drug resistance are not well understood. Drug resistance results from mutations in parasite genes, but it is unknown (or not adequately investigated) whether natural resistance exists in nature (as seen with bacteria, fungi, and other microorganisms) before drug exposure. The sexual stage of the parasite that forms male and female gametocytes, which exists in the blood for weeks and does not cause symptoms, is responsible for transmission through the mosquito and has been proposed to be the key phase for drug-resistance development and spread. The high rate of meiotic recombination that occurs during this stage enhances the development of multiple drug resistance, probably permitting concentration of independently acquired resistant traits into a single dose [67, 68].

Rathod et al. [69] hypothesized that resistance to new antimalarials arise at different frequencies in different clones of *P. falciparum* and that previous drug resistance in the past may predispose to acquisition of resistance to unrelated agents. In vitro experiments performed by these investigators using different *P. falciparum* clones with varying numbers of preexisting resistance mechanisms were treated with two new antimalarial agents. All parasites were equally susceptible in small numbers, but large populations of these clones showed significant variation in

Table 6.1 Antimalarial targets, resistance and markers

Drugs	Site of action	Resistance	Genetic markers
Quinolines			
Quinine	Food vacuole, Hb polymerization, blood stage	Southeast Asia, Western Oceania	Pfmdr1
Chloroquine	Food vacuole, Hb polymerization, blood stage	Common worldwide except Caribbean, Central America	Pfcrt, Pfmdr1
Mefloquine	Food vacuole, Hb polymerization, blood stage	Southeast Asia, parts of Africa, South America	Pfmdr1
Primaquine	Unknown target, liver stage and gametocyte	Partial, rare	None
Antifolates			
Sulfadoxine-pyrimethamine	Folate metabolism, blood, stage	Southeast Asia, Africa, South America	Pfdhps/pfdhfr
Malarone			
Atovaquone-proguanil	Mitochondria/antifolate, blood, and liver stages	Southeast Asia, Africa (Rare)	Cytochrome bc/pfdhfr (proguanil)
Artemesinin	? sarco/endoplasmic reticulum Ca Atpase, blood stage, partial gametocyte	Cambodia-Thai-Myanmar borders (Rare)	Unknown

Data obtained from Refs: [70–73]

frequencies of resistance when challenged with either of the two new compounds. Clone D6 from West Africa (sensitive to all traditional antimalarial agents) failed to develop resistance, whereas the Indochina clone W2 (resistant to the traditional antimalarial drugs) acquired resistance to both new compounds as much as 1,000 times more frequently than D6 [69]. These investigators propose that increased plasticity of some falciparum parasite genomes may offer selective advantages beyond drug resistance. Moreover, the ability of certain clones of *P. falciparum* to readily develop resistance to new unrelated compounds may represent a novel evolutionary strategy to survive different chemotherapeutic agents. They call these phenotypes "accelerated resistance to multiple drugs" (ARMD) strains [69].

To understand drug resistance of the malarial parasite, it is essential to analyze the molecular targets of the drugs and the life cycle stages that are affected. Most antimalarial agents eliminate the asexual stage of the erythrocytic forms and target only a small number of biological functions (Table 6.1) [69]. The quinolines (quinine, chloroquine, amodiaquine, mefloquine, halofantrine, lumefantrine) target the parasite metabolism and detoxification of hemoglobin, SP and dapsone are antifolates, atovaquone-proguanil affects the mitochondria function, and artemisinin's mechanism is not well understood but is believed to target the sarco-endoplasmic reticulum

Ca^{++}-ATPase (SERCH) [71, 74]. Primaquine is the only drug that eliminates the hypnozoites of the chronic liver phase (*P. vivax* and *P. ovale*), and the mechanism of action is unknown. Although not used for *P. falciparum* infection, it also has an effect on the gametocyte of this parasite [75].

The gametocytes are usually unaffected by most antimalarial agents that eliminate the asexual trophozoites, and chloroquine may actually induce gametocytogenesis [76]. Artemisinins prevent the development of early-stage gametocytes and reduce gametocyte carriage and thus have the advantage of reducing transmission and preventing the spread of resistance partially [77, 78].

The molecular basis of drug resistance has been reviewed by Olliaro [72] and will be summarized in this chapter. Resistance to chloroquine is multigenic and epistatic (interaction between genes at different loci) and associated with a decrease in the accumulation of the drug within the food vacuole. Studies have identified mutation in the *P. falciparum* chloroquine resistance transporter (PfCRT) gene, associated with decreased chloroquine accumulation and activity [79, 80]. Multiple polymorphisms in the gene are associated with in vivo resistance, but the primary mutation seems to be replacement of lysine with threonine at codon 76 [81]. In addition, mutations in the major P glycoprotein homologue I of the major multidrug transporter, *P. falciparum* multidrug resistance gene (PfMDR), may modulate the extent of chloroquine resistance conferred by mutations in PfCRT. Polymorphisms in PfMDR also predicts partial mefloquine resistance [82].

The antifolate drugs interrupt de novo folate synthesis, which is essential for survival, by targeting two enzymes: dihydrofolate reductase (DHFR) and dihydropteroate synthase (DHPS). Pyrimethamine and proguanil target DHFR, and sulfa drugs (sulfadoxine) target DHPS [70]. Step-wise mutation to DHFR and DHPS genes occur, and cumulative mutations lead to increased resistance to antifolate drugs. Single mutations in one or both genes may not cause clinical failure to SP, whereas double or triple mutations usually result in clinical failure [83]. The highest levels of antifolate resistance are found in Southeast Asia and South America, where polymorphism at DHFR residue 164 is always found [70]. However, in Africa, moderate level of resistance conferred by mutations in DHFR and DHPS genes is typically found, with the absence of I164L polymorphism (associated with 20,000-fold decrease in susceptibility compared to the wild type) [70]. This explains why SP is partially effective in preventing malaria in pregnant women, but ineffective in treating symptomatic disease.

In French Guiana, in 2002–2003, decreased in vitro susceptibility of *P. falciparum* to artemether was reported with the S769N mutation in the PsSERCA gene (gene encoding the sarco-endoplasm reticulum calcium ATPase 6), but this was not correlated with clinical failure [84]. In Cambodia, increased copies of the PfMDRI gene was associated with high failure rates to artesunate-mefloquine therapy [84], but this could be due primarily to high mefloquine resistance. Differences in PfMDR copy numbers are linked to changes in clinical efficiency of several drugs [70]. Although PfMDRI amplification can cause a small decrease in artemisium susceptibility [82], this or other mutations could not account for the decreased parasite clearance recently noted in Pailin, Cambodia [27].

6.8 Vector Factors

It has been estimated that there are about 450 *Anopheles* mosquito species in the world, and 70 of these are vectors of malaria [85]. *Anopheles culicifacies* is largely responsible for malaria transmission in India, Iran, Afghanistan, Pakistan, and Sri Lanka [85]. Although it strives in dry and semi-humid climate, it is a monsoon-associated species, and most of the malaria transmission occurs during the rainy season. In Africa, the *Anopheles gambiae* complex is responsible for transmitting the parasite to hundreds of people [86]. This species has also been imported in Brazil where it has caused malaria epidemic in the past [87]. It is considered a "super vector" as it is easily infected with the malaria parasite, has a long life span, and feeds primarily on humans. The efficacy of malaria transmission may be assessed by using the vectorial capacity. The duration of sporogony of *P. falciparum* in mosquitoes has been postulated to be exponentially related to an increase in vectorial capacity. It has been proposed that deforestation in Kenya led to increased vector transmission of malaria by *A. gambiae* mosquitoes by 77.7%, through decreased duration of sporogony, increased mosquito density, increased biting frequency, and longer survival [88]. Deforestation results in an increased ambient temperature and temperature affects sporogonic development of *P. falciparum* in anophelines by altering kinetics of ookinete maturation [84].

In the past, African highlands (elevation >1,500 m above sea level) were considered low risk for malaria, but there have been reemergence of epidemic malaria in East Africa highlands [89]. Increase in malaria transmission at these high altitudes may be related to a combination of factors: climate change, deforestation, changes in land forms or configuration, surface water, land use, and drug resistance. Malaria transmission in the highlands can be intense, but it is variable with the season (greatest after the rainy season) and the distance from major mosquito breeding habitats in nearby valleys or lowlands [90].

Conhuct et al. [91] hypothesized that the competence and vectorial capacity of *Anopheles* to transmit malaria is the result of constant evolution of mosquitoes due to selection pressures exerted by the parasites (*Plasmodium*), in relationships to adaptation to humans and the changing environment (see Fig. 6.2). This results in the parasites shaping the vector to its benefit – increasing its longevity, shortening the duration of sporogonic development, honing its specialization on feeding on humans, and immune evolution. Evidence to support the theory that *Plasmodium* parasite can modify the behavior of the mosquito host includes the following: (1) vectors show a preference for biting gametocyte-infected humans [94] (2) and pregnant women (generally more heavily infected) [96], and (3) infected vectors are more aggressive toward humans [95].

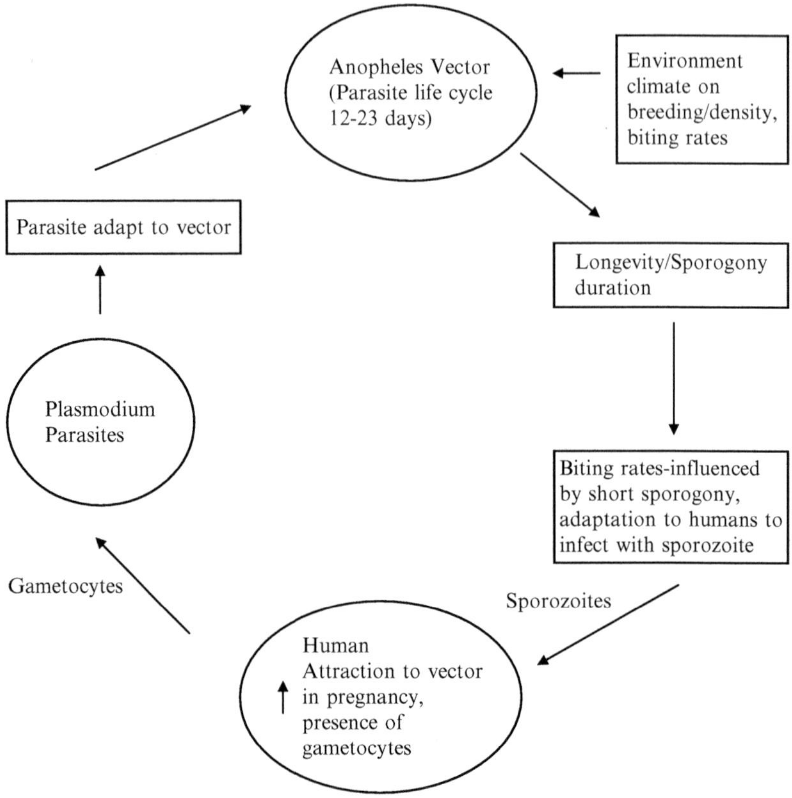

Fig. 6.2 Diagram of the interaction between vectors, parasites environment & humans of the vectorial capacity & competence of the mosquitoes (Derived from data obtained from Refs. [91–95])

6.9 Vector Resistance

Since the 1940s to current times and in the foreseeable future, mosquito vector control with insecticides has and will continue to play a major role in the battle against malaria. Vector control is still considered the mainstay of malaria control programs worldwide.

Africa remains the main focus of WHO malaria control renewed program, and insecticide resistance threatens malaria control in Africa. The main vector *A. gambiae* has developed increasing resistance to DDT and pyrethroids [97]. Control of *Anopheles* mosquitoes relies mainly on the use of pyrethroid-impregnated bednets and DDT residential spraying. A survey of insecticide resistance sponsored by the WHO reported on mosquito resistance to five insecticides (DDT, permethrin and deltamethrin [pyrethroids]; bendiocarb [carbamate]; and fenitrothion [organophosphate]) with discouraging results [97]. Although there were marked variations in resistance levels between sentinel sites (Angola, Burkina Faso, Benin, Chad, and Sudan), in some areas, pyrethroid resistance was found in 80% of vectors and DDT resistance in 70%. Most of the mosquitoes surveyed were susceptible to bendiocarb and fenitrothion, except in Burkina Faso and, to a lesser extent, Benin. In Ghana, the vector was found to be resistant to pyrethroids, the organochlorines, and the carbamates, but susceptible to organophosphates [98]. In Ethiopia, *A. arabiensis* is the primary vector, and genetic studies of 240 mosquito samples from 15 villages found the West African knockdown resistance mutation (61,014 F) in almost all specimens (98.5%), and bioassay confirmed high resistance to DDT and permethrin, but deltamethrin was still lethal in 82.2% of *A. gambiae* s.i [99].

Pyrethroid insecticide resistance in *A. gambiae* is mainly due to target site insensitivity arising from single point mutation, knockdown resistance (Kdr), but metabolic-based resistance has also been implicated in East Africa. This co-occurrence of both resistance mechanisms has been found in *A. gambiae* s.s. from Nigeria [100].

The insecticide resistance of mosquitoes detected by genetic studies and bioassay appears to reflect clinical experience. In a recently published study from Senegal, a longitudinal prospective evaluation of long-lasting insecticidal nets, LLINS (impregnated with deltamethrin), was performed in villages between January 2007 and December 2010 [101]. The incidence density of malaria attacks before distribution of LLINS was 5.45 per 100 person-months, and this declined to 0.41 per 100 person-months for the first 2.5 years. However, by the latter part of 2010, the incidence density of malaria increased back to 4.59 per 100 person-months, just 27–30 months after distribution of the insecticide-impregnated bednets [101]. Thirty-seven percent of *A. gambiae* mosquitoes were resistant to deltamethrin in 2010, and the presence of Leu1014Pho Kdr resistance mutation increased from 8% in 2007 to 48% in 2010.

There are currently several logistical factors that have hampered the progress in vector control in Africa: financial and manpower resources to implement interventions, and universal access to bednets is far from being achieved; lack of communication between researchers and the countries' malaria control programs; inadequate facilities for monitoring and testing of batches of bednets before distribution, to guard against vector resistance due to inadequate insecticide concentration; and lack of communication between the health and agriculture departments, to ensure that farmers and malaria programs use different insecticides for each sector to prevent cross-resistance [102].

6.10 Facing the Challenge

The greatest challenges to malaria conquest and control can be summarized under the two main categories: (1) prevention which has largely centered on vector control but should include development of an effective and inexpensive vaccine and (2) rapidly effective treatment and diagnosis which has been hampered by drug-resistant parasites.

To meet the challenge of insecticide-resistant vectors and to attain adequate prevention of malaria, it is essential to understand the mechanisms of resistance, the entomological and epidemiological impact, and to regularly monitor the development and spread of insecticide resistance. There are two major mechanisms associated with resistance: changes in the insecticide target sites that reduce its binding and increase in the rate of insecticide metabolism that lowers the active compound reaching the target site [103]. Target site resistance is fairly well understood, and molecular diagnostics are integrated into resistance monitoring by malaria control programs. The pyrethroid and organochlorine (DDT) insecticides target the voltage-gated sodium channel on the insects' neurons [103]. Mutations in genes associated with target sites are usually labeled as knockdown resistance (Kdr), and several mutations in the sodium channel have been associated with resistance to pyrethroids, especially amino acid substitutions at codon 1014. It is unclear, however, whether Kdr mutations alone can result in control failure of pyrethroids and DDT [104].

Metabolic resistance is more complex and key enzymes responsible for detoxification have been identified. The cytochrome P450s are the primary enzymes responsible for pyrethroid metabolism in insects, and these P450 genes have been overexpressed in resistant *A. gambiae* mosquitoes. Since establishment of the Innovative Vector Control Consortum in 2005, several promising chemicals are being evaluated in field trials [105]. However, based on the history of evolution of insecticide resistance, we can expect even resistance to these agents in the future. Thus, for future directions it is imperative for investigators to assess the effect on combination of residual insecticides and include noninsecticidal methods for vector control.

Preliminary field trials on limited scale have identified several promising insecticide agents such as HCTELLIC5oE, pirimiphos methyl (an emulsifiable organophosphate) [98], chlorfenapyr (novel mode of action) [106], chlorpyrifos-methyl [107] and insecticide paint Inesfly5A IGR, containing 2 organophosphates (chlorpyrifos and diazinon), and an insect growth regular (pyriproxyfen) [108]. These limited trials demonstrated efficacy against multiresistant vectors with new agents, but it is likely a matter of course before the mosquitoes develop mutations to resist these new chemicals.

The use of "two-in-one" bednets, impregnated with two chemicals of different structure and mechanism of action, may become the standard in the future to delay the spread of insecticide resistance. In one study, a mixture of insect repellant (DEET or KBR) and organophosphate insecticide showed promising results in an area of mosquitoes with multiple insecticide resistance [109].

A previous model of combining zooprophylaxis (using cattle to attract vectors and act as a dead-end host) and insecticide spraying, assessed as useful to control insecticide resistance several years ago [110], have not been adequately tested in field trials. Other novel method to counter insecticide resistance is the use of enteropathogenic fungi (*Beauveria bassiana* or *Metarhizium anisopliae*) to infect mosquitoes to reduce their survival [111]. The feasibility of disseminating fungal bioinsecticide over large geographical forested areas would be challenging.

Some investigators speculate that it may not be possible to eradicate malaria without modifying the mosquitoes [86]. Much of the research in this area has been focused on the dengue vector mosquitoes (*Aedes aegypti*), which is largely an urban vector. Significant advances have been made in the generation of genetically modified mosquitoes that are unable to transmit disease. Progress in this area was made possible by determination of the full length genomic sequences of *A. gambiae* in 2002 and *A. aegypti* in 2007. The genetic modification of *Anopheles stephensi* mosquitoes (the main vector for *P. falciparum* in the Indian subcontinent) has been achieved [112]. Laboratory-based study has produced genetically engineered *A. aegypti* (OX3604C strain) male mosquitoes to mate with wild-type female mosquitoes to produce a flightless female phenotype (effectively lethal) by transgenic mosquitoes carrying a dominant lethal gene [113]. Oxitec, the British biotechnology company, has developed transgenic "sterile" male *A. aegypti* mosquitoes that pass a lethal genetic element to their offsprings and has already conducted trials in the Cayman Islands in 2009/2010 [114]. Field trials in Grand Cayman showed transgenic mosquitoes can survive the wild and mate with wild-type females; results of a large release of transgenic mosquitoes showed about 80% reduction in the numbers of wild mosquitoes about 11 weeks after release [115]. Using sterile insect technique is not unique and has been commonly used in agriculture to control insects by rendering males sterile by radiation.

Some scientists are concerned about unique biosafety issues with release of genetically modified mosquitoes without specific guidelines. Biological innovations with the lowest ecological risks by using natural symbionts, intracellular insect bacteria, have been proposed to be the least harmful alternative. One promising approach that has been used extensively in fruit fly control is *Wolbachia* symbionts. *Wolbachia pipientis* is an intracellular host population, and embryo from *Wolbachia*-uninfected females die when they mate with infected males. *Wolbachia* infection of wild insect population can affect transmission of pathogens by reducing insect lifespan and reducing the insects' ability to combat viruses and other pathogens. *Wolbachia* has been successfully introduced into *A. aegypti* mosquitoes' natural population in Australia in an attempt to suppress dengue transmission [116]. Even if these innovations prove to be successful in controlling transmission of dengue infection, it would be more daunting to achieve success against the malaria vector, which is more widely distributed in and around more wooded or forested areas. However, field trials with these methods should be conducted with *Anopheles* species in malaria-endemic areas.

6.11 Malaria Vaccine

There is substantial data indicating that previous malaria infection produces partial immunity and that parasite multiplication rates during the initial prepatent period in semi-immune individuals are substantially lower than in malaria-naïve subjects [117].

These findings support development of a blood-stage vaccine that may abort clinical illness. However, for a highly effective vaccine to eliminate malaria, it would have to do better than natural infection. Currently, most of the research of malaria vaccines has focused on *P. falciparum* because of its clinical severity. Natural acquired immunity to malaria is not fully understood; it is slow to develop and wanes with time (short-lived) unless there is repeated exposure [118]. Although there is evidence of the presence of memory B cells which boost antibody response to reinfection, there appears to be low frequencies of malaria-specific memory B cells in children exposed to *P. falciparum*, and they may fail to boost antibody response after repeat exposure and after initial good response.

An effective vaccine that would prevent malaria transmission theoretically could be developed to target the two main transmission stages of the malaria cycle in humans. A preerythrocytic stage vaccine to induce immune responses against sporozoites inoculated into the blood stream, and/or infected hepatocytes to prevent development of schizonts in the liver. This early stage of infection lasts only a few days (5–6 days), and for immune response to be protective, specific CD4+ and CD4+ memory cells need to be maintained at high frequencies just before the next mosquito bite to generate enough effector killer cells rapidly [118]. A preerythrocyte stage vaccine based on radiation-attenuated *P. falciparum* sporozoites has been developed (*Sanaria* Pf5PZ vaccine) which, in volunteers, provides protection of >90% against malaria for ≥10 months [119]. However, the main challenge will be the logistics of delivering the vaccine in the field, as the vaccine is administered via bites of mosquitoes carrying the attenuated sporozoites. Another preerythrocytic vaccine in development RTSS (GlaxoSmithKline Biologicals) is an adjuvant recombinant vaccine that targets the circumsporozoite protein of the parasite in the liver. Phase 1/2 trials in children and infants of malarious areas have reported good safety with about 66% efficacy against new infection [120]. Over a 45-month surveillance period, children (aged 1–4 years) receiving this vaccine had a 34% lower prevalence of *P. falciparum* compared to controls [121]. A potential drawback of these vaccines targeting the preerythrocyte stage is that they reduce the exposure to the blood-stage merozoite antigen and may result in reduced immunity to malaria in the long term; as prospective immuno-epidemiological studies demonstrate that antibodies to merozoite antigen prevents invasion of erythrocytes. However, in a recent trial of the RTSS/ASO1E vaccine, anti-merozoite antigen-antibody concentration was induced in young children after vaccination, but these antibodies were not correlates of clinical immunity to malaria [122]. However, a recent phase 3 trial of RTS_1S/AS01 conducted in seven African countries, the first 6,000 children (5–17 months of age) receiving three vaccine doses, showed a vaccine efficiency of 55% against clinical malaria within 14 months after the first dose [123].

A transmission-blocking vaccine (TBV) is the second approach to target the sexual stages of the parasites (gametocytes and gametes) and/or the mosquito stages of the parasites (zygotes and ookinetes) could be effective in eliminating the infection but would not prevent disease in infected subjects or vaccinees. One such vaccine targeted the surface proteins of both *P. falciparum* and *P. vivax* mosquito stages (25 kDa protein of the fertilized zygote in the mosquito midgut) [124].

Weak immune responses in volunteers resulted in combining the antigen with an adjuvant. However, although initial results showed some volunteers produced antibodies that could block 90% of oocyst development in mosquitoes, the study was terminated due to development of severe reactions in two participants [124]. Ongoing research on other candidate vaccines targeting other proteins in the sexual stage is still being investigated.

A promising candidate vaccine being developed is to target a mosquito protein in the insects' gut [125]. Binding of the gut protein would impede development of the parasite, and would be effective against several strains of *Plasmodium.* Antibodies generated in rabbits by vaccination with the antigen (AnPPN1) have shown exciting results by blocking development of *P. vivax* in mosquitoes by 98% and completely blood *P. falciparum* development in mosquitoes in Cameroon [125]. Although the individual vaccinees would not benefit from these TBV, trials could be performed in several dozen communities/villages with similar rates of malaria transmission in controlled design to prove efficacy in the field. An ideal vaccine would be a multicomponent candidate combining components of a TBV with preerythrocytic vaccine such as the RTSS.

Blood-stage vaccines are difficult to develop because of antigenic diversity, high parasitic load at this stage, and evasive mechanisms developed by parasites against host responses [73]. Although merozoite antigens have been considered as prime vaccine candidates, no blood-stage vaccine has shown any success. A recent trial of a blood-stage vaccine (FMP2.1/AS02A) in a randomized, blinded study in 400 Malian children failed to provide clinical protection against malaria [126].

6.12 Challenges to Curb Drug Resistance

Rapid diagnosis and effective treatment of clinical malaria are key components in the campaign to eradicate malaria. A rapid and reliable parasitological diagnosis of severe malaria is essential for appropriate life-saving treatment, but overtreatment of febrile illnesses not due to malaria may lead to drug resistance. It is a common practice in many malaria-endemic regions, where proper diagnostic facilities (good microscopy of stained blood smears) are unavailable, for practitioners or patients to self-treat as presumptive malaria often with readily available over-the-counter medications. The use of empiric treatment for malaria in severe febrile undiagnosed conditions probably plays a role in the evolution of malaria drug resistance, but this aspect has not been properly evaluated and accurate data would be difficult to obtain. Malaria rapid diagnostic tests (RDTs) are now available in many endemic countries and do not require extensive training or expensive well-maintained equipment. These RDTs are immunochromatographic tests that identify malaria antigens (*P. falciparum* histidine-rich protein 2 (PfHRP2) or *Plasmodium* lactate dehydrogenase (PLDH)) but provide only qualitative information [127].

Although malaria RDTs can be used for both uncomplicated and severe malaria, the sensitivity of these tests are relatively low for parasite count < 1,000 parasites/uL

(46–70%) [128]. However, both the PfHRP2- and PLDH-based tests are more sensitive than expert microscopy in a comparative study with somewhat lower (PfHRP2) or similar specificity (PLHD) [128].

Other disadvantages of these RDTs are some of the PLDH-based tests are heat-sensitive, and in general, they can only be performed in a hospital or health-care-based laboratory. Future developments should focus on a rapid dipstick blood tests (similar to the Chemstrip used for urinalysis), which can provide prompt diagnosis in the field or remote areas.

Since the report of artemisinin-resistant malaria from the Thai-Myanmar border and in a province of Vietnam, the WHO launched a plan to stop artemisinin-resistant malaria spreading from Southeast Asia to Africa [129]. Besides some $3 billion spent annually to control malaria, it is estimated that an extra $175 million a year will be required to prevent the global spread of artemisinin-resistant parasites [129]. Intensification of existing programs to decrease malaria transmission will also be deployed, such as increasing the availability and use of insecticide-treated nets, screening and treatment of migrants, and updating more accurate boundaries of the resistant parasites.

Currently, there is no alternative drug available to replace artemisinin-derivatives, and new antimalarials with unique mechanisms of action are urgently needed. Scientists have identified several candidates of natural and synthetic origin to be used in combinations that are being evaluated for efficacy against multidrug-resistant *Plasmodium*. Various parasitic pathways and targets identified for development of novel antimalarials include the purine salvage pathway, pyrimidine biosynthesis pathway, the apicoplast organelle, and the proteases necessary for liver stage development [73, 130]. The apicoplast is essential for lipid, heme, and isoprenoid synthesis, with potentially several drug targets for development [73]. Since the apicoplast is maintained through the parasite life cycle, drugs targeting this organelle may act at both the liver phase and blood stages. It should be noted, however, that the development of a drug to marketing takes several years (average ≥10 years) and costs hundreds of millions of dollars.

A promising fully synthetic trioxolane drug (arterolane) already in phase II trials appears to be more potent than artemisinin and rapidly plasmocidal, may not be effective for artemisinin-resistant malaria [131]. As the mechanism of action is similar, a pharmacophoric peroxide molecule and cross-resistance would likely occur. Other novel chemotherapeutic approaches would include utilization of existing drugs to reverse drug resistance in malaria. The main focus has been on chloroquine resistance reversal agents. Several compounds from different pharmacologic classes have demonstrated the capability of reversing quinolone resistance in vitro, in animal models, and in human malaria parasites [132].

These chloroquine resistance reversal agents include calcium channel blockers, tricyclic antidepressants, antipsychotic calmodulin antagonists, histamine H1-receptor antagonists, xanthines, and others [132]. However, clinical experience with these agents as chloroquine resistance reverser is lacking, and most of the data is based on in vitro studies and limited animal experiments [133].

Despite previous widespread chloroquine-resistant *P. falciparum*, there is renewed interest in using this drug in higher doses or combined with artemisinin. After removal of chloroquine for a decade in Malawi, there is now evidence of restored efficacy of chloroquine for treatment of falciparum malaria [134]. Moreover, resistance to chloroquine may be relative rather than absolute as higher doses (2–3 times usual dose) may be effective for treatment of falciparum malaria in chloroquine-resistant malaria areas [135]. In a recently reported randomized trial from West Africa (Guinea-Bissau), 378 children (6 months–15 years of age) with falciparum malaria were randomized to artemether-lumefantrine or double dose of chloroquine (50 mg/kg), given as 6 doses over 3 days, and results of efficacy at 42 days were similar, 97 vs. 94%, respectively [136]. Parasites with resistance associated pfcrt 76 T allele treated with chloroquine were cleared in 87% at day 28. Moreover, the higher dose of chloroquine was well tolerated. There is a good probability and real concern, however, that reintroduction of chloroquine (at even higher doses) for widespread use will result in the malaria parasite evolution to greater degrees of chloroquine resistance, especially for monotherapy. Clearly, trials with high-dose chloroquine-artemisinin combination are urgently needed in the Myanmar-Cambodia-Thailand border regions.

A global profile of new antimalarial agents under development in 2009 by Olliaro and Wells [137] indicated that the pipeline of new antimalarial drugs was strong with 21 projects underway or planned. Six of the new combination medicines in phase III or registration stages included five artemisinin combinations and one non-ACT combination, azithromycin 250 mg/chloroquine 150 mg. The latter fixed combination (4 tablets daily) is targeted for new treatment in early stages of pregnancy and appears to be effective even when chloroquine resistance is high [137], indicating synergistic effect despite relatively low activity of the individual components. It was estimated that about 300 million treatments for malaria was needed annually, and almost 100 million ACT treatments were used annually of which 75% was in the fixed combination of artemether-lumefantrine (Cortem, Riamet) and the remaining 25% as artesunate-amodiaquine (to be available as a fixed combination from Sanofi-Aventis). The principle behind the pharmacodynamics of the mismatch combination (artemisinins having much shorter half-life than their companion drugs) is that the rapid onset of action of the artemisinins quickly reduces the parasitic load, and the longer-acting drug would eliminate the remaining few parasites and minimize the risk of selecting resistant organisms [138]. The relative resistance of *P. falciparum* documented along the Cambodia-Thailand border, results in delayed clearance of the parasites (from less than 2 days for artemisinin-sensitive parasites to 3–4 days for resistant parasites). This delayed clearance would lead not only to high-level resistance to artemisinins but enhanced risk of developing resistance to the longer-acting companion drugs.

It is evident that in order to curb the spread of artemisinin resistance, immediate information is needed on the extent of resistance beyond the Cambodia-Thailand border region. If resistance is confined to this limited area, then targeting elimination of *P. falciparum* from this region may be the only way to prevent artemisinin resistance from spreading [139]. However, current barriers to achieving this goal must be overcome, and these challenges have been summarized recently by Dondorp et al. [140]. Currently, a full understanding of the mechanism of artemisinin resistance and reliable in vitro tests to detect resistance is unavailable. In vitro tests assessing inhibition of ring-stage parasites appear promising to detect resistance, as the ring-stage parasites may be the phase of artemisinin resistance rather than the trophozoite or schizont stages [141]. Identification of a suitable and reliable molecular marker of artemisinin resistance is urgently needed to facilitate standardized rapid surveillance studies. The WHO's global plan for artemisinin resistance containment [142] may facilitate the discovery of markers of resistance through stimulation of genome-wide association studies. Conventional malaria control measures such as bednets and insect spraying may not be very effective in the Cambodia-Thailand border regions due to the migratory population and forest-dwelling mosquitoes. This fact places greater reliance on drug treatment for containment or elimination, including regional mass-drug administration campaigns and screening and treatment of parasitemic persons [140], which would be a daunting challenge and may predispose to greater risk of drug resistance due to high drug exposure. Primaquine, as a gametocidal agent, although could be used theoretically to prevent transmission, is limited by its toxicity in G6PD deficient subjects, and safer gametocidal agents are urgently needed. Other measures suggested by these experts [140] include actions to remove artemisinin-based monotherapies from the market, elimination of counterfeit or falsified antimalarial drugs from the open market, monitoring drug quality, coordination of research and containment efforts globally, and sharing of data, research tools, and experiences. Currently, WHO national authorities, drug companies, academic groups, the United States Pharmacopeia, and Interpol are collaborating on these actions.

6.13 Conclusion

There are major challenges still ahead for realizing the goal of global elimination or even partial elimination of malaria. There is a sense of urgency voiced by the experts in the field that halting the spread and elimination of artemisinin-resistant *P. falciparum* in the Cambodia-Thailand border as soon as possible is critical to achieve this goal. It is clear that coordinated global efforts through the auspices of the WHO and private organizations (such as the Bill and Melinda Gates Foundation) are essential in the fight against malaria.

Although research and development are crucial to provide new drugs to counteract drug-resistant malaria, these measures have to be combined with efforts to contain the vector – mosquitoes to achieve eradication. However, these efforts alone may not be sufficient, and just as important are the political will and social measures in endemic countries, with adequate funding. Resource-poor countries carry the global burden of malaria, especially in Africa, and these countries face numerous challenges besides infectious diseases (such as AIDS, tuberculosis, diarrheal diseases, etc.) including poverty, war and strife, famine, lack of sanitation and clean water, endemic malnutrition, inadequate shelter, and lack of proper social and health infrastructures.

Models for ranking elimination feasibility between malaria-endemic countries (using spatial data of shared technical and operational factors that enable some countries to eliminate malaria) have concluded that malaria elimination is most feasible in countries in the Americas and Asia and least feasible in countries in central and west Africa [143].

References

1. Kappe SH, Vaughan AM, Boddey JA, Cowman AF (2010) This was then but this is now: malaria research in the time of an eradication agenda. Science 328:862–866
2. Snow RW, Guerra CA, Noor AM, Mywit HY, Hay ST (2005) The global distribution of clinical episodes of *Plasmodium falciparum* malaria. Nature 434:214–217
3. Feachem RG, Philips AA, Hwang J et al (2010) Shrinking the malaria map: progress and prospects. Lancet 376:566–578
4. Schreiber W, Mathys FK (1987) Malaria. In: Infectio. Infectious Diseases in the history of medicine. Hoffman La Roche & Co. Ltd, Basle, pp 213–223
5. Zucker JR (1996) Changing patterns of autochthonous malaria transmission in the United States: a review of recent outbreaks. Emerg Infect Dis 2:37–43
6. Rich S, Ayala FJ (2006) Evolutionary origins of human malaria parasites. In: Dronamraju KR, Arese P (eds) Malaria: Genetic and evolutionary aspects. Springer, New York, pp 125–146
7. Sherman IW (ed) (1998) A brief history of malaria and the discovery of the parasites life cycle. In: Malaria: parasite biology, pathogenesis and protection. American Society of Microbiology, Washington, DC, pp 3–10
8. Miller RL, Ikram S, Armelagos GI et al (1994) Diagnosis of *Plasmodium falciparum* infections in mummies using the rapid manual Parasight™ – F test. Trans R Soc Trop Med Hyg 88:31–32
9. Cox-Singh J, Davis TM, Lee KS et al (2008) *Plasmodium knowlesi* malaria in humans is widely distributed and potentially life threatening. Clin Infect Dis 46:165–171
10. Putaporntip C, Hongsrimuang T, Seethamchai S, Kobasa T, Limkittikul K, Cui L, Jongwatiwes S (2009) Differential prevalence of Plasmodium infections and cryptic *Plasmodium knowlesi* malaria in humans. J Infect Dis 199:1143–1150
11. Price RN, Tjitra E, Guerra CA, Yeung S, White NJ, Anstey NM (2007) Vivax Malaria: Neglected and not benign. Am J Trop Med Hyg 77(6 suppl):79–87
12. Hay SI, Guerra CA, Tatem AJ, Noor AM, Snow RW (2004) The global distribution and population at risk of malaria; past, present and future. Lancet Infect Dis 4:327–336
13. WHO (1999) Making a difference. The world health report 1999. Health Millions 25:3–5
14. Brito I (2001) Eradicating Malaria: high hopes or a tangible goal? Health Policy Harv 2:61–66
15. Roberts DR, Manguin S, Moucher J (2000) DDT house spraying and re-emerging malaria. Lancet Infect Dis 356:330–332
16. Greenwood BM, Fidock DA, Kyle DE, Kappe SH, Alonso PL, Collings FH, Duffy PE (2008) Malaria: progress, perils and prospects for eradication. J Clin Invest 118:1266–1276
17. Wellems TE, Plowe CV (2001) Chloroquine resistant malaria. J Infect Dis 184:770–776
18. Trape JF, Pison G, Preziozi MP et al (1998) Impact of chloroquine resistance on malaria mortality. C R Acad Sci III 32:689–697

19. WHO (2004) The Abija declaration and the plan of action. An extract from the African Summit on Roll Back Malaria, Abija, 25 Apr 2000 (WHO/CDS/RBM/2000.17). http://www.rollbackmalaria.org/docs/abija_declaration_final.htm
20. Sachs JD, McArthur JW (2005) The Millennium Project: a plan for meeting the Millennium Goals. Lancet 365:347–353
21. Global Fund to Fight AIDS, Tuberculosis and Malaria (2009) Commitments and disbursements. http://www.theglobalfund.org/en/commitmentsdisbusements/
22. Snow RW, March K (2010) Malaria in Africa: progress and prospects in the decade since the Abrija declaration. Lancet 376:137–139
23. Ceesay SJ, Casals-Pascual C, Erskine J et al (2008) Changes in Malaria indices between 1999 and 2007 in The Gambia: a retrospective analysis. Lancet 372:1545–1554
24. Kleinschmidt I, Schwadbe C, Benavente L et al (2009) Marked increase in child survival after four years of intensive malaria control. Am J Trop Med Hyg 80:882–888
25. O'Meara WP, Bejoin P, Mwangi TW et al (2008) Effect of a fall in Malaria transmission on morbidity and mortality in Kilifi, Kenya. Lancet 372:1555–1562
26. Enserink M (2010) Redrawing Africa's Malaria map (news). Science 328:842
27. Dundorp AM, Nosten F, Yi P et al (2009) Artemisinin resistance in *Plasmodium falciparum* malaria. N Engl J Med 361:455–467
28. Mehlotra RK, Zimmerman PA (2006) Resistance to antimalarials drugs: parasite and host genetic factors. In: Dronamraju KR, Arese P (eds) Malaria: genetic and evolutionary aspects. Springer, New York, pp 81–124
29. Yeung S, Van Damme W, Socheat D, White NJ, Mills A (2008) Access to artemisinin combination therapy for malaria in remote areas of Cambodia. Malar J 7:96
30. Roper C, Pearce R, Nair S, Sharp B, Nosten F, Anderson T (2004) Intercontinental spread of pyrimethamine-resistant malaria. Science 305:1124
31. Verdragger J (1986) Epidemiology of the emergence and spread of drug-resistant falciparum malaria in South East Asia and Australasia. J Trop Med Hyg 89:277–289
32. Cortese JF, Caraballo A, Contreras CE (2002) Origin and dissemination of *Plasmodium falciparum* drug mutations in South America. J Infect Dis 186:999–1006
33. Pickard AL, Wongsrichanalai C, Pinfied A et al (2003) Resistance to antimalarials in Southeast Asia and genetic polymorphisms in pfmdrl. Antimicob Agents Chemother 47:2418–2423
34. Cerutti CJR, Dunlacher RP, de Alencar FE et al (1999) In vivo efficacy of mefloquine for treatment of falciparum malaria in Brazil J. Infect Dis 180:2077–2080
35. Wichman O, Betschart B, Loscher T et al (2003) Prophylaxis failure due to probably mefloquine resistant *P. falciparum* from Tanzania. Acta Trop 86:63–65
36. Guerin PJ, Olliaro P, Nosten F et al (2002) Malaria: current status of control, diagnosis, treatment, and a proposed agenda for research and development. Lancet Infect Dis 2:569–578
37. Price RN, Douglas NM, Anstey NM (2009) New developments in *Plasmodium vivax* malaria: severe disease and the rise of chloroquine resistance. Curr Opin Infect Dis 22:430–435
38. Campbell CC (1991) Challenges facing antimalarial therapy in Africa. J Infect Dis 163:1207–1211
39. Bjorkman A, Phillips-Howard PA (1990) The epidemiology of drug-resistant malaria. Trans R Soc Trop Med Hyg 84:177–180
40. Wongsrichanalai C, Pickard AL, Wernsdorfer W, Meshnick SR (2002) Epidemiology of drug-resistant malaria. Lancet Infect Dis 2:209–218
41. Aramburu Guarda J, Ramal Asayag C, Witzig R (1999) Malaria reemergence in the Peruvian Amazon Region. Emerg Infect Dis 5:209–215
42. Gosling RD, Cairns ME, Chico RM, Chandramohan D (2010) Intermittent preventive treatment against malaria: an update. Expert Rev Anti Infect Ther 8:589–606
43. Peters W (1987) Resistance of Human Malaria I, III, and IV. In: Chemotherapy and drug resistance in malaria, 2nd edn. Academic Press, London, pp 543–568, 593–658, 659–786
44. Zalis MG, Pang L, Silveria MS, Milhous WK, Wirth DF (1998) Characterization of *Plasmodium falciparum* isolated from the Amazon region of Brazil: evidence for quinine resistance. Am J Trop Med Hyg 58:630–637

45. Jelinek T, Grobusch MP, Loscher T (2001) Patterns of *Plasmodium falciparum* drug resistance in nonimmune travelers to Africa. Eur J Clin Microbiol Infect Dis 20:284–286
46. Shanks GD (1994) The rise and fall of mefloquine as an antimalarial drug in Southeast Asia. Mil Med 159:275–281
47. Wongsrichanalai C, Sirichaisinthop J, Karwacki JJ, Congpuong K, Miller RS, Pang L, Thimassarn K (2001) Drug resistant malaria on the Thai-Myanmar and Thai-Cambodian borders. Southeast Asian J Trop Med Public Health 32:41–49
48. Wernsdorfer WH (1994) Epidemiology of drug resistance in malaria. Acta Trop 56:143–156
49. Looareesuwan S, Viravan C, Webster HK, Kyle DE, Hutchinson DR, Canfield CJ (1996) Clinical studies of atovaquone, alone or in combination with other antimalarial drugs for treatment of acute uncomplicated malaria in Thailand. Am J Trop Med Hyg 54:62–66
50. Muehlen M, Schreiber J, Ehrhardt S, Otchwenah R, Jelinek J, Bienzle U, Mockenkaupt FP (2004) Short communication: prevalence of mutations associated with resistance to atovaquone and to the antifolate effect of proguanil in *Plasmodium falciparum* isolates in Northern Ghana. Trop Med Int Health 9:361–363
51. Happi CT, Ghotosho GO, Folarin OA et al (2006) Confirmation of emergence of mutations associated with atovaquone-proguanil resistance in unexposed *Plasmodium falciparum* isolates from Africa. Malar J 5:82
52. Thimasarn K, Sirichaisinthop J, Vijaykadya S et al (1995) *In vivo* study of the response of *Plasmodium falciparum* to standard mefloquine/sulfadoxine/pyrimethamine (MSP) treatment among gem miners returning to Cambodia. Southeast Asia J Trop Med Public Health 26:204–212
53. Alker AP, Lim P, Sem R et al (2007) Pfmdr1 and *in vivo* resistance to artesunate-mefloquine in falciparum malaria on the Cambodian-Thai border. Am J Trop Med Hyg 76:641–647
54. Wongsrichanalai C, Meshnick SR (2008) Declining artesunate-mefloquine efficacy against falciparum malaria on the Cambodia-Thailand border. Emerg Infect Dis 14:716–719
55. Greenwood B, Marsh K, Snow R (1991) Why do some African children develop severe malaria? Parasitol Today 7:277–281
56. Hastings IM, D'Alessandro U (2000) Modeling a predictable disaster: The rise and spread of drug-resistant malaria. Parasitol Today 16:340–347
57. Molyneux DH, Floyd K, Barnish G, Feure EM (1999) Transmission control and drug resistance in malaria: a crucial interaction. Parasitol Today 15:238–240
58. Draper CG, Brubaker G, Geser A, Kilimali VA, Wernsdorfer WH (1985) Serial studies on the evolution of drug resistance in an area of East Africa, receiving intermittent chemosuppression. Bull World Health Organ 63:109–118
59. Watkins WM, Mosobo M (1993) Treatment of *Plasmodium falciparum* malaria with pyrimethamine-sulfadoxine: selective pressure for resistance is a function of long elimination half-life. Trans R Soc Trop Med Hyg 192:130–134
60. Stepniewska K, White NJ (2008) Pharmacokinetic determinant of selection for antimicrobial drug resistance. Antimicrob Agents Chemother 52:1589–1596
61. Djimde AA, Fofana B, Sagara I et al (2008) Efficacy, safety and selection of molecular markers of drug resistance by two ACTs in Mali. Am J Trop Med Hyg 78:455–461
62. Martensson A, Stromberg J, Sisowath C et al (2005) Efficacy of artesunate plus amodiaquine versus that of artemether-lumefantrine for the treatment of uncomplicated childhood *Plasmodium falciparum* malaria in Zanzibar Tanzania. Clin Infect Dis 41:1079–1086
63. White NJ, Stepniewska K, Barnes K, Price RN, Simpson J (2008) Simplified antimalarial therapeutic monitoring: using the 7-day drug level? Trends Parasitol 24:159–163
64. Simpson JA, Watkins ER, Rn P, Aarons L, Kyle DE, White NJ (2000) Mefloquine pharmacokinetic-pharmacodynamic models: implications for dosing and resistance. Antimicrob Agents Chemother 44:3414–3424
65. Kofoed PE, Lopez F, Johansson P, Sandstrom A, Hedegaard K, Aaby P, Rombo L (2002) Treatment of children with *Plasmodium falciparum* malaria with chloroquine in Guinea-Bissau. Am J Trop Med Hyg 67:28–31

66. Ursing J, Schmidt BA, Lebbad M, Kofoed PE, Dias F, Gill JP, Rombo L (1990) Chloroquine resistant *P. falciparum* prevalence is low and unchanged between 1990 and 2003 in Guinea-Bissan effect of high chloroquine dosage? Infect Genet Evol 7:555–561
67. Walliker D, Quakyi IA, Wellems TE et al (1987) Genetic analysis of the human malaria parasite *Plasmodium falciparum*. Science 236:1661–1666
68. Su X, Ferdig MT, Huang Y et al (1999) A genetic map and recombination parameters of the human malaria parasite *Plasmodium falciparum*. Science 286:1351–1353
69. Rathod PK, McErlean T, Lee PC (1997) Variations in frequencies of drug resistance in *Plasmodium falciparum*. Proc Natl Acad Sci U S A 94:9389–9393
70. Travassos MA, Laufer MK (2009) Resistance to antimalarial drugs: molecular, pharmacological and clinical considerations. Pediatr Res 65:64–70
71. Daily JP (2006) Antimicrobial drug therapy: the role of parasite biology and drug resistance. J Clin Pharmacol 46:1487–1497
72. Olliaro PL (2001) Mode of action and mechanisms of resistance for antimalarial drugs. Pharmacol Ther 89:207–219
73. Koppe SHI, Vaughan AM, Boddey JA, Cowman AF (2010) That was then, but this is now: malaria research in the time of an eradication agenda. Science 328:862–866
74. Eckstein-Ludwig U, Webb RJ, Van Goethem ID et al (2003) Artemisinins target the SERCA of *Plasmodium falciparum*. Nature 424:957–961
75. Bunwag D, Harinasuta T, Pinichpongse S, Suntharasami P (1980) Effect of primaquine on gametocytes of *Plasmodium falciparum* in Thailand. Lancet 2:91
76. Buckling A, Ranford-Cartwright LC, Miles A, Read AF (1999) Chloroquine increases *Plasmodium falciparum* gametocytogenesis *in vitro*. Parasitology 8(pt. 4):339–346
77. Kumar N, Zheng H (1990) Stage-specific gametocystocidal effect *in vitro* of the antimalaria drug qinghaosu on *Plasmodium falciparum*. Parasitol Res 76:214–218
78. Targett C, Drakeley C, Jawara M et al (2001) Artesunate reduces but does not prevent post-treatment transmission of *Plasmodium falciparum* to *Anopheles gambiae*. J Infect Dis 183:1254–1259
79. Wellens TE, Walker-Jonath A, Panton LJ (1991) Genetic mapping of the chloroquine resistance locus on *Plasmodium falciparum* chromosome 7. Proc Natl Acad Sci U S A 88:3382–3386
80. Fidock DA, Nomura T, Talley AK et al (2000) Mutations in the *P. falciparum* digestive vacuole transmembrane protein PfCRT and evidence for their role in chloroquine resistance. Mol Cell 6:861–871
81. Djimde A, Doumbo OK, Cortese JK et al (2001) A molecular marker for chloroquine-resistant falciparum malaria. N Engl J Med 344:257–263
82. Price RN, Uhlemann AC, Brockman A et al (2004) Mefloquine resistance in *Plasmodium falciparum* and increased pfmdr1 gene-copy number. Lancet 364:438–447
83. Nzila AM, Mberu EK, Sulo J et al (2000) Towards an understanding of the mechanism of pyrimethamine-sulfadoxine resistance in *Plasmodium falciparum*: genotyping of dihydrofolate reductase and dihydropteroate synthase of Kenyan parasites. Antimicrob Agents Chemother 44:991–996
84. Jambou R, Legrand E, Niang M et al (2005) Resistance of *Plasmodium falciparum* field isolates to *in vitro* artemether and point mutations of the SERCA-type PfATPase6. Lancet 366:1960–1963
85. Sharma VP (2006) Vector genetics in malaria control. In: Dronamraju KR, Arese P (eds) Malaria: genetic and evolutionary aspects. Springer, New York, pp 147–167
86. Miller LH, Peirce SK (2009) Perspective on malaria eradication: Is eradication possible without modifying the mosquito? J Infect Dis 200:1644–1645
87. Packard RA, Gadelha P (1994) A land filled with mosquitoes: Fred L. Soper, The Rockefeller Foundation, and the *Anopheles gambiae* invasion of Brazil. Parrasitologia 36:197–213
88. Afrane YA, Little TJ, Lawson BW, Githeko AK, Yan G (2008) Deforestation and vectorial capacity of *Anopheles gambiae* Giles mosquitoes in malaria transmission Kenya. Emerg Infect Dis 14:1533–1538

89. Githeco A, Clive S (2005) The history of malaria control in Africa: lessons learned and future perspectives. In: Ebi K, Smith J, Burton I (eds) Integration of public health with adaptation to climate change: lessons learned and new directions. Francis & Taylor, London
90. Munyekenye GO, Githeko AK, Zhou G, Mushinzimana E, Minakawa N, Yan G (2005) *Plasmodium falciparum* spatial analysis in Western Kenya highlands. Emerg Infect Dis 10:1571–1577
91. Cohuet A, Harris C, Robert V, Fontenille D (2009) Evolutionary forces on anopheles: what makes a malaria vector? Trends Parasitol 26:130–136
92. MacDonald G (1957) The epidemiology and control of malaria. Oxford University Press, Oxford
93. Noden BH, Kent MD, Beier JC (1995) The impact of variations in temperature on early *Plasmodium falciparum* development in *Anopheles stephensi*. Parasitology 111:539–545
94. Lacroix R, Mukabana WR, Gouagna LC, Koella JC (2005) Malaria infection increases attractiveness of humans to mosquitoes. PLoS Biol 3:e298
95. Koella JC, Sørensen FL, Anderson RA (1998) The malaria parasite, *Plasmodium falciparum* increases the frequency of multiple feeding of its mosquito vector, *Anopheles gambiae*. Proc Biol Sci 265:763–768
96. Ansell J, Hamilton KA, Pinder M, Walraven GEL, Lindsay SW (2002) Short-range attractiveness of pregnant women to *Anopheles gambiae* mosquitoes. Trans R Soc Trop Med Hyg 96:113–116
97. Baleta A (2009) Insecticide resistance threatens malaria control in Africa (news). Lancet 374:1581–1582
98. Fusein G, Ebsworth P, Jones S, Knight D (2011) The efficacy of ACTELLIC 50E, primiphos methyl for indoor residual spraying in Ahafo, Ghana: an area of high vector resistance to pyrethroids and organochlorines. J Med Entomol 48:437–440
99. Yewhalaw D, Bartel WV, Denis L, Cooseman M, Duchateau L, Speybroeck N (2010) First evidence of high knockdown resistance frequency in *Anopheles arabiensis* (Diptera; Cullicidae) from Ethiopia. Am J Trop Med Hyg 83:122–125
100. Awolola TS, Oduola OA, Strode C, Koekemoer LL, Brook B, Ranson H (2009) Evidence of multiple pyrethroid resistance mechanisms in the malaria vector *Anopheles gambiae* sensustricto from Nigeria. Trans R Soc Trop Med Hyg 103:1139–1145
101. Trape JF, Tall A, Diagne N et al (2011) Malaria morbidity and pyrethroid resistance after the introduction of insecticide-treated bednets and artemisinin-based combination therapies: a longitudinal study. Lancet Infect Dis 11(12):925–932, PMID;21856232
102. Baleta A (2009) Insecticide resistance threatens malaria control in Africa (Word Report). Lancet 374:1581–1582
103. Ranson H, N'Guessan R, Lines J, Moirouxa W, Nkuni Z, Corbel V (2011) Pyrethroid resistance in African anopheline mosquitoes: what are the implications for malaria control? Trends Parasitol 29:91–98
104. Donnelly MJ, Corbel V, Weetman D, Wilding CS, Williamson MS, Blair WC 4th (2009) Does Kdr genotype predict insecticide resistance phenotype in mosquitoes? Trends Parasitol 25:213–219
105. Hemingway J, Beaty BJ, Rowland M, Scott TW, Sharp BC (2006) The innovative vector control consortium: improved control of mosquito-borne diseases. Trends Parasitol 22:308–312
106. Raghavendra K, Barik TH, Sharma P, Bhatt RM, Srivastava HC, Srechhari U, Dash AP (2011) Chlorfenapyr: a new insecticide with novel mode of action can control pyrethroid resistant malaria vectors. Malar J 10:16
107. N'Guessan R, Boko P, Odjo A, Chabi J, Akogbeto M, Rowland M (2010) Control of pyrethroid and DDT resistant *Anopheles gambiae* by application of indoor residual spraying or mosquito nets treated with long-lasting organophosphate insecticide, chlorpyrifos-methyl. Malar J 9:44
108. Mosqueira B, Chabi J, Chandre F, Akogbeto M, Hougard JM, Carnevale P, Mas-Coma S (2010) Efficacy of an insecticide paint against malaria vectors and nuisance in West Africa – Part 2: field evaluation. Malar J 9:340–341

109. Pennetier C, Costantini C, Corbel V et al (2008) Mixture for controlling insecticide-resistant malaria vectors. Emerg Infect Dis 14:1707–1714
110. Kawaguchi I, Sasaki A, Mogi M (2004) Combining zooprophylaxis and insecticide spraying: a malaria control strategy limiting the development of insecticide resistance in vector mosquitoes. Proc R Soc Lond Ser B Biol Sci 271:301–309
111. Farenhorst M, Mouatcho JC, Kikonkie CK et al (2009) Fungal infection counters insecticide resistance in African malaria mosquitoes. Proc Natl Acad Sci U S A 106:17443–17447
112. Corby-Harris V, Drexler A, Watkins de Jong L et al (2010) Activation of Akt signaling reduces the prevalence and intensity of malaria parasite infection and lifespan in *Anopheles stephensi* mosquitoes. PLoS Pathog 6:e1001003
113. Wise de Valdez MR, Nimmo D, Betz J, Gong HF, James AA, Alphey L, Black WC IV (2011) Genetic elimination of dengue vector mosquitoes. Proc Natl Acad Sci U S A 108:4772–4775
114. Subbaraman N (2011) Science snipes at Oxitec Transgenic mosquito trial (News). Nat Biotechnol 29:9–11
115. Ostera GR, Gostin LO (2011) Biosafety concerns involving genetically modified mosquitoes to combat dengue in developing countries. JAMA 305:930–931
116. Hoffmann AA, Montgomery BL, Popovici J et al (2011) Successful establishment of Wolbachia in *Aedes* population to suppress dengue transmission. Nature 476:454–457
117. Douglas AD, Andrews L, Drapner SJ et al (2011) Substantially reduced prepatent parasite multiplication rates are associated with naturally acquired immunity to *Plasmodium falciparum*. J Infect Dis 203:1337–1340
118. Langhorne J, Ndungu FM, Sponaas AM, Marsh K (2008) Immunity to malaria: more questions than answers. Nat Immunol 9:725–732
119. Hoffman SL, Billingsley PF, James E et al (2010) Development of a metabolically active non-replicating sporozoite vaccine to prevent *Plasmodium falciparum* malaria. Hum Vaccin 6:97–106
120. Aponte JJ, Aide P, Renom M et al (2007) Safety of the RTS_1S/AS02D candidate malaria vaccine in infants living in a highly endemic area of Mozambique: a double blind randomized controlled phase I/IIb trial. Lancet 370:1543–1551
121. Sacarlal J, Aide P, Aponte JJ et al (2009) Long-term safety and efficacy of the RTS_1S/AS02A malaria vaccine in Mozambican children. J Infect Dis 200:329–336
122. Bejon P, Cook J, Bergmann-Leitner E et al (2011) Effect of the pre-erythrocytic candidate malaria vaccine RTS_1S/AS01E on blood stage immunity in young children. J Infect Dis 204:9–18
123. Agnandji ST, Lell B, Soulanoudjingar SS et al (2011) The RTS_1S clinical trials partnership. First results of phase 3 trial of RTS_1S/AS01 malaria vaccine in African children. N Engl J Med 365:1163–1175
124. Wu Y, Ellis RD, Shaffer D et al (2008) Phase I trial of malaria transmission blocking vaccine candidates Pfs25 and Pvus25 formulated with montanide ISA51. PLoS One 3:e2636
125. Vogel G (2010) The 'Do Unto Others' malaria vaccine (news). Science 328:847–848
126. Thera MA, Doumbo OK et al (2011) A field trial to assess a blood-stage malaria vaccine. N Engl J Med 365:1004–1131
127. World Health Organization (WHO) (2010) Malaria rapid diagnostic test performance. Results of a WHO product testing of malaria RDTs: round 2. WHO 2009, Geneva, Switzerland. Available at: http//www.finddiagnostics.org/resource-centre-reports-brochures/malaria-diagnostic-test-report-round2.html
128. Hendriksen ICE, Mtove G, Pedro AJ et al (2011) Evaluation of a PfHRP2 and a pLDH-based rapid diagnostic test for the diagnosis of severe malaria in 2 populations of African children. J Infect Dis 52:1100–1107
129. Nebehay S (2011) Drug-resistant malaria could spread fast: expert warns. Malaria. Reuters Health. 12 Jan 2011. http://www.reuters.com/assets/print
130. Choi SR, Mukherjee P, Avery MA (2008) The fight against resistant malaria: novel plasmodial targets and antimicrobial drugs. Curr Med Chem 15:161–171

131. Valechia N, Looareesuwan S, Mortensson A et al (2010) Artenolane, a new synthetic trioxolane for treatment of uncomplicated *Plasmodium falciparum* malaria: a phase II multicenter, randomized, dose-finding clinical trial. Clin Infect Dis 51:684–691
132. Henry M, Alibert S, Orlandi-Pradines E et al (2006) Chloroquine resistance reversal agents as promising antimicrobial drugs. Curr Drug Targets 7:935–948
133. Egan TJ, Kaschula CH (2007) Strategies to reverse drug resistance in malaria. Curr Opin Infect Dis 20:598–604
134. Laufer MK, Thesting PC, Eddington ND et al (2006) Return of chloroquine antimalarial efficacy in Malawi. N Engl J Med 355:1959–1966
135. Hand CC, Meshnick SR (2011) Is chloroquine making a comeback? J Infect Dis 203:11–12
136. Ursing J, Kofoed PE, Rodriques A, Blessborn D, Thoft-Nielsen R, Bjorkman A, Rombo L (2011) Similar efficacy and tolerability of double-dose chloroquine and artemether-lumefantrine for treatment of *Plasmodium falciparum* in Guinea-Bissau.: a randomized trial. J Infect Dis 203:109–116
137. Olliaro P, Wells TN (2009) The global portfolio of new antimalarial medicines under development. Clin Pharmacol Ther 85:584–595
138. White NJ, Olliaro PL (1996) Strategies for the prevention of antimalarial drug resistance: rationale for combination chemotherapy for malaria. Parasitol Today 12:399–401
139. Maude RJ, Pontavornpinyo W, Savalamba S et al (2009) The last man standing is the most resistant: eliminating artemisinin-resistant malaria in Cambodia. Malar J 8:31
140. Dondorp AM, Fairhurst RC, Slutsker L et al (2011) The threat of artemisinin-resistant malaria (perspective). N Engl J Med 365:1073–1075
141. Saralamba S, Pan-Ngum W, Maude RJ et al (2011) Intrahost modeling of artemisinin resistance in *Plasmodium falciparum*. Proc Natl Acad Sci U S A 108:397–402
142. WHO (2011) Global plan for artemisinin resistance containment. World Health Organization, Geneva.http://www.who.int/malaria/publication/atoz/artemisinin-resistance-containment-2011.pdf
143. Tatem AJ, Smith DL, Gething PW, Kabaria CW, Snow RW, Hay SI (2010) Ranking of elimination feasibility between malaria-endemic countries. Malaria elimination 2. Lancet 376:1579–1591

Chapter 7
Lymphatic Filariasis: Progress and Challenges in the Move Toward Elimination

Thomas B. Nutman

7.1 Introduction

Among the eight filarial species of humans (Table 7.1), three closely related parasitic nematodes (*Wuchereria bancrofti, Brugia malayi*, and *Brugia timori*) cause lymphatic filariasis (LF). Unlike most other helminthiases, the burden of infection and disease in lymphatic filariasis occurs primarily during adulthood where the cumulative effects of chronicity and infection intensity manifest themselves.

Because disease due to LF is characterized by disfigurement of the genitalia (hydroceles and other anatomical changes in the male genitalia) and the limbs (elephantiasis), LF has been shown to not only have medical consequences but also have significant economic and psychosexual effects. Indeed, lymphatic filariasis is among the leading health-related impediments to economic and social development worldwide [1, 2].

Lymphatic filariasis can be transmitted in any region of the world where the appropriate mosquito vector breeds. It currently is a significant health problem in tropical and subtropical Africa, Asia, the Indian subcontinent, many islands of the western and southern Pacific, and focal areas of Central and South America. In certain regions of the world the geographic distribution of *W. bancrofti* and *B. malayi* infections is expanding due to increased numbers of breeding sites that appear when large numbers of people migrate from rural to urban areas. These epidemiologic trends are counterbalanced by the recent gains and successes by the Global Program to Eliminate Lymphatic Filariasis using yearly single-dose administration of antifilarial chemotherapy [3].

T.B. Nutman, M.D. (✉)
Helminth Immunology Section, Laboratory of Parasitic Diseases, National Institute of Allergy and Infectious Diseases, Bethesda, MD 20892-0425, USA

Clinical Parasitology Section, National Institutes of Health, Bethesda, MD 20892-0425, USA
e-mail: tnutman@niaid.nih.gov

I.W. Fong (ed.), *Challenges in Infectious Diseases*, Emerging Infectious Diseases of the 21st Century 502, DOI 10.1007/978-1-4614-4496-1_7,

7.2 Current Epidemiology

It is estimated that 120 million people (in 72 countries) are infected with one of the three genera of lymphatic filariae [4]. Among those with LF, more than 90% of infections are due to *W. bancrofti*, and, of these, the greatest numbers are in sub-Saharan Africa, Southeast Asia, and the western Pacific. The infection is prevalent in India, Indonesia, the Philippines, Papua New Guinea, and several Pacific countries. Within Africa, *W. bancrofti* infection is not limited to tropical zones since endemic foci are found as far north as the Nile delta in Egypt and Sudan. In the Americas, endemic foci persist in several islands in the Caribbean (Haiti and the Dominican Republic) and coastal areas of South America (Brazil and Guyana). There are no animal reservoirs of *W. bancrofti.* As can be seen in Table 7.1, however, there is broad geographical overlap between *W. bancrofti* and many of the other non-lymphatic dwelling filarial parasites, with many countries in West and Central Africa being endemic for three or more different genera of filariae.

Infection with *B. malayi* is limited to Asia (China, India, and Malaysia) and several Pacific island groups (e.g., Indonesia and the Philippines). There are fewer than 10–20 million persons in these areas infected with *B. malayi*, infections that may coexist with *W. bancrofti. B. malayi* infection is a zoonosis in that there are feline and primate reservoirs.

B. timori infection is limited in its distribution to the islands comprising Timor-Leste.

Within a given geographic area, the distribution of lymphatic filariasis is highly focal. This heterogeneity of infection patterns, both locally and globally, is due in large part to the peculiarities of the ecological relationships among the mosquito vector, the human host, and the impact of filarial parasites on both. Unlike other common vector-borne infectious diseases of the tropics (e.g., malaria), several genera of mosquitoes are capable of transmitting lymphatic filariae. *W. bancrofti* is transmitted in many rural areas of Africa and the Pacific by *Anopheles* species [5]. The proximity of human dwellings to breeding sites increases the risk of repeated contact with mosquitoes bearing infective larvae. In many urban areas of the world, including India, *Culex* species is the major vector of *W. bancrofti* and *B. malayi* [6]. Unlike anopheline mosquitoes, larvae of these mosquitoes breed readily in small pools of water that form in discarded tires and cans. Other vectors include *Aedes aegypti* in some Pacific islands (e.g., Tahiti) and *Mansonia*, which transmits only *B. malayi.* These various genera of mosquitoes also differ in their efficiency of transmission. In general, anopheline mosquitoes are more efficient vectors of *W. bancrofti* than are culicine mosquitoes.

The pattern of infection increases gradually with age up until the third or fourth decade of life, after which it remains constant or decreases slightly. This epidemiologic pattern is related to the gradual slow accumulation of adult-stage worms over time. The proportion of the entire population or a specific age group with patent infection is remarkably variable in different endemic areas. In addition, there is remarkable variation in the frequency of various disease manifestations based on

Table 7.1 Filarial parasites of humans

Organism	Geographic distribution	Estimated number infected	Associated disease	Control programs[a]
Wuchereria bancrofti	South America, Caribbean, Africa, South Asia, Southeast Asia, Eastern Pacific	120 million	Lymphatic filariasis	Yes (MDA) Alb/Iver DEC/Alb
Brugia malayi	Southeast Asia, Indonesia, India	10 million	Lymphatic filariasis	Yes (MDA) DEC/Alb
Brugia timori	Indonesia, Timor-Leste	???	Lymphatic filariasis	Yes (MDA) DEC/Alb
Onchocerca volvulus	South and Central America, Africa	39 million	Onchocerciasis ("river blindness")	Yes (MDA) Iver
Loa loa	West and Central Africa	~10 million	Loiasis	No
Mansonella ozzardi	South and Central America, Caribbean	???	Mansonelliasis	No
Mansonella perstans	South and Central, America, Africa	???	Perstans filariasis	No
Mansonella streptocerca	West and Central Africa	???	Streptocerciasis	No

[a]MDA using annual dosing of ivermectin/albendazole (Alb/Iver) in Africa and diethylcarbamazine/albendazole (DEC/Alb) elsewhere for LF, annual dosing of ivermectin (Iver) for onchocerciasis

age and geographic area. Lymphatic disease, manifested by persistent lymphedema of the lower extremity or genital disease in males, is rare in children under the age of 10 and tends to increase gradually throughout life. Of the total 120 million persons estimated to be infected in all endemic areas, about one third have clinically overt disease. The likelihood of developing such manifestations appears to be particularly high in some areas of the world, such as India, Pacific islands such as Papua New Guinea, and in equatorial Africa, whereas it is considerably lower in the Caribbean and South America. Local transmission conditions may account for the striking heterogeneity of disease manifestations that may be observed within a given geographic area. Indeed the cumulative exposure to infective larvae may be an important risk factor for lymphatic pathology at the population level [7].

7.3 Biology

The existence of lymphatic filariasis has been recorded in ancient writings, but the causative agents and their life cycles were not described in detail until the late nineteenth century [8, 9]. The microfilariae of *W. bancrofti*, first discovered by Demarquay in hydrocele fluid from a patient in Cuba in 1863 [10], were later identified in the urine by Wucherer in 1868 [11] and in the blood by Lewis in 1872 [12]. Manson described the periodicity of microfilariae in the peripheral blood [13] and also demonstrated that mosquitoes transmit the parasite [14]. Bancroft was the first to describe the adult female worm [15], and the adult male worm was later described by Bourne [16]. Bancroft in 1899 [17] and Low in 1900 [18] established the mode of transmission of the parasite. Lichtenstein, Brug, and Buckley were primarily responsible for the identification of brugian parasites [19].

W. bancrofti, *B. malayi*, and *B. timori* are threadlike nematodes having five morphologically and molecularly distinct stages in their life cycle. Infective or third-stage larvae (L3) are transmitted to humans during blood feeding by mosquitoes. The organisms are deposited from the mouthparts of the mosquito in the vicinity of the skin puncture wound and make their way through the dermis to enter the local lymphatics. Infective larvae shed their cuticle and develop a new surface (a process referred to as molting) that presents novel antigens and other molecules to the mammalian host. These fourth-stage larvae migrate centrally in lymphatic vessels develop into sexually mature adult male or female worms over a 6–9-month period. Adult worms are considerably larger than larval stages (male worms are 20–40 mm in length, and female worms 40–100 mm) and have highly differentiated and complex reproductive and digestive systems. The adult stages of the parasite dwell primarily in the afferent lymphatics. Although each of the anatomical areas in which adult lymphatic filariae live in humans is not known with certainty, there is a predilection for the lymphatics of the lower extremities (inguinal and obturator groups), upper extremities (axillary lymph nodes), and, for *W. bancrofti*, the male genitalia (epididymis, spermatic cord, testicle). The mean life span of adult worms is estimated to be ~5 years.

Following insemination by male worms, fertilized adult female parasites release large numbers (often more than 10,000 per day) of embryonic forms or first-stage larvae (microfilariae). These microfilariae are distinguished by their small size (260 μm in length and approximately 10 μm in width). Microfilariae of the lymphatic filariae have an acellular sheath that is chitin-containing. *W. bancrofti* and *Brugia* microfilariae frequently have a nocturnal periodicity whereby the number present in the peripheral circulation peak at midnight. When absent from the peripheral circulation, microfilariae are believed to be sequestered in deep vascular beds of the lung and other organs. This periodicity represents an adaptation to local ecological conditions in that the time at which peak parasitemia occurs that often coincides with the time when the local mosquito vectors take their blood meal [20].

After ingestion in a blood meal taken by a female mosquito, microfilariae exsheath within 24 h, penetrate the gut wall of the mosquito, and migrate into the thoracic musculature. Over a period of 10 days to 2 weeks, the organisms mature to become third-stage larvae capable of infecting another human.

An important biologic feature of *W. bancrofti* and *Brugia* species relates to the presence in these nematodes of an obligate bacterial endosymbiont *Wolbachia*. Ultrastructure studies performed in the 1970s suggested the presence of intracellular bacteria in adult worms and microfilariae [21, 22], but it was not until the late 1990s when molecular tools became available that *Wolbachiae* were definitively identified in human filarial parasites [23, 24]. These endosymbiotic bacteria appear to effect filariae in several ways that are pertinent to human LF. Incubation of *Brugia* worms with tetracycline and other antibiotics known to kill *Wolbachia* diminishes the release of microfilariae and suppresses larval molting [25, 26]. In the context of human LF, administration of doxycycline to those with *W. bancrofti* or *B. malayi* infection has been shown to have macrofilaricidal activity [27–29].

7.4 Clinical Aspects

Infection with *W. bancrofti*, *B. malayi*, or *B. timori* can cause a wide variety of clinical manifestations, ranging from those without apparent clinical disease to those with lymphedema and/or severe disfigurement of the limbs and genitalia. From the clinical perspective, it should be stressed that there is a great deal of overlap in these symptom complexes, several of which may occur contemporaneously.

7.4.1 Subclinical Patent Infection

The overwhelming majority of filarial-infected people in endemic areas have few overt clinical manifestations of their filarial infection despite large numbers of circulating microfilariae in the peripheral blood [30]. Although they may be clinically asymptomatic, virtually all persons with patent *W. bancrofti* or *B. malayi* infection (microfilaria- and/or circulating filarial antigen-positive) have some degree of subclinical disease that includes microscopic hematuria and/or proteinuria [31], dilated (and tortuous) lymphatics (visualized by lymphoscintigraphy [32–34]), and, in men with *W. bancrofti* infection, scrotal lymphangiectasia (detectable by ultrasound) [35–37].

7.4.2 Acute Adenolymphangitis (ADL)

ADL is often the first manifestation of lymphatic filariasis. It is characterized by the sudden onset of high fever, painful lymph node and lymphatic inflammation (lymphangitis and lymphadenitis), and transient local edema. The lymphangitis is retrograde, extending peripherally from the lymph node draining the area where the adult parasites reside—the retrograde nature of the lymphadenitis distinguishes filarial-induced disease from bacterial-induced lymphangitis. Regional lymph nodes are often enlarged, and the entire lymphatic channel can become indurated and inflamed. Concomitant local thrombophlebitis can occur as well. In brugian filariasis, a single local abscess may form along the involved lymphatic tract and subsequently ulcerate. The lymphadenitis and lymphangitis can involve both the upper and lower extremities in both bancroftian and brugian filariasis, but involvement of the genital lymphatics occurs almost exclusively with *W. bancrofti* infection [38]. This genital involvement can be manifested by funiculitis (inflammation of the spermatic cord), epididymitis, scrotal pain, and tenderness, as well as a condition-termed lymph scrotum [39].

7.4.3 Dermatolymphangioadenitis

In endemic areas, another type of acute disease—dermatolymphangioadenitis (DLA) [40, 41]—is recognized as a syndrome that includes high fever, chills, myalgias, and headache. Edematous inflammatory plaques clearly demarcated from normal skin are seen. Vesicles, ulcers, and hyperpigmentation may also be noted. There is often a history of trauma, burns, radiation, insect bites, punctiform lesions, or chemical injury. Entry lesions, especially in the interdigital area, are common. DLA is often diagnosed as cellulitis.

7.4.4 Lymphedema of the Arms, Legs, and Breasts

Swelling of the upper or lower extremities is the most common chronic manifestation of lymphatic filarial infection. Disease of the lower extremities is more prevalent.

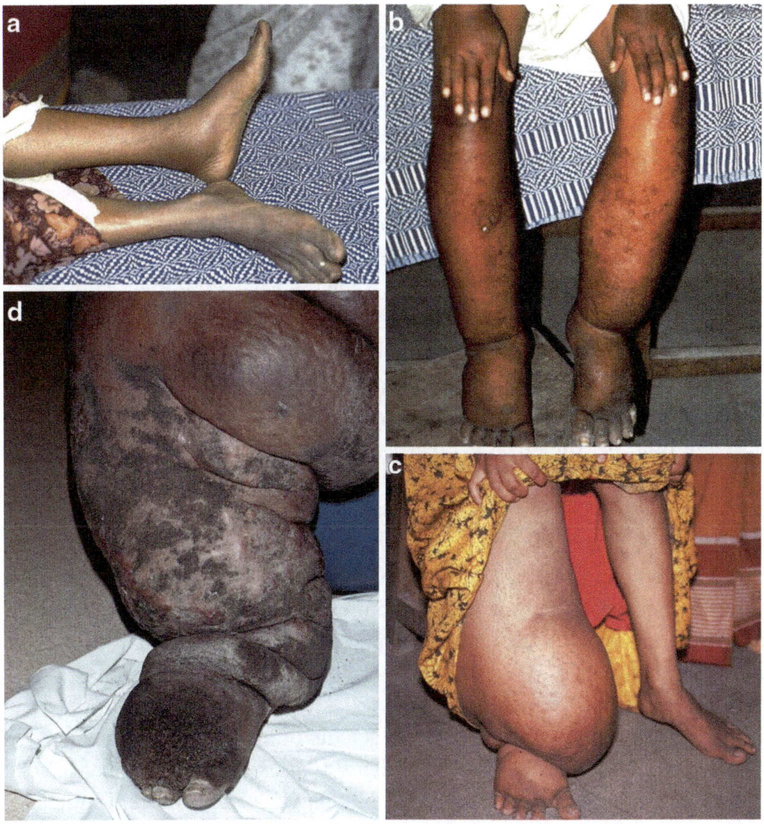

Fig. 7.1 The range of lymphedema of the lower extremities in its progression from reversible mild lymphedema (*Panel A*) to lymphedema with mild secondary changes (*Panel B*) to marked lymphedema with significant secondary changes (*Panel C*) to elephantiasis (*Panel D*)

Leg involvement in bancroftian filariasis may include the entire limb, whereas only the area below the knee is usually involved in brugian filariasis. The World Health Organization has developed a grading system to quantify the severity of involvement [42], and other grading schemes have also been proposed [43]. These range from pitting edema that is reversible to elephantiasis (Fig. 7.1). Although both lower extremities may be involved, asymmetry is the rule.

In some persons with filarial-associated edema, the overlying skin may exude serous fluid suggestive of lymph. Although it is possible that this sign occurs as a result of increased hydrostatic pressure in the lymphatics draining the skin, skin turgor alone cannot reliably be used to distinguish between edema due to lymphatic disease and that from other causes, such as cardiac failure and liver disease.

Unilateral or bilateral involvement of the female breast occurs in adult residents of filarial endemic areas. This should be distinguished from chronic mastitis and other causes of chronic breast inflammation.

7.4.5 Disease Involving the Genitourinary System

Along with lymphatic disease of the lower extremities, disease of the male genitalia is the most common manifestation of bancroftian filariasis. Indeed, in many endemic areas, its prevalence is greater than that of lymphedema. Genital involvement is uncommon in *Brugia* infection. The prevalence of disease of the female genitalia is not known. Anecdotal evidence suggests that the frequency of vulvar disfigurement is low.

Chronic disease of the male genitals mostly produces hydroceles, which vary in diameter from less than 5 to over 30 cm. As is the case with other causes of hydrocele, the scrotal contents appear translucent when transilluminated. Hydroceles are usually not painful unless they are complicated by acute epididymitis or funiculitis. Thickening of the spermatic cord commonly accompanies hydroceles. The skin of the scrotum may also be thickened and have a "brawny" character on palpation. If hydrocele fluid is drained, it is clear and straw colored. Parasites are usually not found in this fluid. Inguinal lymph nodes and other nearby lymph nodes may also be enlarged.

Swelling of the scrotum when accompanied by thickened scrotal or penile skin may have a characteristic "peau d'orange" appearance [38]. In long-standing cases, verrucous lesions and lymphorrhea are common [39], the latter being a condition in which lymph oozes out to the exterior directly from dilated ruptured lymphatic vessels in the scrotal wall.

Chyluria, resulting from obstruction or physiologic impairment of the renal lymphatics with passage of lymph from the lacteals draining the genitourinary tract, is a rare but serious manifestation of lymphatic filariasis. Chyluria may have serious nutritional consequences in that large amounts of fat and protein are lost in the urine. Its precise frequency in filarial endemic areas has not been established but is exceedingly low compared to lymphedema of the extremities and hydroceles [44].

7.4.6 Tropical Pulmonary Eosinophilia

Tropical pulmonary eosinophilia (TPE) is a distinct syndrome that develops in some individuals infected with either *W. bancrofti* or *B. malayi* [45, 46]. The majority of cases have been reported from India, Pakistan, Sri Lanka, Brazil, Guyana, and Southeast Asia. The main clinical features include paroxysmal cough and wheezing that are usually nocturnal (and probably related to the nocturnal periodicity of microfilariae), weight loss, low-grade fever, adenopathy, and pronounced blood eosinophilia (>3,000 eosinophils/μL). Tests of pulmonary function show restrictive abnormalities in most cases and obstructive defects in half. Chest radiographs often show increased bronchovascular markings. Total serum IgE levels (10,000–100,000 ng/mL) and antifilarial antibody titers are characteristically elevated. Typically those with TPE do not have microfilaremia. If patients with TPE are not treated appropriately, the disease may progress to chronic restrictive lung disease with interstitial fibrosis [47].

7.5 Present Treatment/New Developments

7.5.1 Drug Regimens

Diethylcarbamazine (DEC, 6 mg/kg daily for 12 days), which has both macro- and microfilaricidal properties, remains the treatment of choice for the individual with active lymphatic filariasis (microfilaremia, antigen positivity, or adult worms on ultrasound), although albendazole (400 mg twice daily for 21 days) has also demonstrated macrofilaricidal efficacy. The use of a 4–6-week course of doxycycline (targeting the intracellular *Wolbachia*) has also been demonstrated to have significant macrofilaricidal activity [28, 29] as has daily DEC/albendazole used for 7 days [48]. Adding diethylcarbamazine to a 3-week course of doxycycline has also been shown to be efficacious [27].

Regimens that utilize combinations of single doses of albendazole (400 mg) and either DEC (6 mg/kg) or ivermectin (200 μg/kg) have all been demonstrated to have a sustained microfilaricidal effect [49–52] and are the mainstay of control programs in Africa (albendazole/ivermectin) or elsewhere (albendazole/DEC) for the eradication of lymphatic filariasis (see below).

7.5.2 Morbidity Control

In persons with chronic manifestations of lymphatic filariasis, treatment regimens that emphasize hygiene, prevention of secondary bacterial infections, and physiotherapy have gained wide acceptance for morbidity control. These regimens are similar to those recommended for lymphedema of most non-filarial causes and are known by a variety of names, including *complex decongestive physiotherapy* and *complex lymphedema therapy*. Drainage of hydroceles provides immediate relief, though they recur in the absence of drug therapy or surgical removal of the *tunica albuginea*.

In severe cases of deforming elephantiasis, surgical approaches involving lymphatic-venous and nodal-venous anastomoses have been somewhat successful in diminishing the degree of leg swelling [53] as has reconstructive surgery for genital involvement. The long-term effects of these expert surgical techniques have not been determined.

7.6 Potential for Vaccines

Vaccines against filarial infections were felt to be a potential tool for their elimination and eradication for several different reasons. First, reinfection after chemotherapy occurs if transmission in ongoing. Secondly, there is the remote possibility of the emergence of drug resistance. Thirdly, control of the vectors involved in transmission (e.g., mosquitoes in lymphatic filarial parasites) has been difficult to achieve for both logistical and economic reasons; the emergence of pesticide resistance is also problematic. Thus, vaccination could ultimately provide the most efficacious way to both prevent parasitic disease and interrupt transmission. However, there are no currently available candidates in late preclinical testing.

With rapid advances in the parasite genomics and proteomics as well the newer, better vaccine delivery systems offering better and more rapid assessment development, prospects for newer antifilarial vaccines are possible, although the potential lack of commercial markets imposes a significant impediment to their development.

7.7 Advances in Control/Prevention

Individual protection against filarial infection may be achieved by avoiding contact with infected mosquitoes. This can be done by use of personal protective measures including bednets, particularly those impregnated with insecticides such as permethrin.

Created in 1997, the global program to eliminate lymphatic filariasis (GPELF) was based on mass drug administration (MDA) with single annual doses of diethylcarbamazine plus albendazole (non-African regions) or albendazole plus ivermectin in Africa [50, 54–58]. Information at the end of 2010 (halfway toward the elimination goals set for 2020) indicates that >695 million persons in 53 countries have thus far participated [4]. Not only has there been success in eliminating lymphatic filariasis in some defined areas, but also the collateral benefit in averting disability (estimated 32 million disability adjusted life years [DALYs] averted [56]) and treating intestinal helminths and other conditions (e.g., scabies, lice).

The strategy of the global program is being refined but has been set forth in a series of recent position statements and publications [59–65]. Moreover these strategies are being guided by ongoing research aimed at understanding the ecology and transmission efficiency of the various mosquito vector species and integration with other mass treatment strategies (e.g., deworming programs, malaria control, trachoma control) [66–73].

Reaching the two target goals—interruption of transmission through MDA and the reduction of suffering by the disease through morbidity control—of elimination of LF as a public health problem by 2020 has a number of major obstacles to overcome [64, 65, 73–80]. These include:

1. The failure to start MDA in 18 countries including 40% of LF-endemic countries in Africa
2. The presence of *Loa loa* in Central and West Africa that, because of potential life-threatening adverse reactions following MDA for LF, has precluded treatment with ivermectin
3. The lack of good endpoints to determine how to stop MDA and/or to verify that transmission has been interrupted

4. The relative paucity of disability management programs within LF-endemic countries
5. The reliance on a single strategy (MDA) for transmission interruption without addition of additional strategies (e.g., vector control)
6. The relative lack of integration with other control programs often ongoing within the same geographical area
7. The reliance on existing models to determine when to stop MDA.

7.8 Future

The march toward elimination of LF is at its halfway point, and it is certain that—like the several countries in which LF has already been eliminated—many more will have achieved elimination by the target date of 2020. Whether it be because of civil unrest, concomitant coinfections (particularly *Loa loa*), lack of political will or resources, or failure to integrate with other public health programs, there are likely to be countries or regions that may fail to meet this very ambitious target date. Nevertheless, the tremendous progress (both economic and health-related) made to date [81, 82] by the GPELF provides the most compelling argument in favor of overcoming whatever barriers that may exist to achieve the ambitious goals of elimination of LF.

References

1. Mathers CD, Ezzati M, Lopez AD (2007) Measuring the burden of neglected tropical diseases: the global burden of disease framework. PLoS Negl Trop Dis 1(2):e114
2. Haddix AC, Kestler A (2000) Lymphatic filariasis: economic aspects of the disease and programmes for its elimination. Trans R Soc Trop Med Hyg 94(6):592–593
3. Ottesen EA (2006) Lymphatic filariasis: treatment, control and elimination. Adv Parasitol 61:395–441
4. WHO (2011) Meeting of the international task force for disease eradication – October 2010. Wkly Epidemiol Rec 86(7):53–59
5. Bockarie M et al (1996) Transmission dynamics of *Wuchereria bancrofti* in East Sepik Province, Papua New Guinea. Am J Trop Med Hyg 54(6):577–581
6. Sasa M (1976) Human filariasis. University Park Press, Baltimore, pp 1–819
7. Kazura JW et al (1997) Transmission intensity and its relationship to infection and disease due to *Wuchereria bancrofti* in Papua New Guinea. J Infect Dis 176(1):242–246
8. Routh HB, Bhowmik KR (1993) History of elephantiasis. Int J Dermatol 32(12):913–916
9. Rajan TV (2000) Lymphatic filariasis: a historical perspective. In: Nutman TB (ed) Lymphatic filariasis, vol 1. Imperial College Press, London, pp 1–4
10. Demarquay J-N (1863) Helminthologie. Gazette Medicale de Paris 18:665–667
11. Wucherer OEH (1868) Noticia preliminar sobrevermes de uma especie ainda nao descripta, encontrados na urina de donentes de hematuria intertropical no Brazil. Gazetas Medica de Bahia 3:97–99

12. Lewis TR (1872) On a hematozoan inhabiting human blood, its relation to chyluria and other diseases. In: Microscopic organisms found in the blood of man an animals and its relationship to disease. Office of the Superintendent of the Sanitary Commissioner with the Government of India, Calcutta, pp 75–79
13. Manson P (1899) On filarial periodicity. Br Med J 2:644–646
14. Manson P (1884) Further observations on filaria sanguinis hominis in an epitome of the reports of the medical officers to the China imperial maritime customs, from 1871–1882. Balliere, Tindall and Cox., London, pp 203–206
15. Cobbold TS (1877) Discovery of the adult representative of a microscopic Filariae. Lancet 2:70–71
16. Bourne AG (1888) A note on filaria Filaria Sanguinis Hominis (with description of a male specimen). Br Med J 1:1050–1051
17. Bancroft TL (1899) On the metamorphosis of the young form of Filaria bancrofti Cobbold (Filaria sanguinis hominis Lewis; Filaria nocturna Manson) in the body of Culex ciliaris, the house mosquito of Australia. J Trop Med 2:91–94
18. Low GC (1900) A recent observation on Filaria nocturna in Culex; probable mode of infection of man. Br Med J 1:1456–1457
19. Buckley JJ (1960) On *Brugia gen. nov.* for *Wuchereria spp.* of the inverted question markmalayl' group, i.e., W. malayi (Brug, 1927), W. pahangi Buckley and Edeson, 1956, and W. patei Buckley, Nelson and Heisch, 1958. Ann Trop Med Parasitol 54:75–77
20. O'Connor FW (1931) Filarial periodicity with observations and on the mechanisms of migration of the microfilariae and from parent worm to the blood stream. PR Public Health Trop Med 6:263
21. Kozek WJ, Marroquin HF (1977) Intracytoplasmic bacteria in *Onchocerca volvulus*. Am J Trop Med Hyg 26(4):663–678
22. McLaren DJ et al (1975) Micro-organisms in filarial larvae (Nematoda). Trans R Soc Trop Med Hyg 69(5–6):509–514
23. Sironi M et al (1995) Molecular evidence for a close relative of the arthropod endosymbiont Wolbachia in a filarial worm. Mol Biochem Parasitol 74(2):223–227
24. Taylor MJ, Hoerauf A (1999) Wolbachia bacteria of filarial nematodes. Parasitol Today 15(11):437–442
25. Hise AG, Gillette-Ferguson I, Pearlman E (2004) The role of endosymbiotic Wolbachia bacteria in filarial disease. Cell Microbiol 6(2):97–104
26. Rajan TV (2004) Relationship of anti-microbial activity of tetracyclines to their ability to block the l3 to L4 molt of the human filarial parasite *Brugia malayi*. Am J Trop Med Hyg 71(1):24–28
27. Mand S et al (2009) Macrofilaricidal activity and amelioration of lymphatic pathology in bancroftian filariasis after 3 weeks of doxycycline followed by single-dose diethylcarbamazine. Am J Trop Med Hyg 81(4):702–711
28. Taylor MJ et al (2005) Macrofilaricidal activity after doxycycline treatment of *Wuchereria bancrofti*: a double-blind, randomised placebo-controlled trial. Lancet 365(9477):2116–2121
29. Supali T et al (2008) Doxycycline treatment of *Brugia malayi*-infected persons reduces microfilaremia and adverse reactions after diethylcarbamazine and albendazole treatment. Clin Infect Dis 46(9):1385–1393
30. Ottesen EA (1992) Infection and disease in lymphatic filariasis – an immunological perspective. Parasitology 104:571
31. Dreyer G et al (1992) Renal abnormalities in microfilaremic patients with Bancroftian filariasis. Am J Trop Med Hyg 46(6):745–751
32. Freedman DO et al (1994) Lymphoscintigraphic analysis of lymphatic abnormalities in symptomatic and asymptomatic human filariasis. J Infect Dis 170(4):927–933
33. Case T et al (1991) Vascular abnormalities in experimental and human lymphatic filariasis. Lymphology 24(4):174–183
34. Witte MH et al (1993) Lymphatic abnormalities in human filariasis as depicted by lymphangioscintigraphy. Arch Intern Med 153(6):737–744

35. Mand S et al (2003) Animated documentation of the filaria dance sign (FDS) in bancroftian filariasis. Filaria J 2(1):3
36. Noroes J et al (1996) Ultrasonographic evidence of abnormal lymphatic vessels in young men with adult *Wuchereria bancrofti* infection in the scrotal area. J Urol 156(2 Pt 1):409–412
37. Noroes J et al (1996) Occurrence of living adult *Wuchereria bancrofti* in the scrotal area of men with microfilaraemia. Trans R Soc Trop Med Hyg 90(1):55–56
38. Dreyer G et al (2000) Pathogenesis of lymphatic disease in bancroftian filariasis: a clinical perspective. Parasitol Today 16(12):544–548
39. Aguiar-Santos AM et al (2009) Lymph scrotum: an unusual urological presentation of lymphatic filariasis. A case series study. Rev Inst Med Trop Sao Paulo 51(4):179–183
40. Addiss DG, Brady MA (2007) Morbidity management in the Global Programme to Eliminate Lymphatic Filariasis: a review of the scientific literature. Filaria J 6:2
41. Dreyer G et al (1999) Acute attacks in the extremities of persons living in an area endemic for bancroftian filariasis: differentiation of two syndromes. Trans R Soc Trop Med Hyg 93(4):413–417
42. WHO (1984) Lymphatic filariasis. Fourth report of the WHO Expert Committee on Filariasis. World Health Organ Tech Rep Ser 702:3–112
43. Dreyer G et al (2002) Basic lymphoedema management: treatment and prevention of problems associated with lymphatic filariasis. Hollis Publishing Co, Hollis, p 112
44. Dreyer G, Mattos D, Noroes J (2007) Chyluria. Rev Assoc Med Bras 53(5):460–464
45. Ottesen EA, Nutman TB (1992) Tropical pulmonary eosinophilia. Annu Rev Med 43:417–424
46. Coutinho AD et al (1998) Tropical filarial pulmonary eosinophilia and its differential diagnosis. Rev Hosp Clin Fac Med Sao Paulo 53(1):42–51
47. Rom WN et al (1990) Persistent lower respiratory tract inflammation associated with interstitial lung disease in patients with tropical pulmonary eosinophilia following conventional treatment with diethylcarbamazine. Am Rev Respir Dis 142(5):1088–1092
48. El Setouhy M et al (2004) A randomized clinical trial comparing single- and multi-dose combination therapy with diethylcarbamazine and albendazole for treatment of bancroftian filariasis. Am J Trop Med Hyg 70(2):191–196
49. Horton J et al (2000) An analysis of the safety of the single dose, two drug regimens used in programmes to eliminate lymphatic filariasis. Parasitology 121(Suppl):S147–S160
50. Molyneux DH et al (2003) Mass drug treatment for lymphatic filariasis and onchocerciasis. Trends Parasitol 19(11):516–522
51. Ottesen EA (2002) Major progress toward eliminating lymphatic filariasis. N Engl J Med 347(23):1885–1886
52. Addiss D, et al (2004) Albendazole for lymphatic filariasis. Cochrane Database Syst Rev (1): CD003753
53. Jamal S (1981) Lymphovenous anastomosis in filarial lymphedema. Lymphology 14(2):64–68
54. Ottesen EA et al (1997) Strategies and tools for the control/elimination of lymphatic filariasis. Bull World Health Organ 75(6):491–503
55. Molyneux DH, Zagaria N (2002) Lymphatic filariasis elimination: progress in global programme development. Ann Trop Med Parasitol 96(Suppl 2):S15–S40
56. Ottesen EA et al (2008) The global programme to eliminate lymphatic filariasis: health impact after 8 years. PLoS Negl Trop Dis 2(10):e317
57. Bockarie MJ, Molyneux DH (2009) The end of lymphatic filariasis? BMJ 338:b1686
58. Molyneux D (2003) Lymphatic filariasis (elephantiasis) elimination: a public health success and development opportunity. Filaria J 2(1):13
59. Addiss DG (2010) Global elimination of lymphatic filariasis: addressing the public health problem. PLoS Negl Trop Dis 4(6):e741
60. Schneider MC et al (2011) Elimination of neglected diseases in latin america and the Caribbean: a mapping of selected diseases. PLoS Negl Trop Dis 5(2):e964
61. Ramaiah KD et al (2011) Effect of annual mass administration of diethylcarbamazine and albendazole on bancroftian filariasis in five villages in south India. Trans R Soc Trop Med Hyg 105(8):431–437

62. Hoerauf A et al (2011) Filariasis in Africa-treatment challenges and prospects. Clin Microbiol Infect 17(7):977–985
63. Simonsen PE et al (2010) Lymphatic filariasis control in Tanzania: effect of repeated mass drug administration with ivermectin and albendazole on infection and transmission. PLoS Negl Trop Dis 4(6):e696
64. Gyapong JO et al (2010) Integration of control of neglected tropical diseases into health-care systems: challenges and opportunities. Lancet 375(9709):160–165
65. Bockarie MJ, Deb RM (2010) Elimination of lymphatic filariasis: do we have the drugs to complete the job? Curr Opin Infect Dis 23(6):617–620
66. Brady MA, Hooper PJ, Ottesen EA (2006) Projected benefits from integrating NTD programs in sub-Saharan Africa. Trends Parasitol 22(7):285–291
67. Smits HL (2009) Prospects for the control of neglected tropical diseases by mass drug administration. Expert Rev Anti Infect Ther 7(1):37–56
68. Blackburn BG et al (2006) Successful integration of insecticide-treated bed net distribution with mass drug administration in Central Nigeria. Am J Trop Med Hyg 75(4):650–655
69. Richards FO Jr et al (2006) Integration of mass drug administration programmes in Nigeria: the challenge of schistosomiasis. Bull World Health Organ 84(8):673–676
70. Haddad D et al (2008) Health care at the end of the road: opportunities from 20 years of partnership in onchocerciasis control. Glob Public Health 3(2):187–196
71. Tadesse Z, Hailemariam A, Kolaczinski JH (2008) Potential for integrated control of neglected tropical diseases in Ethiopia. Trans R Soc Trop Med Hyg 102(3):213–214
72. Matthews GA et al (2009) Preliminary examination of integrated vector management in a tropical rainforest area of Cameroon. Trans R Soc Trop Med Hyg 103(11):1098–1104
73. Addiss D (2010) The 6th Meeting of the Global Alliance to Eliminate Lymphatic Filariasis: a half-time review of lymphatic filariasis elimination and its integration with the control of other neglected tropical diseases. Parasit Vectors 3(1):100
74. Shriram AN et al (2011) Diurnally subperiodic filariasis in India-prospects of elimination: precept to action? Parasitol Res 109(1):1–8
75. Bhullar N, Maikere J (2010) Challenges in mass drug administration for treating lymphatic filariasis in Papua, Indonesia. Parasit Vectors 3:70
76. Ramaiah KD (2009) Lymphatic filariasis elimination programme in India: progress and challenges. Trends Parasitol 25(1):7–8
77. Bockarie MJ, Taylor MJ, Gyapong JO (2009) Current practices in the management of lymphatic filariasis. Expert Rev Anti Infect Ther 7(5):595–605
78. Streit T, Lafontant JG (2008) Eliminating lymphatic filariasis: a view from the field. Ann N Y Acad Sci 1136:53–63
79. Pedersen EM et al (2009) The role of monitoring mosquito infection in the Global Programme to Eliminate Lymphatic Filariasis. Trends Parasitol 25(7):319–327
80. Stolk WA, de Vlas SJ, Habbema JD (2006) Advances and challenges in predicting the impact of lymphatic filariasis elimination programmes by mathematical modelling. Filaria J 5:5
81. Hooper PJ et al (2009) The Global Programme to Eliminate Lymphatic Filariasis: health impact during its first 8 years (2000–2007). Ann Trop Med Parasitol 103(Suppl 1):S17–S21
82. Chu BK et al (2010) The economic benefits resulting from the first 8 years of the Global Programme to Eliminate Lymphatic Filariasis (2000–2007). PLoS Negl Trop Dis 4(6):e708

Chapter 8
Leishmaniasis: Challenges in the Control and Eradication

Shyam Sundar and Jaya Chakravarty

8.1 Introduction

8.1.1 The Organism

Leishmaniasis is one of the world's most neglected diseases, affecting largely the poorest of the poor, mainly in developing countries. It is a vector-borne disease caused by obligate intracellular protozoa of the genus *Leishmania*. It is endemic in large areas of the tropics, subtropics and the Mediterranean basin. Infection in humans is caused by more than 20 *Leishmania* species and is transmitted by ~30 different species of phlebotomine sandflies [1]. It broadly manifests as visceral leishmaniasis (VL, also known as kala-azar), cutaneous leishmaniasis (CL) and muco-cutaneous leishmaniasis (MCL).

VL is typically caused by the *Leishmania donovani* complex: *L. donovani*, the causative organism of VL in the Indian subcontinent and Africa and *L. infantum (L. chagasi)* which causes VL in the Mediterranean basin and Central and South America [2].

CL is caused by various *Leishmania* species. Based on its geographical distribution, CL can be divided into Old World (including southern Europe, the Middle East, parts of southwest Asia and Africa) caused mainly by *L. tropica*, *L. major* and *L. aethiopica* and New World leishmaniasis (from Mexico and Latin America) caused predominantly by *L. mexicana complex* and *Viannia subgenus*. MCL is caused by New World *Leishmania* species *L. braziliensis* and *L. panamensis* (both species of the subgenus *Viannia*) [2].

S. Sundar, M.D. (✉) • J. Chakravarty, M.D.
Department of Medicine, Institute of Medical Sciences, Banaras Hindu University, Varanasi 221005, India
e-mail: drshyamsundar@hotmail.com

I.W. Fong (ed.), *Challenges in Infectious Diseases*, Emerging Infectious Diseases of the 21st Century 502, DOI 10.1007/978-1-4614-4496-1_8,

Diffuse cutaneous leishmaniasis is caused by *L. aethiopica* in the Old World and *L. mexicana* and *L. amazonensis in the New World.*

8.1.2 Disease Burden

Leishmaniasis is endemic in 98 countries and three territories, with more than 350 million people at risk. An estimated incidence of 2 million new cases occur per year (0.5 million of visceral leishmaniasis and 1.5 million of cutaneous leishmaniasis) [3]. Ninety per cent of VL occur in the endemic areas of India, Nepal, Bangladesh, Sudan, Ethiopia and Brazil and cause an estimated 50,000–60,000 deaths annually [4].

8.1.3 Transmission

The leishmaniases can be grouped into two broad categories according to the source of human infection: zoonotic leishmaniases, in which the reservoir hosts are wild animals, commensals or domestic animals, and anthroponotic leishmaniases, in which the reservoir host is human. In South Asia and the Horn of Africa, the predominant mode of transmission of VL is anthroponotic, and humans with kala-azar or post-kala-azar dermal leishmaniasis provide the major reservoir for ongoing transmission [4, 5]. In the Mediterranean, the Middle East and Brazil, VL is zoonotic, with the domestic dog as the most important reservoir host sustaining transmission [5]. Most cutaneous leishmaniases have zoonotic transmission except those caused by *L. tropica* which in a predominantly anthroponotic.

8.1.4 The Disease

In cutaneous leishmaniasis, the patient generally presents with one or several ulcer(s) or nodule(s) in the skin. The ulcers heal spontaneously in immunocompetent individuals but cause disfiguring scars.

Diffuse cutaneous leishmaniasis is characterised by widely disseminated cutaneous macules, papules, nodules or plaques or by diffuse infiltration of the skin, especially on extensor surfaces of the limbs and on the face. This disease does not heal spontaneously, and relapses are frequent after treatment.

In muco-cutaneous leishmaniasis, patients suffer from progressively destructive ulcerations of the mucosa, extending from the nose and mouth to the pharynx and larynx. These lesions are not self-healing and are usually seen months or years after a first episode of cutaneous leishmaniasis, when the macrophages of the naso-oropharyngeal mucosa become colonised.

VL is the systemic and most severe form of leishmaniasis, characterised by prolonged fever, splenomegaly, lymphadenopathy, hepatomegaly, pancytopenia, progressive anaemia and weight loss. If untreated, VL is uniformly fatal. Some patients with VL may develop a chronic form of dermal leishmaniasis characterised by indurated nodules or depigmented macules, and is called post-kala-azar dermal leishmaniasis (PKDL) [6]. PKDL is quite common (occurring in >50% patients with VL) in Sudan, where it may occur concurrently with VL and heals spontaneously in most patients [6]. In the Indian subcontinent, it occurs only in a small proportion of patients, 6 months to several years after an episode of VL, and treatment is necessary [7]. Patients with PKDL serve as an important reservoir of infection.

8.2 Leishmaniasis: The Challenges

8.2.1 Increase in the Risk Factors for Leishmaniasis

Migration, civil war and environmental changes like deforestation and urbanisation cause introduction of nonimmune people into areas with existing endemic or enzootic transmission cycles. This has been associated with epidemics of both visceral and cutaneous leishmaniasis as exemplified by the severe epidemic of VL in southern Sudan which led to the death of 100,000 patients [8].

The other emerging risk factor is the human immunodeficiency virus (HIV) pandemic, which has modified the natural history of leishmaniasis [9]. Both diseases exert a synergistic detrimental effect on the cellular immune response because they target similar immune cells [10, 11]. HIV infection increases the risk of developing VL in areas of endemicity, reduces the likelihood of a therapeutic response, and greatly increases the probability of relapse [12–15]. At the same time, VL promotes the clinical progression of HIV disease and the development of acquired immunodeficiency syndrome (AIDS) defining conditions. These factors make HIV/VL co-infected patients a potential source for the emergence of drug resistance [9, 16]. Further, reports of transmission of the infection via needle sharing in HIV/VL co-infected patients in southern Europe threaten to convert an apparently zoonotic disease into the anthroponotic form [9, 17, 18].

HIV/VL co-infection has been reported from more than 35 countries; initially most of these cases were from south-western Europe, but the number of cases are increasing in sub-Saharan Africa, Brazil and South Asia [9, 19, 20]. The spread and overlap of both leishmaniasis and HIV infections in the major foci of leishmaniasis (India, Brazil and Eastern Africa) make VL-HIV co-infection a serious worldwide concern.

8.2.2 Diagnosis

8.2.2.1 Visceral Leishmaniasis

The clinical features of VL are shared by a number of commonly occurring diseases like malaria, typhoid, tuberculosis, etc. The gold standard for the diagnosis of VL is demonstration of parasites. The sequestration of parasites in spleen, bone marrow or lymph nodes necessitates embarking upon invasive procedures, making it difficult to perform in the prevailing field conditions. Although the specificity of microscopy is high, its sensitivity varies, being higher for spleen (93–99%) than for bone marrow (53–86%) or lymph node (53–65%) aspirates. The detection of parasite DNA by PCR in blood or bone marrow aspirates is highly sensitive for the diagnosis of VL, but these techniques remain restricted to referral hospitals and research centres, despite efforts to simplify them.

Antigen-based tests like the latex agglutination test detecting a heat-stable, low-molecular-weight carbohydrate antigen in the urine of VL patients have shown good specificity but only low to moderate (48–87%) sensitivity in East Africa and the Indian subcontinent [21–24].

Serological tests though widely used have some drawbacks. Antibodies remain detectable up to several years after cure; therefore, VL relapse cannot be diagnosed by serology [25, 26].

In endemic areas, a significant proportion of healthy individuals with no history of VL are positive for anti-leishmanial antibodies owing to asymptomatic infections. The seroprevalence in healthy populations varies from <10% in low to moderate endemic areas [27–29] to >30% in high-transmission foci or in household contacts [30–32]. A recent study from the endemic region showed that almost half of healthy population were positive for signatures of infection, either serology or PCR positive (Sundar et al., unpublished data). This makes the diagnosis of VL in the endemic region difficult. What remains to be clarified is whether these asymptomatic persons play a role in the transmission of the disease.

Another drawback of antibody-based tests is that over 40% of HIV co-infected individuals have no detectable specific antibody levels against *Leishmania* [9]. Therefore, antibody-based tests must always be used in combination with a standardised clinical case definition for visceral leishmaniasis.

The direct agglutination test (DAT) and the rK39-based immunochromatographic test (ICT) are the two serological tests which have been extensively validated in the field. In a meta-analysis, DAT had a sensitivity of 94.8% (95% confidence intervals (CI), 92.7–96.4) and specificity of 97.1% (95% CI, 93.9–98.7), respectively [24]. The performance of DAT was not influenced by region or by species of *Leishmania*. Its main drawbacks are requirement of well-equipped laboratory, need for the storage of the antigen at 2–8 °C once it has been dissolved and prolonged incubation time. rK39 is a 39-amino acid repeat that is part of a kinesin-related protein and is conserved within the *L. donovani* complex [33]. rK39 immunochromatographic strip tests (ICTs) are easy to perform, rapid and cheap and give reproducible results. A meta-analysis that included 13 validation studies of the rK39 ICT showed sensitivity and specificity estimates of 93.9% (95% CI, 87.7–97.1) and 95.3% (95% CI, 88.8–98.1), respectively [24]. However, this test shows a regional variation and has been shown to be less accurate in East Africa [34–37].

The need of the hour is the development of a sensitive and easy to use non-invasive antigen-detection test for the diagnosis of primary VL (particularly in HIV co-infected patients), which would be able to diagnose relapses and differentiate between asymptomatic infection.

8.2.2.2 Cutaneous Leishmaniasis

Parasitological diagnosis obtained by scraping, fine-needle aspiration or biopsy of lesions remains the gold standard in diagnosis of cutaneous leishmaniasis because of its high specificity. The sensitivity varies over a broad range, depending on geographical location, species and stage of the lesion.

Serological diagnosis is of limited use in cutaneous leishmaniasis because of its low sensitivity and variable specificity. The leishmanin skin test may be useful in epidemiological studies but is of little value in the diagnosis of cutaneous leishmaniasis. Neither serological tests nor the leishmanin skin test distinguishes between past and present infections.

As parasites are scarce in mucosal lesions because of the strong local immune reaction, demonstration of parasite DNA by PCR has proved to be the most sensitive approach to confirm cutaneous and mucosal leishmaniasis [38–40]. However, molecular-based diagnosis requires substantial laboratory infrastructure and technical expertise, limiting their use to reference laboratories.

8.2.3 Treatment

8.2.3.1 Visceral Leishmaniasis

The treatment of VL is far from satisfactory. All anti-leishmanials with the exception of miltefosine have to be administered parenterally. The duration of treatment is long, drugs are toxic, and hospitalisation is required for monitoring, making the treatment costly and beyond the reach of most patients. Moreover, emergence of drug resistance further complicates the treatment. Table 8.1 summarises the treatment of VL and PKDL.

Pentavalent Antimonials (Sb^v)

Sodium stibogluconate and meglumine antimoniate daily injection of 20 mg/kg body weight for 28–30 days have been standard first-line medicines in most parts of the world. However, drug resistance is a major concern in India, and Nepal, where unresponsiveness is as high as 60% [41, 42].

Large-scale misuse of anti-leishmanial drugs was the main reason behind the emergence of widespread resistance in this region. Sb^v was freely available in India; almost 73% patients consulted unqualified practitioners first [43]. It was a common practice to start with a small dose and gradually build up to the full dose over a week; it was also advocated to have drug-free periods to minimise the toxicity, and physicians split the daily dose in two injections. These practices resulted in build-up of subtherapeutic blood levels and increased tolerance of parasites to Sb^v. There were several manufacturers of Sb^v in India, and quality of products was inconsistent, resulting in occasional batches being substandard and toxic; this added to the problems

Table 8.1 Recommended treatment regimens for visceral leishmaniasis, ranked by preference

Anthroponotic visceral leishmaniasis caused by *L. donovani* in Bangladesh, Bhutan, India and Nepal

1. Liposomal amphotericin B: 3–5 mg/kg per daily dose by infusion given over 3–5 days period up to a total dose of 15 mg/kg[a] by infusion or 10 mg/kg as a single dose by infusion[a]
2. Combinations (co-administered)[a]
   - Liposomal amphotericin B (5 mg/kg by infusion, single dose) plus miltefosine (daily for 7 days, as below)
   - Liposomal amphotericin B (5 mg/kg by infusion, single dose) plus paromomycin (daily for 10 days, as below)
   - Miltefosine plus paromomycin, both daily for 10 days, as below
3. Amphotericin B deoxycholate: 0.75–1.0 mg/kg/day by infusion, daily or on alternate days for 15–20 doses[a]
4. Miltefosine: for children aged 2–11 years, 2.5 mg/kg/day; for people aged ≥12 years and <25 kg body weight, 50 mg/day; 25–50 kg body weight, 100 mg/day; >50 kg body weight, 150 mg/day; orally for 28 days[a]
   or
   Paromomycin: 15 mg (11 mg base) per kg body weight per day intramuscularly for 21 days[a]
5. Pentavalent antimonials: 20 mg Sb^{5+}/kg/day intramuscularly or intravenously for 30 days in areas where they remain effective: Bangladesh, Nepal and the Indian states of Jharkhand, West Bengal and Uttar Pradesh[a]

Rescue treatment in case of non-response: conventional amphotericin B deoxycholate infusions or liposomal amphotericin B at higher doses

Visceral leishmaniasis caused by *L. donovani* in East Africa (Ethiopia, Eritrea, Kenya, Somalia, Sudan and Uganda) and Yemen

1. Combination: pentavalent antimonials (20 mg Sb^{5+}/kg/day intramuscularly or intravenously) plus paromomycin (15 mg [11 mg base] per kg body weight per day intramuscularly) for 17 days[a]
2. Pentavalent antimonials: 20 mg Sb^{5+}/kg/day intramuscularly or intravenously for 30 days[a]
3. Liposomal amphotericin B: 3–5 mg/kg per daily dose by infusion given over 6–10 days up to a total dose of 30 mg/kg[b]
4. Amphotericin B deoxycholate: 0.75–1 mg/kg/day by infusion, daily or on alternate days, for 15–20 doses[a]
5. Miltefosine orally for 28 days at dosage as above[a]

Post-kala-azar dermal leishmaniasis

East Africa

1. Pentavalent antimonials: 20 mg Sb^{5+}/kg/day intramuscularly or intravenously for 30–60 days, when indicated[c]
2. Liposomal amphotericin B: 2.5 mg/kg/day by infusion for 20 days, when indicated[c]

Bangladesh, India, Nepal

1. Amphotericin B deoxycholate: 1 mg/kg/day by infusion, up to 60–80 doses over 4 months[c]
2. Miltefosine orally for 12 weeks at dosage as above[a]

Visceral leishmaniasis caused by *L. infantum*: Mediterranean Basin, Middle East, Central Asia, South America

1. Liposomal amphotericin B: 3–5 mg/kg per daily dose by infusion given over a 3–6 days period, up to a total dose of 18–21 mg/kg[b]
2. Pentavalent antimonials: 20 mg Sb^{5+}/kg/day intramuscularly or intravenously for 28 days[b]
3. Amphotericin B deoxycholate: 0.75–1.0 mg/kg/day by infusion, daily or on alternate days for 20–30 doses, for a total dose of 2–3 g[c]

Adapted from WHO [2]

[a]Evidence obtained from at least one properly designed randomised controlled trial

[b]Evidence obtained from well-designed trials without randomization

[c]Opinions of respected authorities, based on clinical experience, descriptive studies or reports of expert committees

associated with Sb^v therapy, causing serious toxicity and deaths related to the drug [44]. Another reason for the growing resistance to Sb^v in the Indian subcontinent could be due to the fact that transmission is largely anthroponotic. In an anthroponotic cycle, once Sb^v resistance gets established, it spreads exponentially, and organisms sensitive to the drug get eliminated quickly.

Amphotericin B Deoxycholate

Amphotericin B deoxycholate is the drug most commonly used for the treatment of refractory VL in India [45, 46]. Amphotericin B has high cure rate (~100%) at a dose of 0.75–1 mg/kg for 15–20 intravenous infusions. However, this drug has many adverse effects, which necessitates close monitoring and hospitalisation for 4–5 weeks which ultimately increases the cost of therapy.

Lipid formulations of amphotericin B have lower toxicity and shorter duration of therapy. The total dose requirements for treatment of visceral leishmaniasis vary by region. In India (*L. donovani*), a total dose of ≥10 mg/kg results in a cure rate of >95%, while a total dose of 18–21 mg/kg has 90–100% efficacy in southern Europe. However, their cost is extremely prohibitive. A preferential pricing agreement with WHO (agreement between Gilead and WHO of 14 March 2007) has recently reduced the price of liposomal amphotericin B (LAmB) (AmBisome®) for endemic regions to $18 per 50-mg vial [47]. Recently, an open-label study in India, randomly assigned 412 patients in a 3:1 ratio to receive either liposomal amphotericin B (at a dose of 10 mg/kg of body weight) as a single dose or the conventional amphotericin B deoxycholate administered in 15 infusions of 1 mg/kg, was given every other day during a 29-day hospitalisation. Cure rates at 6 months were similar in the two groups: 95.7% (95% confidence interval [CI], 93.4–97.9) in the liposomal-therapy group and 96.3% (95% CI, 92.6–99.9) in the conventional-therapy group [48].The preferential pricing, along with a single day of hospitalisation, makes a single infusion of the liposomal preparation an excellent option for the Indian subcontinent.

Miltefosine

It is the first oral anti-leishmanial agent registered for use in India in March 2002. At the dose of 50–100 mg for 28 days, the long-term cure rate was 94% [49]. The limitations are its high cost, need for monitoring of gastrointestinal side effects and occasional hepatic- and nephrotoxicity. As miltefosine is teratogenic, women of child-bearing potential have to observe contraception for the duration of treatment and for an additional 3 months, due to its half-life of approximately 1 week. Its long half-life also makes it vulnerable to the rapid development of drug resistance. Free availability and quick recovery (within 10 days most patients feel better) coupled with the high cost of the drug may motivate patients to prematurely discontinue treatment, and suboptimal compliance will ultimately lead to the development of parasite resistance [50]. In a recent phase IV trial of the drug in India, the final cure rate was only 82% by intention to treat and 95% by per protocol analysis [51].

Paromomycin (Aminosidine)

It is an aminoglycoside–aminocyclitol antibiotic, which has been used for the treatment of VL in a parenteral formulation and CL in both topical and parenteral formulations. In the phase III trial of paromomycin in the Indian subcontinent, a dose of 15 mg/kg paromomycin sulphate (11 mg base) for 21 days gave a cure rate of 95% and was shown to be non-inferior to amphotericin B and was approved by the Indian government in August 2006 for the treatment of patients with visceral leishmaniasis [52]. The efficacy was 85% in East Africa at an increased dose of 20 mg/kg (15 mg base) per day for 21 days. One of the advantages of this agent is its low cost (approximately US$10 per patient) [53]. The disadvantages are need for administering intramuscular injection, monitoring of serum transaminases and inadequate data regarding its use in pregnancy.

Combination Therapy

The growing resistance of the parasite to anti-leishmanial drugs suggests that the currently used monotherapy needs to be reviewed. Multidrug combination therapy has been used successfully in tuberculosis, leprosy and malaria. The rationale behind combination therapy are increased activity through use of compounds with synergistic or additive activity, preventing the emergence of drug resistance, lower dose requirement thereby reducing chances of toxic side effects and cost, and increased spectrum of activity.

A randomised, noncomparative, group-sequential, triangular design study assigned 181 subjects to treatment with 5 mg/kg of LAmB alone, 5 mg/kg of LAmB followed by miltefosine for 10 days or 14 days or 3.75 mg/kg of LAmB followed by miltefosine for 14 days. When it became apparent that all regimens were effective, 45 additional, nonrandomised patients were assigned to receive 5 mg/kg of LAmB followed by miltefosine for 7 days. Final cure rates were similar in all the groups with combinations. These results suggest that single infusion of LAmB (in most instances, administered in an outpatient setting) followed by a brief self-administered course of miltefosine could be an excellent option against Indian kala-azar [54].

In another phase 3 study in the Indian subcontinent, the three drug combinations: single injection of 5 mg/kg LAmB and 7-day 50-mg oral miltefosine, single 10-day 11 mg/kg intramuscular paromomycin or 10 days each of miltefosine and paromomycin, showed an excellent cure rate and were non-inferior to the standard treatment [55].

Combination drug therapy is expected to reduce the probability of development of resistant parasites, thereby prolonging the useful therapeutic lifespan of these drugs, which are needed for the elimination of VL. As the pipeline for the anti-leishmanial drug is empty, it is imperative that we try and protect and prolong the effective life of the existing drugs. The high cost of the anti-leishmanial drugs coupled with easy, over-the-counter availability often leads to under dosing and incomplete treatment. This has been the major factor for antimony resistance and could lead to resistance to other drugs as well especially the novel oral agent miltefosine. Considering that majority of the population cannot afford to purchase and complete a full course of treatment, it is recommended that anti-leishmanials should be made available free of cost to be distributed through public and/or private health care providers like antitubercular and antiretroviral drugs, and anti-leishmanial drugs should be withdrawn from the open market.

Post-Kala-azar Dermal Leishmaniasis (PKDL)

In India, treatment of PKDL patients for up to 4 months with intermittent amphotericin B deoxycholate (20 days on, 20 days off) or 12 weeks of continuous miltefosine proved successful—disappearance of the lesion being taken as the criterion of cure [2]. In East Africa, PKDL is not treated routinely, as the majority of cases (85%) heal spontaneously within 1 year. However, patients with severe (grade 3) or disfiguring disease, those with lesions that have remained for >6 months, those with concomitant anterior uveitis and young children with oral lesions that interfere with feeding are treated, with either sodium stibogluconate (20 mg/kg Sb^v per day) for up to 2 months or a 20-day course of LAmB at 2.5 mg/kg/day [2].

8.2.3.2 Cutaneous Leishmaniasis

In cutaneous leishmaniasis, the infecting species and geographical region affect the efficacy of treatment. Mucosal involvement is exceptional in the Old World and is generally restricted to *L. braziliensis* and *L. panamensis* infections in the New World. Some species (especially *L. major*) are associated with a self-cure rate >50% at 6 months.

In Old World cutaneous leishmaniasis local therapy in the form of paromomycin ointment, thermotherapy, cryotherapy or intralesional pentavalent antimonials is given if it is a confirmed or strongly suspected infection with *L. major*, there are fewer than four lesions requiring immediate treatment, lesions are <5 cm in diameter, there is no potentially disfiguring or disabling lesion (face, joints, toes, fingers) and no immunosuppression, and there is a possibility for follow-up. In patients in whom systemic treatment is the only option, the schedule of pentavalent antimonials generally used is 20 mg/kg Sb^v per day intramuscularly or intravenously for 10–20 days.

The New World form tends to be more severe and to last longer than that of the Old World; some patients infected by *L. amazonensis, L. mexicana* and *L. panamensis* develop diffuse disease where systemic therapy needs to be given. The *systemic treatment* options are pentavalent antimonials, pentamidine, paromomycin sulphate, miltefosine and ketoconazole (Table 8.2).

Table 8.2 Treatment of cutaneous and mucosal leishmaniasis

Disease	Species	Drug and route[a] (or procedure)	Regimen
Cutaneous	*L. major*	Few, small lesions on non-visible parts of body	
		No anti-leishmanial treatment	Not applicable
		Few, large, visible lesions	
		Paromomycin topical	2 applications per day × 10–30 days
		Cryotherapy topical + Sb intralesional	0.5–6 applications/ week × 1–10 weeks
		Photodynamic topical therapy	1 application/week × 4 weeks
		Other lesions or failure of topical therapy	
		Sb systemic	15–20 mg Sb/kg/ day × 15–20 days
	L. tropica	Sb intralesional	1 application per week × 5 weeks
		Thermotherapy topical	1 session of > or =1 application
	L. mexicana	No anti-leishmanial treatment (For few small lesions)	Not applicable
		Ketoconazole oral	600 mg/day × 28 days
	L. braziliensis	Sb systemic	20 mg Sb/kg × 10–20 days
		Miltefosine oral	~2.5 mg/kg/day × 28 days
	L.panamensis/L. guyanensis	Miltefosine oral	~2.5 mg/kg/day × 28 days
		Pentamidine im or iv	2–7 mg/kg × 1–7 injections (7–14 mg/kg total dose over 1–7 days)
		Sb systemic	20 mg Sb/kg × 10–20 days
Mucosal	*L. braziliensis*	Sb systemic	20 mg Sb/kg/ day × 28–40 days
		Miltefosine oral	2.5 mg/kg/day × 28–42 days 2,250 mg total dose
		Amphotericin B deoxycholate iv	3 infusions/week × 15 weeks
		Liposomal amphotericin B iv	2,000–5,300 mg (30–105 mg/ kg) total dose
		Amphotericin B cholesterol dispersion iv	2,000–2,600 mg (35–50 mg/ kg) total dose

[a]Abbreviations: *im* intramuscular, *iv* intravenous

In mucosal leishmaniasis, high cure rates are obtained when the lesions are limited to the nose and mouth; when the larynx, vocal cords and trachea are involved; however, the cure rates after therapy with systemic antimonials are low, and relapse and recurrence are frequent after clinical improvement and apparent cure. The scarcity of amastigotes and the difficulty of culture usually complicate parasitological monitoring.

8.2.3.3 HIV/VL Co-infection

Another potential source for the emergence of drug resistance are the HIV/VL co-infected patients. These patients have high parasite burden, a weak immune response, respond poorly to treatment and have a high relapse rate. Therefore, they are ideal candidates to harbour drug-resistant parasites. All anti-leishmanial therapies are less effective in HIV-positive patients. There is a high mortality rate due to concurrent illness, complications and drug toxicity. Pentavalent antimonials and amphotericin B are more toxic to HIV patients, who require close monitoring for pancreatitis, cardiotoxicity and nephrotoxicity [20]. In Ethiopia, miltefosine was found to be less effective than antimonials in co-infected patients, and side effects were worse in these patients [56]. The best option for these patients is LAmB. Secondary prophylaxis with liposomal amphotericin B, 5 mg/kg every three weeks, has shown a beneficial effect [20]. Initiation of highly active antiretroviral therapy (HAART) dramatically decreases the incidence of VL co-infection. Therefore, HAART in combination with anti-leishmanials should be advocated strictly in these patients.

8.2.4 Vaccine

Leishmaniasis is unique among parasitic diseases because a single vaccine has the potential to protect against more than one species and be successful at both treating and preventing disease. Therefore, development of a vaccine would go a long way in the control of this disease. Although progress in developing a protective vaccine against the different human leishmaniases has been limited, therapeutic (or immunochemotherapeutic) vaccines may be achievable.

'Leishmanization', which simulates live infection by inoculation of live *L. major* as a vaccine for protection against cutaneous leishmaniasis, has been carried out in Uzbekistan, Iran and Israel [57, 58]. However, the vaccine preparations are not standardised or widely available and can cause persistent cutaneous lesions.

A trial of a killed *L. major* vaccine that was administered with the tuberculosis vaccine bacille Calmette–Guérin (BCG) failed [59]. A novel immunochemotherapeutic agent using alum-precipitated autoclaved *L. major* plus BCG together with pentavalent antimonials showed encouraging results in persistent PKDL in Sudan [60]. The use of such a therapeutic vaccine could reduce the dose and duration of chemotherapy and be an important control tool.

Second-generation vaccines consist of recombinant proteins and genetic vaccines. A second-generation vaccine is now in clinical development as a therapeutic or prophylactic vaccine against VL; it contains a recombinant protein, comprising three leishmanial antigens (LEISH-F1) [61] and a defined adjuvant (MPL-SE) [62]. In Brazil, the LEISH-F1+MPL-SE vaccine was safe and immunogenic in CL patients and appeared to shorten their time to cure when used in combination with meglumine antimoniate chemotherapy. Eighty per cent of vaccine recipients were clinically cured, compared to 50 and 38% of adjuvant alone and placebo recipients [63]. In patients with mucosal leishmaniasis in Peru and healthy adults in India, this vaccine was safe, well tolerated and immunogenic [64, 65].

8.2.5 Control of Reservoir Hosts

Control of reservoir hosts has been recommended as a component of control strategies for zoonotic visceral and cutaneous leishmaniasis. This is a complex undertaking, as less than half of infected dogs show signs of leishmaniasis, and asymptomatic infected dogs have been shown to be infective to sandflies. In Brazil, screening and mass culling of seropositive dogs has not proved uniformly effective in control programmes. Even after anti-leishmanial treatment, a large percentage of treated dogs recover their infectivity to sandflies despite being clinically cured; thus treating infected dogs may not be an effective control strategy [66]. The use of deltamethrin-treated collars reduced the risk of infection in dogs (by 54%) and children (by 43%) in a study conducted in Iran [67]; however, this approach has not been tested in mass campaign.

Wild animal reservoir hosts like the great gerbil, the fat sand rat, can be dealt with by destroying the burrow systems by ploughing with a subsoil plough followed by planting or poisoning them with zinc phosphide (12%) mixed with wheat grains and vegetable oil (2.3%) and the anticoagulant dicoumarol. However, reinvasion is common, and the agents are toxic and may harm humans and other animals. In the New World, few rational measures for the control of reservoir hosts are available. An integrated environmental management approach might be effective, combining clearance of primary forest around villages and spraying of the cleared areas with insecticides to remove both the reservoir hosts and the vector, thus creating a vector- and reservoir-free zone around villages.

8.2.6 Vector Control

Vector control is an important strategy to reduce or interrupt transmission of disease. An integrated vector management approach including chemicals, environmental management and personal protection should be taken for sandfly control.

Chemical control can be done by indoor residual spraying, spraying of resting sites of sylvatic species, use of insecticide-impregnated materials such as bednets and curtains and pyrethroid-impregnated dog collars. Residual insecticide spraying of houses and animal shelters was shown to be efficacious in India [68], where the vector (*Phlebotomus argentipes*) is restricted to areas in and around the home. However, in Sudan and other endemic countries in East Africa, transmission occurs mainly outside villages [69]; therefore, indoor residual spraying for disease control is therefore unlikely to be as efficient in this region. Case-control studies conducted in Bangladesh and Nepal showed that sleeping under a non-impregnated bednet during the warm months was a protective factor against VL [70, 71]. However, in a recent large-scale study on long-lasting insecticide-impregnated bednets in India and Nepal, nets had no significant effect on the incidence of either the infection or the disease [72]. Thus, a blanket strategy of vector control will not work, and it should be designed after careful study of vector behaviour (resting place, breeding sites, feeding pattern, etc.) for each endemic region. The mass distribution of insecticide-treated nets (ITNs) in Sudan was accompanied by a 27% reduction in the incidence of VL in an observational study [73].

A recent study showed that VL was associated with housing conditions like living in a thatched house or in a house with damp floors which suggests that improving living conditions could decrease the incidence of VL [74]. Insecticide spraying, use of insecticide-treated nets and improving housing conditions could be used for decreasing VL transmission.

8.3 VL Elimination Programme

India, Nepal and Bangladesh harbour an estimated 67% of the global VL disease burden [75], and the governments of these countries have launched a regional VL elimination programme. The target of this programme is to eliminate VL as a public health problem in these countries by 2015 by using a local approach to reduce the annual incidence of VL to less than 1 case per 10,000 individuals.

The rationale for VL elimination in the Indian subcontinent are as follows: the disease in this area is anthroponotic, with humans being the only reservoir and *Phlebotomus argentipes* sandflies the only known vector; new and more effective drugs and a rapid diagnostic test, the rk39 immunochromatographic test, are available that can be used in the field; there is strong political commitment and inter-country collaboration, and the disease is endemic in only a limited number of districts.

The five main strategies for this programme are early diagnosis and complete treatment of cases, integrated vector management, effective disease surveillance through passive and active case detection, social mobilisation and partnership building at all levels and clinical and operational research.

8.4 Conclusion

Inventory of anti-leishmanial drugs is very small, and emergence of drug resistance is further complicating the control of leishmaniasis. Combination therapy by reducing the duration of therapy and decreasing the chances of developing resistance should be encouraged. Till the time combination therapy is available, countries should adopt the best monotherapy. Innovative research to generate better therapeutic regimens for CL, MCL and PKDL should be encouraged. The development of prophylactic as well as therapeutic vaccines and immunomodulators would go a long way in the control of the disease.

In diagnostics, markers of disease and parasite resistance, tests of cure and antigen-based tests for diagnosis of HIV/VL co-infection should be developed.

In areas with zoonotic transmission, elimination of animal reservoir is almost impossible, and this is a big hurdle in control and ultimate eradication of the disease. Cost-effective integrated vector control measures suitable for the region should be implemented. Leishmaniasis should be designated as a notifiable disease in all endemic countries, and effective national control programmes should be supported. Efforts should be made to make the diagnosis and treatment of leishmaniasis free of cost and improve access to these facilities.

References

1. Pearson RD, Sousa AQ (1996) Clinical spectrum of leishmaniasis. Clin Infect Dis 22:1–13
2. Sundar S (2012) Leishmaniases. In: Longo DL, Fauci AS, Kasper DL, Hauser SL, Jameson JL, Loscalzo J (eds) Harrisons's Priniciples of Internal Medicine, 18th edn. McGraw Hill, New York, pp 1709–1716
3. Control of the Leishmaniasis. Report of a meeting of the WHO Expert Committee on the Control of Leishmaniases, Geneva, 22–26 Mar 2010. http://whqlibdoc.who.int/trs/WHO_TRS_949_eng.pdf. Accessed on 29 May 2011
4. Chappuis F, Sundar S, Hailu A, Ghalib H, Rijal S, Peeling RW, Alvar J, Boelaert M (2007) Visceral leishmaniasis: what are the needs for diagnosis, treatment and control? Nat Rev Microbiol 5:873–882
5. Pearson RD, Jeronimo SMB, de Queiroz Sousa A (1999) Leishmaniasis. In: Guerrant RL, Walker DH, Weller PF (eds) Tropical infectious diseases: principles, pathogens and practice. Churchill Livingstone, Philadelphia, pp 797–813
6. Zijlstra EE, Musa AM, Khalil EA, el-Hassan IM, el-Hassan AM (2003) Post-kala-azar dermal leishmaniasis. Lancet Infect Dis 3:87–98
7. Thakur CP, Kumar K (1992) Post kala-azar dermal leishmaniasis: a neglected aspect of kala-azar control programmes. Ann Trop Med Parasitol 86:355–359
8. Seaman J, Mercer AJ, Sondorp E (1996) The epidemic of visceral leishmaniasis in western Upper Nile, southern Sudan: course and impact from 1984 to 1994. Int J Epidemiol 25:862–871
9. Alvar J, Canavate C, Gutierrez-Solar B, Jimenez M, Laguna F, Lopez-Velez R, Molina R, Moreno J (1997) Leishmania and human immunodeficiency virus coinfection: the first 10 years. Clin Microbiol Rev 10:298–319
10. Olivier M, Badaro R, Medrano FJ, Moreno J (2003) The pathogenesis of Leishmania/HIV co-infection: cellular and immunological mechanisms. Ann Trop Med Parasitol 97:79–98
11. Tremblay M, Olivier M, Bernier R (1996) Leishmania and the pathogenesis of HIV infection. Parasitol Today 12:257–261
12. Gradoni L, Scalone A, Gramiccia M, Troiani M (1996) Epidemiological surveillance of leishmaniasis in HIV-1-infected individuals in Italy. AIDS 10:785–791
13. Lopez-Velez R, Perez-Molina JA, Guerrero A, Baquero F, Villarrubia J, Escribano L, Bellas C, Perez-Corral F, Alvar J (1998) Clinicoepidemiologic characteristics, prognostic factors, and survival analysis of patients coinfected with human immunodeficiency virus and Leishmania in an area of Madrid, Spain. Am J Trop Med Hyg 58:436–443
14. Pintado V, Martin-Rabadan P, Rivera ML, Moreno S, Bouza E (2001) Visceral leishmaniasis in human immunodeficiency virus (HIV)-infected and non-HIV-infected patients. A comparative study. Medicine (Baltimore) 80:54–73

15. Rosenthal E, Marty P, Poizot-Martin I, Reynes J, Pratlong F, Lafeuillade A, Jaubert D, Boulat O, Dereure J, Gambarelli F, Gastaut JA, Dujardin P, Dellamonica P, Cassuto JP (1995) Visceral leishmaniasis and HIV-1 co-infection in southern France. Trans R Soc Trop Med Hyg 89:159–162
16. Laguna F, Videla S, Jiménez-Mejías ME, Sirera G, Torre-Cisneros J, Ribera E, Prados D, Clotet B, Sust M, López-Vélez R, Alvar J, Spanish HIV-Leishmania Study Group (2003) Amphotericin B lipid complex versus meglumine antimoniate in the treatment of visceral leishmaniasis in patients infected with HIV: a randomized pilot study. J Antimicrob Chemother 52:464–468
17. Alvar J, Gutiérrez-Solar B, Pachón I, Calbacho E, Ramírez M, Vallés R et al (1996) AIDS and Leishmania infantum. New approaches for a new epidemiological problem. Clin Dermatol 14:541–546
18. Molina R, Gradoni L, Alvar J (2003) HIV and the transmission of Leishmania. Ann Trop Med Parasitol 97:29–45
19. Desjeux P, Alvar J (2003) LeishmaniaIHIV co-infections: epidemiology in Europe. Ann Trop Med Parasitol 97:3–15
20. Alvar J, Aparicio P, Aseffa A, Den Boer M, Cañavate C, Dedet JP, Gradoni L, Ter Horst R, López-Vélez R, Moreno J (2008) The relationship between leishmaniasis and AIDS: the second 10 years. Clin Microbiol Rev 21:334–359
21. Rijal S, Boelaert M, Regmi S, Karki BM, Jacquet D, Singh R, Chance ML, Chappuis F, Hommel M, Desjeux P, Van der Stuyft P, Le Ray D, Koirala S (2004) Evaluation of a urinary antigen-based latex agglutination test in the diagnosis of kala-azar in eastern Nepal. Trop Med Int Health 9:724–729
22. Sundar S, Singh RK, Bimal SK, Gidwani K, Mishra A, Maurya R, Singh SK, Manandhar KD, Boelaert M, Rai M (2007) Comparative evaluation of parasitology and serological tests in the diagnosis of visceral leishmaniasis in India: a phase III diagnostic accuracy study. Trop Med Int Health 12:284–289
23. Sundar S, Agrawal S, Pai K, Chance M, Hommel M (2005) Detection of leishmanial antigen in the urine of patients with visceral leishmaniasis by a latex agglutination test. Am J Trop Med Hyg 73:269–271
24. Chappuis F, Rijal S, Soto A, Menten J, Boelaert M (2006) A meta-analysis of the diagnostic performance of the direct agglutination test and rK39 dipstick for visceral leishmaniasis. BMJ 333:723
25. De Almeida SL, Romero HD, Prata A, Costa RT, Nascimento E, Carvalho SF, Rodrigues V (2006) Immunologic tests in patients after clinical cure of visceral leishmaniasis. Am J Trop Med Hyg 75:739–743
26. Hailu A (1990) Pre- and post-treatment antibody levels in visceral leishmaniasis. Trans R Soc Trop Med Hyg 84:673–675
27. Koirala S, Karki P, Das ML, Parija SC, Karki BM (2004) Epidemiological study of kala-azar by direct agglutination test in two rural communities of eastern Nepal. Trop Med Int Health 9:533–537
28. Schenkel K, Rijal S, Koirala S, Koirala S, Vanlerberghe V, Van der Stuyft P, Gramiccia M, Boelaert M (2006) Visceral leishmaniasis in southeastern Nepal: a cross-sectional survey on Leishmania donovani infection and its risk factors. Trop Med Int Health 11:1792–1799
29. Schaefer KU, Kurtzhals JA, Gachihi GS, Muller AS, Kager PA (1995) A prospective seroepidemiological study of visceral leishmaniasis in Baringo District, Rift Valley Province, Kenya. Trans R Soc Trop Med Hyg 89:471–475
30. Sundar S, Singh RK, Maurya R, Kumar B, Chhabra A, Singh V, Rai M (2006) Serological diagnosis of Indian visceral leishmaniasis: direct agglutination test versus rK39 strip test. Trans R Soc Trop Med Hyg 100:533–537
31. Sundar S, Maurya R, Singh RK, Bharti K, Chakravarty J, Parekh A, Rai M, Kumar K, Murray HW (2006) Rapid, noninvasive diagnosis of visceral leishmaniasis in India: comparison of two immunochromatographic strip tests for detection of anti-K39 antibody. J Clin Microbiol 44:251–253

32. Ibrahim ME, Lambson B, Yousif AO, Deifalla NS, Alnaiem DA, Ismail A, Yousif H, Ghalib HW, Khalil EA, Kadaro A, Barker DC, El Hassan AM (1999) Kala-azar in a high transmission focus: an ethnic and geographic dimension. Am J Trop Med Hyg 61:941–944
33. Burns JM Jr, Shreffler WG, Benson DR, Ghalib HW, Badaro R, Reed SG (1993) Molecular characterization of a kinesin-related antigen of *Leishmania chagasi* that detects specific antibody in African and American visceral leishmaniasis. Proc Natl Acad Sci U S A 90:775–779
34. Ritmeijer K, Melaku Y, Mueller M, Kipngetich S, O'keeffe C, Davidson RN (2006) Evaluation of a new recombinant K39 rapid diagnostic test for Sudanese visceral leishmaniasis. Am J Trop Med Hyg 74:76–80
35. Veeken H, Ritmeijer K, Seaman J, Davidson R (2003) Comparison of an rK39 dipstick rapid test with direct agglutination test and splenic aspiration for the diagnosis of kala-azar in Sudan. Trop Med Int Health 8:164–167
36. Diro E, Techane Y, Tefera T, Assefa Y, Kebede T, Genetu A, Kebede Y, Tesfaye A, Ergicho B, Gebre-Yohannes A, Mengistu G, Engers H, Aseffa A, Desjeux P, Boelaert M, Hailu A (2007) Field evaluation of FD-DAT, rk-39 dipstick and KATEX (urine latex agglutination) for diagnosis of visceral leishmaniasis in northwest Ethiopia. Trans R Soc Trop Med Hyg 101:908–914
37. Boelaert M, El-Safi S, Hailu A, Mukhtar M, Rijal S, Sundar S, Wasunna M, Aseffa A, Mbui J, Menten J, Desjeux P, Peeling RW (2008) Diagnostic tests for kala-azar: a multi-centre study of the freeze-dried DAT, rK39 strip test and KAtex in East-Africa and the Indian subcontinent. Trans R Soc Trop Med Hyg 102:32–40
38. Faber WR, Oskam L, van Gool T, Kroon NC, Knegt-Junk KJ, Hofwegen H, van der Wal AC, Kager PA (2003) Value of diagnostic techniques for cutaneous leishmaniasis. J Am Acad Dermatol 49:70
39. Medeiros AC, Rodrigues SS, Roselino AM (2002) Comparison of the specificity of PCR and the histopathological detection of leishmania for the diagnosis of American cutaneous leishmaniasis. Braz J Med Biol Res 35(4):421
40. Weigle KA, Labrada LA, Lozano C, Santrich C, Barker DC (2002) PCR-based diagnosis of acute and chronic cutaneous leishmaniasis caused by Leishmania (Viannia). J Clin Microbiol 40(2):601–606
41. Sundar S, More DK, Singh MK, Singh VP, Sharma S, Makharia A, Kumar PC, Murray HW (2000) Failure of pentavalent antimony in visceral leishmaniasis in India: report from the center of the Indian epidemic. Clin Infect Dis 31:1104–1107
42. Rijal S, Chappuis F, Singh R, Bovier PA, Acharya P, Karki BM, Das ML, Desjeux P, Loutan L, Koirala S (2003) Treatment of visceral leishmaniasis in south-eastern Nepal: decreasing efficacy of sodium stibogluconate and need for a policy to limit further decline. Trans R Soc Trop Med Hyg 97:350–354
43. Sundar S, Thakur BB, Tandon AK, Agrawal NR, Mishra CP, Mahapatra TM, Singh VP (1994) Clinico-epidemiological study of drug resistance in Indian kala-azar. BMJ 308:307
44. Sundar S, Sinha PR, Agrawal NK, Srivastava R, Rainey PM, Berman JD, Murray HW, Singh VP (1998) A cluster of severe antimony cardiotoxicity in kala-azar due to high osmolality lot. Am J Trop Med Hyg 59:139–143
45. Thakur CP, Singh RK, Hassan SM, Kumar R, Narain S, Kumar A (1999) Amphotericin B deoxycholate treatment of visceral leishmaniasis with newer modes of administration and precautions: a study of 938 cases. Trans R Soc Trop Med Hyg 93:9–23
46. Mishra M, Biswas UK, Jha DN, Khan AB (1992) Amphotericin versus pentamidine in antimony-unresponsive kala-azar. Lancet 340:1256–1257
47. Olliaro P, Sundar S (2009) Anthropometrically derived dosing and drug costing calculations for treating visceral leishmaniasis in Bihar, India. Trop Med Int Health 14:88–92
48. Sundar S, Chakravarty J, Agarwal D, Rai M, Murray HW (2010) Single-dose liposomal amphotericin B for visceral leishmaniasis in India. N Engl J Med 362:504–512
49. Sundar S, Jha TK, Thakur CP, Engel J, Sindermann H, Fischer C, Junge K, Bryceson A, Berman J (2002) Oral miltefosine for Indian visceral leishmaniasis. N Engl J Med 347:1739–1746

50. Sundar S, Murray HW (2005) Availability of miltefosine for the treatment of kala-azar in India. Bull World Health Organ 83:394–395
51. Bhattacharya SK, Sinha PK, Sundar S, Thakur CP, Jha TK, Pandey K, Das VR, Kumar N, Lal C, Verma N, Singh VP, Ranjan A, Verma RB, Anders G, Sindermann H, Ganguly NK (2007) Phase IV trial of miltefosine in the treatment of Indian visceral leishmaniasis. J Infect Dis 196:591–598
52. Sundar S, Jha TK, Thakur CP, Sinha PK, Bhattacharya SK (2007) Injectable paromomycin for visceral leishmaniasis in India. N Engl J Med 356:2571–2581
53. Sundar S, Rai M (2005) Treatment of visceral leishmaniasis. Expert Opin Pharmacother 6:2821–2829
54. Sundar S, Rai M, Chakravarty J, Agarwal D, Agrawal N, Vaillant M, Olliaro P, Murray HW (2008) New treatment approach in indian visceral leishmaniasis: single-dose liposomal amphotericin b followed by short-course oral miltefosine. Clin Infect Dis 47:1000–1006
55. Sundar S, Sinha PK, Rai M, Verma DK, Nawin K, Alam S, Chakravarty J, Vaillant M, Verma N, Pandey K, Kumari P, Lal CS, Arora R, Sharma B, Ellis S, Strub-Wourgaft N, Balasegaram M, Olliaro P, Das P, Modabber F (2011) Comparison of short-course multidrug treatment with standard therapy for visceral leishmaniasis in India: an open-label, non-inferiority, randomised controlled trial. Lancet 377:477–486
56. Ritmeijer K, Dejenie A, Assefa Y, Hundie TB, Mesure J, Boots G, den Boer M, Davidson RN (2006) A comparison of miltefosine and sodium stibogluconate for treatment of visceral leishmaniasis in an Ethiopian population with high prevalence of HIV infection. Clin Infect Dis 43:357–364
57. Nadim A, Javadian E, Tahvildar-Bidruni G, Ghorbani M (1983) Effectiveness of leishmanization in the control of cutaneous leishmaniasis. Bull Soc Pathol Exot Filiales 76:377–383
58. Greenblatt CL (1988) Cutaneous leishmaniasis: the prospects for a killed vaccine. Parasitol Today 4:53–54
59. Khalil EA, El Hassan AM, Zijlstra EE, Mukhtar MM, Ghalib HW, Musa B, Ibrahim ME, Kamil AA, Elsheikh M, Babiker A, Modabber F (2000) Autoclaved *Leishmania major* vaccine for prevention of visceral leishmaniasis: a randomised, double-blind, BCG-controlled trial in Sudan. Lancet 356:1565–1569
60. Musa AM, Khalil EAG, Ismail A, Elhassan IM, Fesharki H, Khamesipour A, Modabber F, Zijlstra EE, El-Hassan AM (2005) Safety, immunogenicity and possible efficacy of immunochemotherapy of persistent post kala-azar dermal leishmaniasis. Sudan J Dermatol 3: 63–72
61. Skeiky YA, Coler RN, Brannon M, Stromberg E, Greeson K, Crane RT, Webb JR, Campos-Neto A, Reed SG (2002) Protective efficacy of a tandemly linked, multi-subunit recombinant leishmanial vaccine (Leish-111f) formulated in MPL adjuvant. Vaccine 20:3292–3303
62. Reed SG, Coler RN, Campos-Neto A (2003) Development of a leishmaniasis vaccine: the importance of MPL. Expert Rev Vac 2:239–252
63. Nascimento E, Fernandes DF, Vieira EP, Campos-Neto A, Ashman JA, Alves FP, Coler RN, Bogatzki LY, Kahn SJ, Beckmann AM, Pine SO, Cowgill KD, Reed SG, Piazza FM (2010) A clinical trial to evaluate the safety and immunogenicity of the LEISH-F1 + MPL-SE vaccine when used in combination with meglumine antimoniate for the treatment of cutaneous leishmaniasis. Vaccine 28(40):6581–6587
64. Llanos-Cuentas A, Calderón W, Cruz M, Ashman JA, Alves FP, Coler RN, Bogatzki LY, Bertholet S, Laughlin EM, Kahn SJ, Beckmann AM, Cowgill KD, Reed SG, Piazza FM (2010) A clinical trial to evaluate the safety and immunogenicity of the LEISH-F1 + MPL-SE vaccine when used in combination with sodium stibogluconate for the treatment of mucosal leishmaniasis. Vaccine 28(46):7427–7435
65. Chakravarty J, Kumar S, Trivedi S, Rai VK, Singh A, Ashman JA, Laughlin EM, Coler RN, Kahn SJ, Beckmann AM, Cowgill KD, Reed SG, Sundar S, Piazza FM (2011) A clinical trial to evaluate the safety and immunogenicity of the LEISH-F1 + MPL-SE vaccine for use in the prevention of visceral leishmaniasis. Vaccine 29(19):3531–3537

66. Alvar J, Molina R, San Andrés M, Tesouro M, Nieto J, Vitutia M, González F, San Andrés MD, Boggio J, Rodriguez F (1994) Canine leishmaniasis: clinical, parasitological and entomological follow-up after chemotherapy. Ann Trop Med Parasitol 88:371–378
67. Gavgani AS, Hodjati MH, Mohite H, Davies CR (2002) Effect of insecticide-impregnated dog collars on incidence of zoonotic visceral leishmaniasis in Iranian children: a matched-cluster randomised trial. Lancet 360:374–379
68. Kaul SM, Sharma RS, Dey KP, Rai RN, Verghese T (1994) Impact of DDT indoor residual spraying on Phlebotomus argentipes in a kala-azar endemic village in eastern Uttar Pradesh. Bull World Health Organ 72:79–81
69. Hassan MM, Elraba'a FM, Ward RD, Maingon RD, Elnaiem DA (2004) Detection of high rates of in-village transmission of *Leishmania donovani* in eastern Sudan. Acta Trop 92:77–82
70. Bern C, Hightower AW, Chowdhury R, Ali M, Amann J, Wagatsuma Y, Haque R, Kurkjian K, Vaz LE, Begum M, Akter T, Cetre-Sossah CB, Ahluwalia IB, Dotson E, Secor WE, Breiman RF, Maguire JH (2005) Risk factors for kala-azar in Bangladesh. Emerg Infect Dis 11:655–662
71. Bern C, Joshi AB, Jha SN, Das ML, Hightower A, Thakur GD, Bista MB (2000) Factors associated with visceral leishmaniasis in Nepal: bed-net use is strongly protective. Am J Trop Med Hyg 63:184–188
72. Picado A, Singh SP, Rijal S, Sundar S, Ostyn B, Chappuis F, Uranw S, Gidwani K, Khanal B, Rai M, Paudel IS, Das ML, Kumar R, Srivastava P, Dujardin JC, Vanlerberghe V, Andersen EW, Davies CR, Boelaert M (2010) Longlasting insecticidal nets for prevention of Leishmania donovani infection in India and Nepal: paired cluster randomised trial. BMJ 341:c6760. doi:10.1136/bmj.c6760
73. Ritmeijer K, Davies C, van Zorge R, Wang SJ, Schorscher J, Dongu'du SI, Davidson RN (2007) Evaluation of a mass distribution programme for fine-mesh impregnated bednets against visceral leishmaniasis in eastern Sudan. Trop Med Int Health 12:404–414
74. Singh SP, Hasker E, Picado A, Gidwani K, Malaviya P, Singh RP, Boelaert M, Sundar S (2010) Risk factors for visceral leishmaniasis in India: further evidence on the role of domestic animals. Trop Med Int Health 15:29–35
75. Hotez PJ, Remme JH, Buss P, Alleyne G, Morel C, Breman JG (2004) Combating tropical infectious diseases: report of the Disease Control Priorities in Developing Countries Project. Clin Infect Dis 38:871–878

Chapter 9
Challenges in Controlling and Eliminating Schistosomiasis

Donald P. McManus, Yuesheng Li, Gail M. Williams, Robert Bergquist, and Darren J. Gray

9.1 Introduction

Schistosomiasis, or bilharzia, is a parasitic, intravascular, trematode worm infection that causes disease through the deposition of eggs in host tissues outside the circulatory system. The main lesions are due to inflammatory responses against these trapped eggs. With more than 200 million people infected globally and close to 800 million at risk [1], it is one of the most prevalent of the tropical infectious diseases [1–4].

D.P. McManus (✉)
Molecular Parasitology Laboratory, Infectious Diseases Division, Queensland Institute of Medical Research, 300 Herston Road, Herston, Brisbane, QLD 4029, Australia
e-mail: donm@qimr.edu.au

Y. Li
Molecular Parasitology Laboratory, Infectious Diseases Division, Queensland Institute of Medical Research, 300 Herston Road, Herston, Brisbane, QLD 4029, Australia

Hunan Institute of Parasitic Diseases, WHO Collaborating Centre for Research and Control on Schistosomiasis in Lake Region, Yueyang, People's Republic of China

G.M. Williams
School of Population Health, University of Queensland, Brisbane, QLD, Australia

R. Bergquist
WHO Special Program for Research & Training in Tropical Diseases, Ingerod, Brastad, Sweden

D.J. Gray
Molecular Parasitology Laboratory, Infectious Diseases Division, Queensland Institute of Medical Research, 300 Herston Road, Herston, Brisbane, QLD 4029, Australia

School of Population Health, University of Queensland, Brisbane, QLD, Australia

School of Public Health, Griffith University, Meadowbrook, QLD, Australia

I.W. Fong (ed.), *Challenges in Infectious Diseases*, Emerging Infectious Diseases of the 21st Century 502, DOI 10.1007/978-1-4614-4496-1_9,

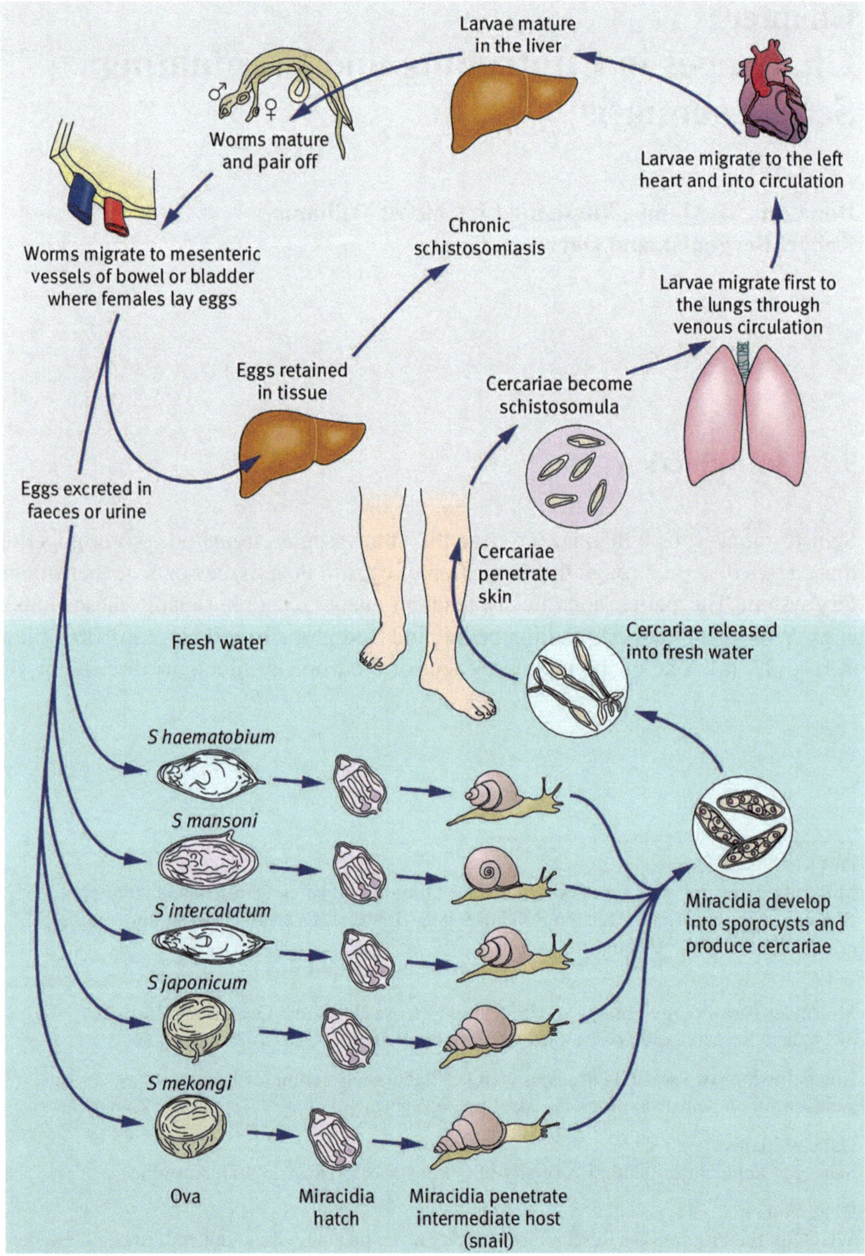

Fig. 9.1 Schistosome lifecycle. Schistosomes have a complex life cycle that involves infection of freshwater molluscs that act as intermediate hosts, and the bloodstream of higher order vertebrate definitive hosts. Adult male and female worms pair up, and the latter produce numerous eggs.

Despite major advances in control and substantial decreases in morbidity and mortality, schistosomiasis continues to spread to new geographic areas. The current disease burden remains high and may exceed 70 million disability-adjusted life years (DALYs) when subtle pathology is taken into account [5, 6]. Established schistosome infections are associated with chronic tissue inflammation leading to obstructive disease in the urinary system (in urinary schistosomiasis, which is caused by *Schistosoma haematobium*) or hepatosplenic inflammation, and liver fibrosis (in intestinal disease, which is caused by the four other schistosome species, i.e. *S. mansoni*, *S. intercalatum, S. japonicum and S. mekongi*) pathogenic to humans [2–4].

The schistosome life cycle is shown in Fig. 9.1. Transmission requires contamination of surface water by faeces or urine containing eggs from an infected human host, presence of a specific freshwater snail as intermediate host and continuous water contact by other humans [2–4]. The intermediate snail hosts are more likely to inhabit still to moderately flowing freshwater, and infection increases exponentially with length of time of water contact – peaking at 30 min [4]. Infection is usually acquired through behavioural and occupational activities such as swimming, bathing, fishing, farming and washing clothes [2, 3].

Fig. 9.1 (continued) Mating and subsequent cohabitation occur when the longer, more slender female schistosome is embraced within the ventral gynaecophoric canal of the male. The shape of the eggs and the location of their excretion differentiate the various species. Eggs are deposited in the capillaries of the target organ that is parasitized by the breeding pair of worms. With *S. haematobium*, this is the urinary system as well as the sacral and pelvic vessels, whereas with the intestinal schistosomes, parasitisation occurs in the intestinal mucosa. Once deposited, a proportion of the eggs then enter the lumen of the bladder or intestines. A small amount of bleeding occurs as eggs perforate the bladder (*S. haematobium*) or intestinal mucosa en route to the urine or faeces. Eggs that do not breach the mucosa are retained in the target organ tissue (specific to the species of worm) or are carried downstream in the portal circulation and, in the case of an *S. mansoni* or *S. japonicum* infection, are trapped in the liver. Once excreted, an ovum hatches in contact with freshwater, and a free-living motile form, called the miracidium, is released. Each schistosome species infects a specific freshwater snail intermediate host – for example, with *S. mansoni*, this is generally *Biomphalaria glabrata* (Americas) or *B. pfeifferi* (Africa). After approximately 30 days, infected snails begin to release cercariae in response to sunlight. The cercariae possess a forked tail and are free-swimming. Because cercariae are non-feeding, using their endogenous nutrient stores for energy production, they must contact with the skin of a human being (or other mammalian hosts, notably bovines, in the case of *S. japonicum*) within 12–24 h after emerging from the snail. Once contact with the skin has occurred, percutaneous penetration is achieved by mechanical activity and by the production of proteolytic enzymes. The cercariae shed their tails, invade the lymphatic system and are transported to the lungs via the blood circulation. After a short-lived residency in the lungs, the developing schistosomula then re-enter the circulation and are carried to the portal or vestibule circulation to complete the life cycle. Once there, the schistosomula mature, form mating pairs and migrate to the final target organ (Reprinted from Gray et al. [4]. With permission from the BMJ group)

9.2 Current Epidemiology

The epidemiology of schistosomiasis is complicated being determined by many biological, ecological, social and economic factors, which involves interaction between the various hosts, life cycle stages and external environment. Consequently, despite major advances in control and substantial decreases in morbidity and mortality, the disease continues to spread to new geographic areas. Figure 9.2 shows the current, global distribution of schistosomiasis. The majority (close to 85%) of *S. haematobium*, *S. mansoni* and *S. intercalatum* infections are found in sub-Saharan Africa [2–4]. *S. mansoni* remains endemic in large parts of Brazil and is also found in Surinam, Venezuela, the Caribbean, lower and middle Egypt and the Arabic peninsula. In many areas, this species coexists with *S. haematobium*, which is spread in much of sub-Saharan Africa, the Nile valley in Egypt and Sudan, the Maghreb and the Arabian Peninsula, whilst *S. intercalatum* is found in pockets in west and central Africa. *S. japonicum* infection occurs mainly in the vast lake and marshland areas in the south of P.R. China and in the Philippines. However, despite substantial and largely successful control measures, it exists also in a few, small pockets in Indonesia [2–4]. *S. mekongi* is only found in Cambodia and Laos, along the Mekong River [2–4, 7]. Important *Schistosoma* transmission sites include Lake Malawi and Lake Victoria in Africa, the Poyang and Dongting Lakes in China and along the Mekong River in Laos [2, 3].

Schistosomiasis transmission arises from agricultural practices and water resource manipulation in areas which are otherwise suitable for the parasite and

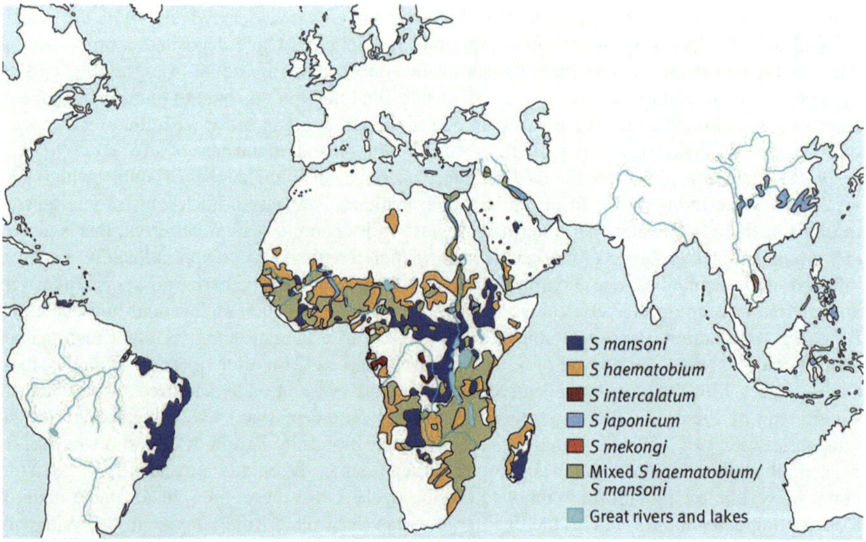

Fig. 9.2 Global distribution of schistosomiasis (Reprinted from Gray et al. [4]. With permission from the BMJ group)

its intermediate host, particularly if there is poor sanitation, and wherever there is substantial water contact such as fishing, washing and recreational activities. Environmental changes linked to water resource development, population growth, migration and disease can facilitate the spread of schistosomiasis into new areas [8]. For example, the potential impact of the recently completed Three Gorges Dam built on China's Yangtze River between two areas where the disease is endemic has invoked considerable global concerns [9]. Schistosomiasis emergences or re-emergences have resulted from other large-scale hydroprojects such as the Diama Dam on the Senegal River at the Senegal–Mauritania border, the Gezira-Managil Dam in Sudan, the Aswan Dam in Egypt, the Melkasadi Dam in Ethiopia and the Danling and Huangshi Dams in China [2].

9.3 Clinical Aspects

Schistosomiasis has three phases of disease progression – acute, chronic and advanced – which present clinically differently and require separate medical approaches.

9.3.1 Early Manifestations and Acute Disease

Often, there is little evidence of the percutaneous schistosome cercarial penetration, which marks the entry of the infection, but a maculopapular eruption may arise at the site. When migrants or tourists who are immunologically naive to the infection, skin reactions may develop within a few hours after contact, although a rash may appear up to 1 week later. The dermatitis is similar to, but less severe than, 'swimmers' itch, which develops in sensitised persons when reinfected by species of schistosomes that do not colonise humans (usually the types that infect birds; e.g. *Trichobilharzia* spp.) [2–4]. This serves to illustrate how specific the various schistosome species are to their hosts – only *S. bovis* is known to sometimes infect humans despite bovines being its definitive host.

Acute schistosomiasis (Katayama syndrome), which is a problem for travellers, is common in areas with high transmission rates [10] and in areas which have been brought under control but where there is still a low level of transmission. In the case of *S. japonicum*, it is also associated with either a superinfection or a hypersensitivity reaction in previously infected people [10].

Symptoms are mediated by immune complex formation [11–14], and the majority of cases begin with the deposition of a schistosome egg into host tissues. Symptoms may include fever, malaise, myalgia, fatigue, non-productive cough, diarrhoea (with or without the presence of blood), haematuria (*S. haematobium*) and right upper quadrant pain [10].

9.3.2 *Chronic and Advanced Disease*

9.3.2.1 Gastrointestinal and Liver Disease

The symptoms of clinical schistosomiasis result from the host's immune response to schistosome eggs and the granulomatous reaction evoked by the antigens they secrete [15, 16]. The granulomas destroy the ova but result in fibrotic deposition in host tissues [15–19]. Most granulomas develop at the sites of maximal accumulation of eggs – the intestine and the liver (in the case of *S. mansoni* and *S. japonicum*) and the genitourinary tract (in the case of *S. haematobium*) [2–4]. Schistosomes may even partially depend on the inflammatory response as an adjunct to the migration of eggs into the lumen of the gut or urinary tract to be discharged eventually into water to hatch there [20]. Murine models of schistosomiasis have proved extremely useful for deciphering the mechanism of granuloma formation and the resulting fibrogenesis [15, 16, 21, 22].

Eggs retained in the gut wall induce inflammation, hyperplasia, ulceration, microabscess formation and polyposis. Colicky hypogastric pain or pain in the left iliac fossa is frequent. Diarrhoea is common, particularly in children, and may alternate with constipation. Occult (or sometimes visible) blood in the faeces is usual. Blood loss due to schistosomiasis can be substantial. Indeed, heavy infection with *S. mansoni* has been shown to surpass that associated with hookworm infection [23].

Severe chronic intestinal disease may result in colonic or rectal stenosis. Colonic polyposis may be manifested as a protein-losing enteropathy. Inflammatory masses in the colon may even mimic cancer [2–4]. Eggs of *S. mansoni* and *S. japonicum* embolise to the liver, where the granulomatous inflammatory response induces presinusoidal inflammation and periportal or clay-pipe-stem fibrosis [2–4]. It takes many years to develop and is associated with sustained heavy infection [2–4, 24–28]. Hepatomegaly reflects the presence of granulomatous inflammation and occurs early in the evolution of chronic disease. Periportal collagen deposits lead to the progressive obstruction of blood flow, portal hypertension and, ultimately, varices, variceal bleeding, splenomegaly and hypersplenism [2, 4]. This periportal fibrosis can be seen on ultrasonography, computed tomography or magnetic resonance imaging and is characteristic of schistosomiasis.

9.3.2.2 Genitourinary Disease

Urinary tract disease is a specific trait of *S. haematobium* where again the pathology is due to granulomatous inflammation in response to tissue egg deposition [2–4, 29]. Haematuria is the first sign of established disease, appearing 10–12 weeks after infection. Dysuria and haematuria are frequent in early and late disease. Late manifestations also include proteinuria (often of the nephrotic type), bladder calcification, ureteric obstruction, renal colic, hydronephrosis and renal failure [2–4, 29]. Secondary bacterial infection is frequent. Cystoscopy generally shows 'sandy patches' (areas of roughened bladder mucosa surrounding egg deposits) which are pathognomonic for the disease. Structural urinary tract abnormalities can occur in children [29].

The association between *S. haematobium* infection and squamous cell carcinoma (SCC) of the bladder has been the subject of intense research and debate [30–34]. *S. haematobium* bladder SCCs tend to be well-differentiated and metastasize locally. Chronic urinary schistosomiasis is epidemiologically associated with squamous bladder cancer. This was typically seen in Egypt before the last few decades of successful schistosomiasis control [2–4, 35] and is still commonly seen in sub-Saharan, African foci [30–34]. Nitrosamines, β-glucuronidase and inflammatory gene damage have been put forward as possible carcinogenic factors [34]. However, another explanation is that schistosomiasis lesions intensify the exposure of the bladder epithelium to mutagenetic substrates from tobacco or chemicals [31]. At present, there is sufficient evidence favouring *S. haematobium* in the aetiology of some human bladder cancer [3]. Recent work suggests a link between metastasis-associated protein 1 – a chromatin-bound component of the NuRD (nucleosome remodelling and deacetylase) complex – schistosomiasis haematobia, granulomatous-specific inflammation in liver and incidence of schistosome-associated bladder cancer [36].

S. haematobium causes genital disease in approximately one-third of women infected [2–4]. Vulval schistosomiasis may also facilitate the transmission of the human immunodeficiency virus (HIV) [2–4, 37, 38].

9.3.2.3 Neurological and Other Clinical Outcomes

Neuroschistosomiasis is one of the most severe clinical outcomes associated with schistosome infection [2–4]. Neurological complications can occur early during the course of infection and are thought to develop following in situ egg deposition following aberrant migration of adult worms to the brain or spinal cord. The mass effect of thousands of eggs and the large granulomas concentrated within the brain or spinal cord explain the signs and symptoms of increased intracranial pressure, myelopathy, radiculopathy and subsequent clinical sequelae [2–4, 39–41]. Myelopathy (acute transverse myelitis and subacute myeloradiculopathy) of the lumbosacral region is the most common neurological manifestation of *S. mansoni* or *S. haematobium* infection, whereas acute encephalitis of the cortex, subcortical white matter, basal ganglia or internal capsule is typical of infection by *S. japonicum* [39, 40]. Cerebral complications include encephalopathy with headache, visual impairment, delirium, seizures, motor deficits and ataxia, whereas spinal symptoms comprise lumbar pain, lower limb radicular pain, muscle weakness, sensory loss and bladder dysfunction [39, 40].

Schistosome infection in childhood causes substantial growth retardation and anaemia [2–4, 42]. Successful chemotherapy leads to appreciable but incomplete catch-up growth and improvement in haemoglobin levels [2–4, 42, 43]. Additionally, these children may have cognitive impairment and memory deficits which can significantly limit human potential. Schistosome infection appears to adversely affect both maternal health and the unborn foetus. Chronic *S. mansoni* and (rarely) *S. haematobium* but not *S. japonicum* infection may cause pulmonary hypertension, cor pulmonale, glomerulonephritis or transverse myelitis [43–48].

9.4 Diagnosis

Despite some limitations, microscopic examination of excreta remains the 'gold diagnostic standard' [2–4]. Schistosome eggs are easy to detect and identify by microscopy owing to their size and shape and their characteristic lateral or terminal spine (Fig. 9.1). Examination of stool or urine should not be undertaken until at least 2 months after the latest known water contact as a patent infection takes this long to start producing eggs [2–4, 49–54]. The rapid, simple and inexpensive Kato–Katz thick smear stool examination [55] requires 40–50 mg of faeces and is used globally to determine the burden of eggs in faeces, although this is generally unnecessary in order to provide clinical care [3]. The use of formalin-based techniques for sedimentation and concentration increases the diagnostic yield somewhat, but may not be sufficient in returned travellers with few eggs [3, 56]. The sensitivity of microscopic detection of eggs in stool or organ biopsies is variable due to the fluctuation of egg shedding, the prevalence and intensity of infection and the number of stool specimens collected and slides prepared for microscopy [57–60].

S. haematobium eggs are generally detected by microscopy in a urine sample concentrated by sedimentation, centrifugation or filtration using a paper or nitrocellulose filter [2–4]. Self-reported blood in the urine and/or microhaematuria on reagent strips indicates potential infection in those living in endemic areas [61–63]. The sensitivity of microscopic detection of eggs in stool or organ biopsies is variable due to the fluctuation of egg shedding, the prevalence and intensity of infection and the number of stool specimens collected and slides prepared for microscopy [57–60]. Questionnaires are often also used for schistosomiasis screening purposes, particularly with schoolchildren [62, 63].

The miracidium-hatching test has been used by public health workers in China to rule out *S. japonicum* infection [3]. The test is initiated by the concentration of eggs from faeces through a nylon tissue bag and suspension in distilled water. Miracidia that hatch are visualised macroscopically and their presence is diagnostic of infection. Detection of *S. mansoni* eggs in faeces through their interaction with paramagnetic beads in a magnetic field may significantly improve diagnosis of infections with low burdens in areas of recent introduction of the parasite, in areas under successful control of transmission or in infected travellers; it may also improve the evaluation of new treatments and vaccines [64]. In patients with a typical clinical presentation but negative urine and faeces specimens, a biopsy of bladder or rectal mucosa should be considered for diagnosis [3, 4].

Specific and highly sensitive polymerase chain reaction (PCR)-based assays have been developed for the detection of schistosome DNA in faeces, urine or sera/plasma [65–68]. This approach has the potential, in appropriately equipped facilities, to provide a test for diagnosing schistosomiasis in all phases of clinical disease, including the capacity to diagnose Katayama syndrome and active disease, and for therapy evaluation in humans. Another promising, highly sensitive assay based on loop-mediated isothermal amplification (LAMP) has recently been developed for the detection of *S. japonicum* DNA [69]. The test, which uses a sequence of the highly repetitive retrotransposon SjR2, can detect 0.08 fg *S. japonicum* DNA, which is considerably more sensitive than conventional PCR.

Indirect methods for diagnosing schistosome infection by the detection of clinical, subclinical or biochemical morbidity markers are generally not very specific given the generalised presentation of the disease. Current indirect methods include the use of clinical assessment of the patient coupled with ultrasound, liver biopsy and subsequent histological examination and the measurement of biochemical markers [2–4]. Additional supportive laboratory evidence of schistosomiasis might include evidence of peripheral-blood eosinophilia, anaemia (iron-deficiency anaemia, anaemia of chronic disease or macrocytic anaemia), hypoalbuminemia, elevated urea and creatinine levels and hypergammaglobulinemia [2–4]. Splenomegaly develops in some patients with pancytopenia [3, 4]. Biochemical markers of liver fibrosis (pro-collagen peptides type III and IV, the P1 fragment of laminin, hyaluronic acid, fibrosin, TNF-αR-II, sICAM-1, tissue inhibitor of matrix-metalloprotease-1 (TIMP-1), cytokeratin 18 and aspartate aminotransferase to platelet ratio index (APRI)) measured in serum have potential to provide a highly sensitive and cost-effective method for the assessment of schistosome-induced fibrosis [3, 4, 60, 70–74]. A biopsy of the liver may be necessary in some patients with co-infection (e.g. with hepatitis virus) [3, 4]. Liver involvement in patients with schistosomiasis is often suggested by the characteristic appearance of the organ on abdominal imaging [2–4].

Antibody detection is highly sensitive and can be useful in specific circumstances. However, its application is limited in practice because antibodies persist after cure [2–4, 75]. A positive serologic test may be diagnostic in patients in whom there are no eggs, such as those with Katayama syndrome. Furthermore, serologic screening is valuable in field studies for defining regions of low-level endemicity where individual patients have low egg burdens. Serologic testing may also be useful in determining whether infection has re-emerged in a region after an apparently successful elimination programme and is important for diagnosis in travellers. Commercially available immunodiagnostic kits are generally not as sensitive as multiple faecal examinations and are less specific, due to antibody cross-reactivity with antigens from other helminths [2–4, 11, 75–77]. Most techniques detect IgG, IgM or IgE against soluble worm antigen or soluble egg antigen (SEA) by ELISA, indirect haemagglutination (IHA) or immunofluorescence [2–4, 78]. A cercarial antigen ELISA equivalent to the SEA assay for serodiagnosis of schistosomiasis has been developed that may be preferred for routine clinical use [79].

Steady advances have been made in detection of circulating egg or adult worm components – especially circulating *Schistosoma* anodic and cathodic antigens (CAA and CCA) [80] – with labelled monoclonal or polyclonal antibodies in serum, urine or sputum in infected individuals, and this promising approach may eventually supersede traditional diagnostic methods. As CAA and CCA are released by viable adult worms, these assays are specific for current infections and can also provide information on infection intensity [81]. A commercially produced diagnostic test – the urine-CCA strip – is available for detecting schistosomiasis [82], and it may be useful for screening schistosome infections, especially in areas with high prevalence [81, 83, 84].

9.5 Present Treatment/New Developments

Praziquantel (PZQ), a pyrazinoisoquinoline derivative, is a safe and effective oral drug that is active against all schistosome species [85, 86]. It is the mainstay of treatment and a critical part of community-based schistosomiasis control programmes, although it does not prevent re-infection. The drug is as safe and efficacious in children aged 1–5 years as it is in older children aged 6–10 years [87]. Since its discovery in the mid-1970s [88], its safety and efficacy have ensured its widespread use. It is absorbed well but undergoes extensive first-pass hepatic clearance. PZQ is secreted in breast milk, it is metabolised by the liver and its (inactive) metabolites are excreted in the urine. Side effects are mild, and it can be used to treat young children and pregnant women. The drug acts within 1 h of ingestion, and it appears to cause titanic contractions and tegumental vacuoles, causing worms to detach from the wall of the vein and die. Schistosome calcium ion (Ca^{2+}) channels are the only moiety so far identified as the molecular target of PZQ, but the evidence remains indirect and its precise mechanism of action remains unknown. ABC transporter genes in schistosomes may play a role in fine-tuning the susceptibility to PZQ; disruption of their function may therefore provide a strategy for enhancing drug action or overcoming or attenuating drug resistance [89]. In animal models, the presence of host antibodies has been shown to be critical for the efficacy of PZQ [85, 86].

Standard human treatment for chronic schistosomiasis is 60 mg/kg of PZQ orally in divided doses over 1 day for *S. japonicum* and *S. mekongi* and 40 mg/kg orally in divided doses over 1 day for the African schistosomes [4]. There is some evidence from experimental laboratory studies, albeit controversial, that resistance to PZQ may be emerging in Africa where there has been heavy exposure to the drug. Worryingly, there are reports from African sites of schistosome infections that are either not responsive or produce incomplete cures in populations given the routine treatment [2, 4, 90, 91]. So far, however, patients in many other communities have undergone multiple courses of treatment over a period of 10 or more years without a demonstrable loss of efficacy.

As worm reproduction in the mammalian definitive host is sexual and the generation time is relatively long, resistance is unlikely in the short term and will take many years to become an important clinical and public health issue. Nevertheless, resistance against PZQ in the future cannot be ruled out, and it is important that research be continued towards development of alternative compounds, such as 4-phenyl-1,2,5-oxadiazole-3-carbonitrile-2-oxide (shown to inhibit a crucial parasite enzyme, thioredoxin glutathione reductase) [92], inhibitors of phytochelatin synthase, an enzyme which is involved in the synthesis of phytochelatins from glutathione [93] and approved cancer drugs, such as inhibitors of protein kinases [94], as novel candidate anti-schistosome agents. Other drugs that have been used in the treatment of schistosomiasis are oxamniquine (Vansil) for *S. mansoni* and metrifonate (trichlorfon) for *S. haematobium*, but both are ineffective against *S. japonicum* [2, 3]. Miltefosine, which is primarily used in the treatment of leishmaniasis, is another anti-schistosomal drug that has shown promise [95]. Combinations of the anti-malarial drug mefloquine and praziquantel may also have clinical utility in the treatment of schistosomiasis [96].

Other drugs that have been used in the treatment of schistosomiasis are oxamniquine (Vansil) for *S. mansoni* and metrifonate (trichlorfon) for *S. haematobium*, but both are ineffective against *S. japonicum* [2, 3]. Corticosteroids (e.g. prednisone 1.5–2.0 mg/kg/day for 3 weeks) and anticonvulsants are needed as possible adjuvants to praziquantel in neuroschistosomiasis, which needs specialised care [2, 97].

PZQ cannot be used for chemoprophylaxis because of its short half-life (1–1.5 h) and because it cannot kill schistosomula (the migrating larvae) that are 3–21 days old. Artemether (ART), which is an artemisinin compound available from the leaves of the Chinese medicinal plant *Artemisia annua*, is not only effective against malaria, but also against juvenile schistosomes during the first 21 days of infection in animals and humans [98]. ART would kill all new infections through its action against immature schistosomula if given every 2 weeks. Accordingly, it has been used as a chemoprophylactic in schistosomiasis-endemic areas in high-risk groups, such as flood relief workers and fishermen in China [99]. The doses required are lower than those required for treatment of malaria, but it is unlikely that ART would be used in other regions, such as Africa, where malaria is endemic because such use might lead to the selection of ART-resistant *Plasmodium falciparum*.

In animals, combination therapy with PZQ plus ART is safe and results in higher worm reduction rates than PZQ alone [98, 99]. However, a randomised, double-blind, placebo-controlled trial for evaluating combined chemotherapy with PZQ and ART at two different dosages (60 and 120 mg/kg) in the treatment of acute schistosomiasis japonica in China failed to improve treatment efficacy compared with PZQ alone [100]. As well, the standard treatment with praziquantel was shown to be more effective than artesunate (another artemisinin) with sulfalene plus pyrimethamine in the treatment of children with *S. mansoni* infection in western Kenya [101]. A recent randomised, exploratory open-label trial of mefloquine–artesunate showed promising efficacy against *S. haematobium* [102], but overall, it is an open question whether artemisinin-based combination therapy will play a significant role in the future treatment of schistosomiasis [103].

9.6 Potential for Vaccines

9.6.1 The Immune Response in Schistosomiasis

Although the modern schistosomiasis control approach [104] has shown that chemotherapy alone is capable of reducing morbidity in humans, rapid re-infection is a reminder that the impact of drug treatment on transmission is marginal. An important feature of schistosome parasites is that they do not replicate in their mammalian hosts so that a naturally acquired or vaccine-induced partial, non-sterilising immunity could potentially decrease human/animal pathology and transmission in areas where schistosomiasis is endemic. In order to report on progress towards the development of anti-schistosome vaccines, a description of some basic details of the immunology of schistosomiasis is necessary.

Much of our knowledge on the immunobiology of schistosomiasis, including the nature of the host innate and adaptive responses to schistosomes, on strategies these parasites use to manipulate such responses and on the mechanisms of schistosome-induced pathogenesis has resulted from studies on murine models of schistosomiasis [16, 105–110]. A valuable review by Allen and Maizels [111] discusses recent advances in defining the immune cell types and molecules that are mobilised in response to helminth, including schistosome infection, and considers how these immunological players are blended and regulated in order to accommodate persistent infection or to mount a vigorous protective response and achieve sterile immunity.

In general, the murine studies have established that T-cell-mediated immunity is fundamental in acquired resistance to schistosomes. Much of this protection has been shown to be mediated by activated macrophages and, together with studies of cytokines, suggests that a vaccine that can induce macrophage-activating Th1 cytokines (interferon-γ and interleukin (IL)-2) may be beneficial in preventing schistosomiasis. However, repeated vaccination with irradiated cercariae produces incremental increases in Th2-mediated protection, which is transferable to non-vaccinated animals. The central player in this type 2 immunity in helminths is the CD4+ T helper 2 (Th2) cell, which produces a broad range of cytokines, including interleukin-4 (IL-4) and IL-13; these act on target cells expressing the IL-4 receptor α-chain [112]. Target cells include most cells of the immune system but also local tissue cells such as epithelial cells that line mucosal surfaces [112]. Data from experimental schistosomiasis models suggest that immunity is also influenced by regulatory T cells [113].

Studies using B-cell-deficient and cytokine-deficient mice have demonstrated that successful anti-schistosome vaccination requires induction of strong Th1 and Th2 responses [113]. Following infection by normal or radiation-attenuated cercariae, the predominant early immune response is Th1-mediated and aimed at the adult worm. Following egg deposition in tissues (6 weeks p.i. for *S. mansoni* or 4–5 weeks for *S. japonicum*), the Th1 response is diminished, being replaced by a prominent Th2-mediated phase. Indeed, it appears that egg antigens are able to directly suppress the Th1 response, a phenomenon which may also occur in humans. Th2 response results in an increase in serum interleukin-5 (IL-5), massive bone and blood eosinophilia and the characteristic granulomatous response aimed at the egg, resulting in collagen deposition, tissue fibrosis and disease manifestations of schistosomiasis, already described.

In human schistosomiasis, longitudinal cohort studies of re-infection rates following curative drug treatment have shown that people living in schistosome-endemic areas acquire some form of protective immunity after years of exposure [113]. However, age-related innate resistance mechanisms may also play an important part in the epidemiology of schistosomiasis. Immune correlative studies in various parts of the world suggest that acquired anti-schistosome protective immunity after curative drug therapy is mediated (although not exclusively) by a Th2 response, orchestrated by IgE against adult and larval antigens, which stimulate eosinophils to release cytotoxins targeting schistosomula [113–115].

Despite the protective role of IgE, high levels of IgG4 are also produced during schistosome infection [113, 116], potentially blocking the protective effects of other immunoglobulins. It has been shown that immunity to re-infection is more closely related to the IgE/IgG4 balance than to the absolute level of each isotype. The clinical expression of immunity to schistosome infection is obviously not simply determined by the mere balance between IgE and IgG4 antibodies. It cannot exclude the participation of additional mechanisms such as a potential protective role of IgA antibodies in human schistosomiasis; the effector functions of IgA antibodies may be associated with as decrease in female worm fecundity and egg viability [113]. The relative proportions of regulatory T cells may influence or reflect different stages of the development of protective schistosome acquired immunity and immunopathogenesis in humans [117].

It is important to emphasise that the development of a vaccine for schistosomiasis that is dependent on IgE would be potentially problematic and would likely be impeded by regulatory and safety issues due to potential anaphylaxis induced by vaccination [113]. Caution is necessary when looking to the immune responses of chronically infected individuals and even those who become refractory by producing IgE after drug treatment.

Although we still know very little about the protective mechanisms required to engineer an efficacious recombinant vaccine for human schistosomiasis, the analysis of human antibody and cytokine responses to candidate antigens has potential for identifying new vaccine targets [113]. The studies that have been undertaken of immune responses against panels of schistosome antigens determined in cohorts of humans living in areas where they were regularly exposed to *S. mansoni* or *S. japonicum* infection and the results compared with parasitological diagnosis indicate that cellular and humoral immune responses were significantly associated with either apparent resistance or with apparent susceptibility to re-infection following chemotherapy [113]. However, only a minority of these responses produced consistent associations, and the results have been shown to be seldom clear-cut. One reason may be the numerous and complex factors that influence *Schistosoma* infection intensity and prevalence within endemic communities, including exposure-related features such as local environment and behaviour, and genetic and other factors that affect an individual's susceptibility to infection and the resulting immune response [113, 118].

Nonetheless, the discovery of the surface-located tetraspanins Sm-TSP-1 and TSP-2 as major candidate vaccine antigens in *S. mansoni* resulted from a combination of protective efficacy data obtained in the murine challenge model with their recognition by IgG1 and IgG3 antibodies from humans exposed but resistant to schistosomiasis [113]. Human studies are thus instructive not only for identifying the few antigens directly and exclusively associated with resistance but also for indicating which of these components can be formulated with adjuvants to generate protective responses in animal models [113].

In the case of *S. japonicum*, zoonotic transmission adds to the complexity of control programmes, but provides a unique opportunity to develop a transmission blocking veterinary vaccine to help prevent human infection and disease [42, 113, 119]. However, there are relatively few studies of protective immunity in bovine schistosome infections; consequently, our knowledge of the immunology of schistosome infections in water buffaloes and cattle is extremely limited. This is particularly the case for water buffaloes although immunological reagents for studying appropriate immune responses are improving. Additional studies on the immunology of bovines represent an important area for future research and will be useful in selecting *S. japonicum* vaccine antigens and in defining the optimum route of immunisation.

9.6.2 Current Vaccine Development

The feasibility of developing vaccines for schistosomiasis has been extensively reviewed [113, 120, 121]. Humans living in endemic areas can become resistant or partially immune to re-infection over time. As well, irradiated cercariae can elicit high levels of protective immunity in laboratory animals, and several recombinant-protein vaccines have been shown to elicit comparable levels of protective immunity in immunised animals that were subsequently challenged with cercariae [113]. Vaccination can be targeted either towards the prevention of schistosome infection or to the reduction of parasite fecundity. A reduction in worm numbers is the gold standard for anti-schistosome vaccine development, with the migrating schistosomulum stage likely to be the major vaccine target of protective immune responses [113]. However, as schistosome eggs are responsible for both pathology and transmission, a vaccine targeted at parasite fecundity and egg viability is also relevant [113].

9.6.2.1 Vaccine Candidates for *S. mansoni* and *S. haematobium*

Vaccine development against *S. mansoni* and *S. haematobium* will necessitate the use of clinical vaccines for human application [113, 120, 121]. Despite there being very little reported work in this area for *S. haematobium*, a vaccine for urinary schistosomiasis has entered clinical trials [16, 113, 122]. Known as Bilhvax, this is a recombinant 28 kDa GST cloned from *S. haematobium* which, adjuvanted with aluminium hydroxide, has been reported to be immunogenic and safe after testing in healthy adults [122]. With regard to intestinal schistosomiasis, a 14 kDa fatty acid-binding protein (Sm14–FABP) has been shown in experimental animals to elicit protection against *S. mansoni* [123, 124]. Recently, the molecule was successfully stabilised by replacing a crucial cysteine residue in order to prevent dimerisation [124], and, as it also protects against *Fasciola hepatica*, Sm14-FABP is being developed in Brazil for use against both fascioliasis in livestock and human schistosomiasis caused by *S. mansoni* [120, 123]. The new construct provides a highly purified protein in large yields with preserved protective activity for both parasites. This has opened the way to veterinary clinical trial as well as the first human phase I safety trial, initiated in June 2011.

Sm-p80, a DNA vaccine, encoding the large subunit of a calcium-dependent neutral protease [125–128] and a 9 kDa fragment of the second extracellular domain of Sm-TSP2, an integral membrane tetraspanin, crucial for tegument development [129, 130], have also shown potential for moving into clinical development for schistosomiasis mansoni. Other molecules that have recently been identified/tested as potential vaccine targets against *S. mansoni* include saposin-like proteins (SAPLIPS) [131], aldolase [132], Sm29 [133], dynein light chains [134], Sm21.6 [135], SmIg [136], annexin [137, 138] and stomatin-like protein 2 [139].

9.6.2.2 Vaccine Candidates for *S. japonicum*

As with the African schistosomes, coordinated laboratory and field research has identified a set of well-defined *S. japonicum* molecules with protective potential, with a view to developing a recombinant-protein, synthetic-peptide or DNA vaccine [113]. Of the leading vaccine candidates, the majority are membrane proteins, muscle components or enzymes and include paramyosin, calpain, GSTs, fatty acid-binding protein and serpin [113]. Other molecules recently identified/tested as potential vaccine targets in *S. japonicum* are methionine aminopeptidase 2 [140], proteasome subunit alpha type 5 protein [141], peroxiredoxin-1 [142], 8-kDa calcium-binding protein [143] and insulin receptors and other signal transduction components [144, 145].

As indicated earlier, *S. mansoni* tetraspanin 2 (Sm-TSP-2) is considered a lead target for vaccine development against schistosomiasis mansoni, but vaccine/challenge experiments in mice with homologous proteins from *S. japonicum* (Sj-TSP-2) by several different groups have provided inconsistent and contradictory results [146–148]. Unlike Sm-TSP-2, which appears to be conserved [148], molecular characterisation studies have shown the *Sj-TSP-2* gene is highly polymorphic at the transcriptional level [147–149], and this may limit the value of Sj-TSP-2 as a target for future *S. japonicum* vaccine development.

In contrast to the African schistosomes, the zoonotic transmission of schistosomiasis japonica allows for the development and deployment of a transmission blocking veterinary vaccine in livestock animals, particularly bovines, prior to developing a human vaccine should this be necessary [113]. The vaccine would be used in reservoir hosts of *S. japonicum* to potentially reduce transmission to humans. Bovines (cattle and water buffaloes) are the major reservoirs for *S. japonicum* infection in China with estimates that 75–90% of egg contamination comes from this source through drug intervention studies and mathematical modelling underpinning the rationale for developing a veterinary vaccine against *S. japonicum* [42, 113, 119]. The possibility that this strategy could pay off already is supported by Chinese studies showing that the animal–snail– human transmission cycle is more prominent than the human–snail–human one in sustaining the infection [150]. Studies of the protection afforded by *S. japonicum* recombinant proteins (e.g. paramyosin (Sj-97), GST-26 (Sj-GST26)) and DNA plasmids (triose-phosphate isomerase (SjC-TP1-Hsp-70), 23-kDa integral membrane (tetraspanin) protein (SjC-23-Hsp70)) [113, 151] in water buffaloes have yielded encouraging results, adding support for the feasibility of developing a vaccine that blocks transmission for use in these reservoir hosts.

9.6.2.3 Future Directions for Vaccine Development

The current schistosome vaccine candidates may prove not to be the most effective, and it is, therefore, important to continue to identify new target antigens [113]. Complete sequencing of the *S. japonicum* [152] and *S. mansoni* [153] genomes and the generation of large schistosome transcriptome databases [154–157] and postgenomic technologies, including DNA microarray profiling [155, 156, 158–161], proteomics [162–167], glycomics [168, 169], metabonomics [170], immunomics [171], whole mount in situ hybridization methodology [172], genetic manipulation, RNA interference (RNAi), mRNA silencing and transgene expression [173–175], can provide the necessary ancillary information. These new approaches in antigen discovery have the potential to identify a new generation of vaccine target molecules that may induce greater potency than the current candidate schistosome antigens [113]. The selection of a suitable adjuvant and delivery system to aid in the stimulation of the appropriate immune response is a critical step in the path to the development and employment of successful anti-schistosome vaccines, and a number of different approaches have been tested with some success [113]. Immunogenicity relies on antigenic access to particular pathways promoting the secretion of cytokines from antigen-presenting and other cells. This can now be achieved artificially by using immunomodulating agents, live microbiological carriers or DNA technology [176–179], and these approaches could provide clues as to how future vaccines might be formulated [113]. Other methodologies such as codon optimization of current schistosome vaccine candidates to enhance immunogenicity [180] or the development of cocktail epitope/protein/multivalent vaccines [120, 181–183] are also relevant and are being actively pursued.

9.7 Advances in Control/Prevention

9.7.1 Current Control Strategies

Schistosomiasis is a focal disease requiring interaction between the human host and the snail intermediate host in an environment conducive to snail inhabitation. Generally, schistosomiasis transmission consists of two major transmission pathways – based on the parasite's lifecycle (Fig. 9.1) – that can be targeted by interventions and control programmes: the parasites' path from humans (the definitive hosts) to snails (the intermediate hosts) and their path from snails to humans (Fig. 9.3) [184, 185]. However, for *S. japonicum* and *S. mekongi*, there are additional pathways of transmission due to their zoonotic nature. Bovines have been identified as the major reservoir for *S. japonicum* transmission [186], whilst dogs are important hosts in the transmission of *S. mekongi* [187]. These additional pathways complicate control, but also provide additional intervention targets.

Schistosomiasis control programmes can be categorised as (1) morbidity control, which aims to reduce morbidity in infected persons/communities; this is achieved through chemotherapy acting upon the human to snail transmission pathway; (2) transmission control, which aims to interrupt transmission by targeting the intermediate host and/or multiple transmission pathways; and (3) elimination, which aims to interrupt transmission to the point where the prevalence is <1%.

The general strategy for schistosomiasis control has shifted since the discovery of PZQ in the 1970s with the result that population-based chemotherapy programmes (morbidity control) have now mostly replaced previous programmes targeting the intermediate snail host (transmission control) [3]. Morbidity control has gained further momentum over the last 5–10 years with a renewed interest in

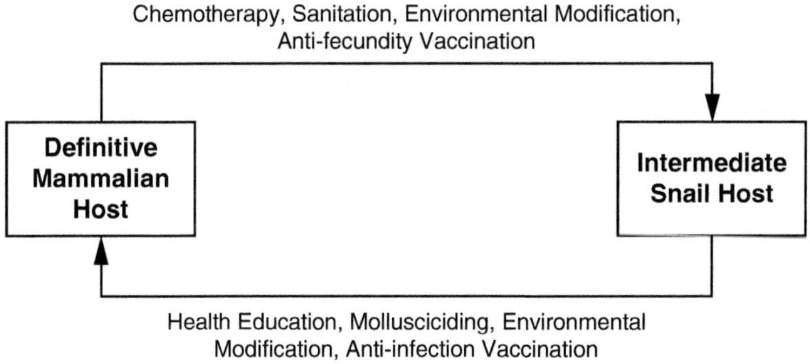

Fig. 9.3 Transmission pathways and various control measures acting on these (Reprinted from Gray et al. [184]. With permission from Elsevier)

the neglected tropical diseases, a reduction in the cost of PZQ and an increased availability of funding [184]. The current WHO strategy for schistosomiasis control focuses on reducing morbidity through mass or targeted drug administration (PZQ 40 mg/kg) now termed 'preventive chemotherapy'. WHO specifically advocates targeting at-risk groups, which include school-aged children, at-risk adults in endemic areas (e.g. pregnant and breastfeeding women and people with occupationally or socially driven contact with infested water) and entire communities living in endemic areas. Frequency of treatment is determined by the prevalence of infection or visible haematuria (*S. haematobium*) in school-aged children (Table 9.1) [188]. It is noteworthy that this strategy is primarily focused on schistosomiasis in Africa as 85% of all cases occur there.

In 2001 the World Health Assembly (WHA Resolution 54.19) recommended that by 2010, member states should attain a minimum target of regularly treating 75–100% of school-aged children at risk of schistosome infection [3, 189, 190]. In 2009, 21 of the 76 countries endemic for schistosomiasis reported that 19,570,971 people were treated with PZQ. This is a 7.8% increase from 2008, although only 10,789,205 (55.1%) of those treated were school-aged children [191]. Whilst this is a great achievement, it falls considerably short of the WHA Resolution 54.19 target. Utzinger and colleagues have predicted that 128 million school-aged children would need to be treated annually to achieve the target and have raised the question on whether enough PZQ could ever be produced [189, 190]. Furthermore, this strategy – with such a large focus on population-based chemotherapy – diverts emphasis away from preventive control measures such as snail control, health education/promotion, access to clean water and improved hygiene and sanitation [189, 190].

Snail control can be a powerful intervention tool as it essentially removes the intermediate host from the parasite's life cycle, thus breaking transmission. This was used extensively prior to the advent of PZQ through widespread chemical mollusciciding and environmental modification but met with many complications, notably environmental toxicity and high-cost implications [3, 42, 119]. Today more environmentally friendly chemicals have been developed, and mollusciciding has become targeted to specific foci, which is now commonly used for schistosomiasis control in China [3, 42, 119]. Environmental modification (e.g. the concreting of irrigation ditches in Japan and China, thus creating an ecosystem uninhabitable by snails) has been used with success in Asia, although it is very expensive [3, 42, 119].

Health education/promotion programmes can increase community knowledge on schistosome transmission and prevention, although effecting behavioural change can be more challenging. Access to clean water and to improved sanitation and hygiene was a major component of the elimination of schistosomiasis from Japan [3, 42] and, coupled with behavioural change, can in principle eliminate schistosomiasis worldwide [3, 42]. Schistosomiasis, however, is linked with poverty, and major economic growth and investment are required to improve sanitation in many endemic communities.

Table 9.1 Recommended preventive chemotherapy strategy for schistosomiasis

Category	Prevalence among school-aged children	Action to be taken	
High risk community	≥50 % by parasitological methods (intestinal and urinary schistosomiasis) or ≥30 % by questionnaire for visible haematuria (urinary schistosomiasis)	Treat all school-age children (enrolled and not enrolled) once a year	Also treat adults considered to be at risk (e.g. pregnant and breastfeeding women and people with occupationally or socially driven contact with infested water; and entire communities living in endemic areas)
Moderate-risk community	≥10 % but <50 % by parasitological methods (intestinal and urinary schistosomiasis) or <30 % by questionnaire for visible haematuria (urinary schistosomiasis)	Treat all school-age children (enrolled and not enrolled) once every 2 years	Also treat adults considered to be at risk (e.g. pregnant and breastfeeding women and people with occupationally or socially driven contact with infested water; and entire communities living in endemic areas)
Low-risk community	<10 % by parasitological methods (intestinal and urinary schistosomiasis)	Treat all school-age children (enrolled and not enrolled) twice during their primary schooling age (e.g. once on entry and once on exit)	Praziquantel should be available in dispensaries and clinics for treatment of suspected cases.

Modified from Ref. [188]

9.7.2 Spatial and Mathematical Modelling

The modelling of schistosomiasis has important implications when considering different geographical targets and options for control.

9.7.2.1 Spatial Modelling

Spatial clustering of parasite infections in high-prevalence communities is a well-described phenomenon [192–197]. Utilising epidemiological data, geographic information systems (GIS) and remote sensing (RS), spatial modelling can provide an evidence base for large-scale control programmes by producing risk maps for the geographical targeting of interventions [192, 195, 198]. For example, Clements and colleagues were able to predict the geographical distribution of *S. haematobium* in northwest Tanzania, thereby providing targets for the national schistosomiasis and soil-transmitted helminth control programme with support from the Schistosomiasis Control Initiative (SCI) [104]. Parasitological and geographic data were collected from at least 60 children in each of 143 primary schools in northwest Tanzania for the purpose of developing the risk maps (Fig. 9.4A). Spatially explicit binomial regression and Bayesian geostatistical modelling were then performed to produce maps of predicted *S. haematobium* prevalence (Fig. 9.4B) [195]. Yang et al. [199] carried out similar studies based on climate factors in China illustrating the risk for spread of schistosomiasis to large areas north of the current limits.

9.7.2.2 Mathematical Modelling

The conventional approach to evaluating the effectiveness of a disease control programme is to conduct a randomised-controlled field trial. Results from such trials are considered the gold standard for evidence-based medicine and are normally required for translation into policy and practice. However, this approach has some shortcomings in many public health settings, as randomised-controlled trials are often of a limited duration and do not capture long-term effects of the control strategy. Additionally, the number of alternatives that can be assessed is restricted because they are extremely expensive and time-consuming to conduct. Also, for infectious diseases, external uncontrollable factors such as climate and weather can disturb the most meticulously planned studies and confound findings. Mathematical models have often been used as a cost-effective, flexible alternative that allow for the prediction of short-, medium- and long-term impacts of control programmes.

Transmission dynamics mathematical models can be specifically used to simulate schistosome transmission, predict the spread of disease and simulate various strategies for control and control programme coverage. Simulations can also be undertaken in the context of control, sustainable control and elimination. This is determined by the parasite reproduction ratio (R_0) where >1 = control, ≥ 1 = sustainable control and <1 = elimination.

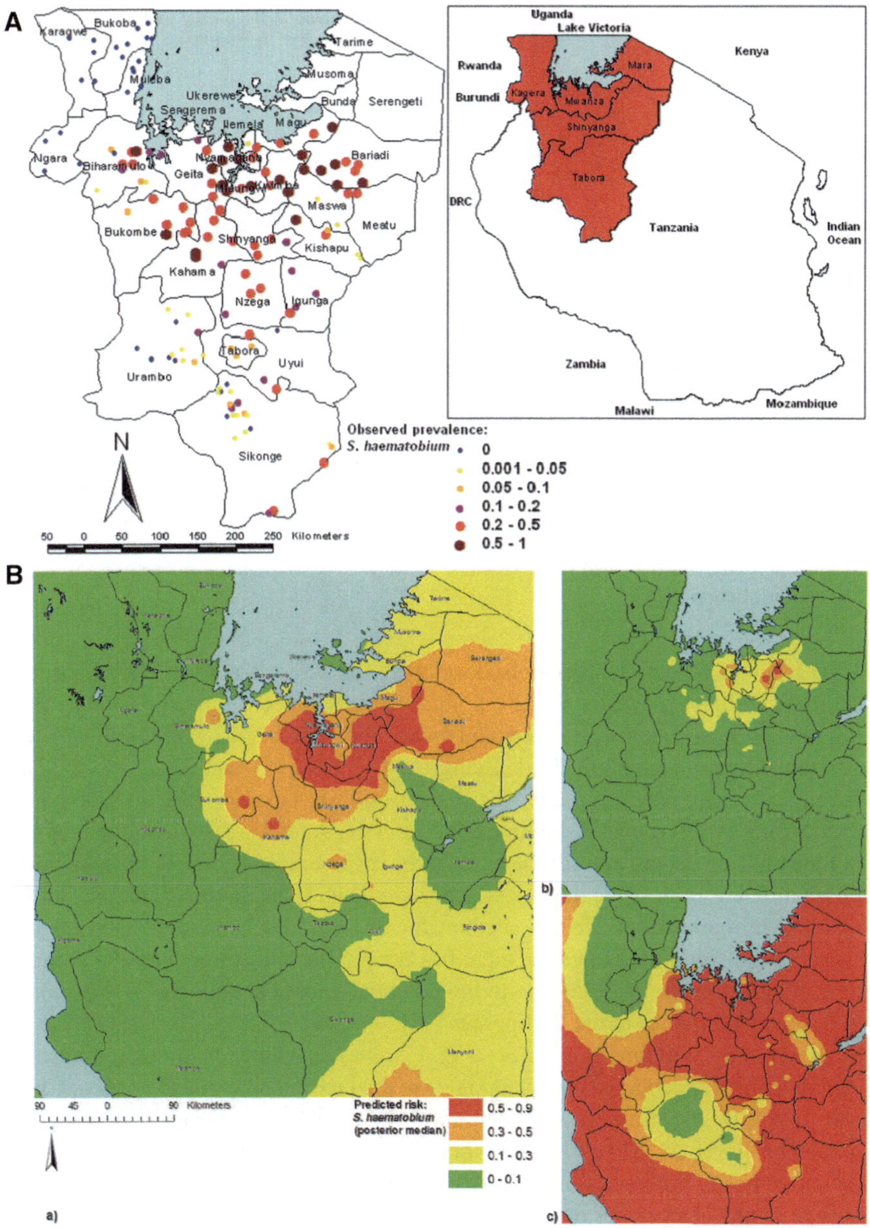

Fig. 9.4 (**A**) Location and *S. haematobium* prevalence of surveyed schools in northwest Tanzania. (**B**) Predicted *S. haematobium* prevalence in northwest Tanzania: (*a*) posterior median, (*b*) *lower* 95% Bayesian credible interval limit, (*c*) *upper* 95% Bayesian credible interval limit (Reprinted from Clements et al. [195]. With permission from Blackwell Publishing Ltd.)

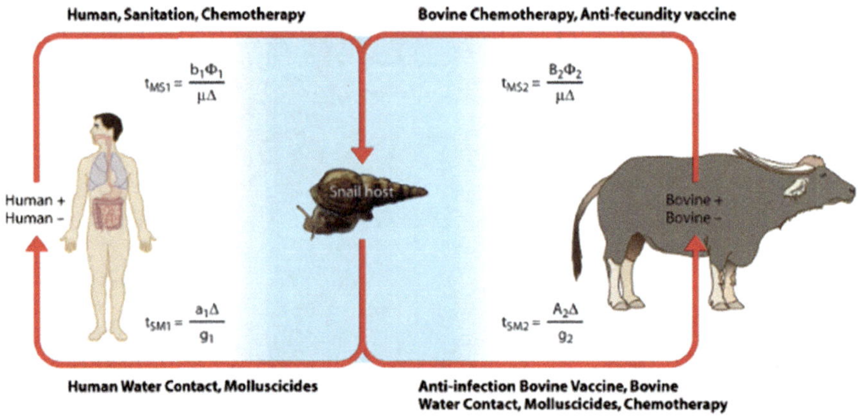

Fig. 9.5 *Left panel*. Mathematical model for *S. japonicum* transmission, showing parameters and intervention pathways. *Right panel* shows model predictions of the bovine vaccine. Effect on human prevalence: (a) vaccine alone, (b) vaccine + initial bovine treatment + annual human treatment (10 years). Effect on bovine prevalence: (c) vaccine + initial bovine treatment + annual human treatment (10 years) (Reprinted from McManus et al. [42]. With permission from the American Society for Microbiology)

The first mathematical models developed for schistosomiasis were those by Hairston [200] and MacDonald [201]. Since then, a number of transmission dynamics models have been developed and published, the majority focussing on the African schistosomes [202–209]. Liang et al. [210, 211] and Spear et al. [212] developed mathematical models for schistosomiasis japonica in China, although they did not model transmission in the lake and marshland areas where the majority of transmission occurs nor did they model the involvement of bovine hosts in transmission. Riley et al. [213] developed a *S. japonicum* transmission dynamics model for the Philippines that tried to account for the additional mammalian hosts and zoonotic transmission. However, there has been some conjecture over the parameterization of the model [185] due to the potential underestimation of *S. japonicum* prevalence in bovines in the Philippines [42].

A model by Williams et al. [214] (Fig. 9.5) was developed to simulate transmission dynamics of schistosomiasis japonica in the lake and marshland areas of China and to predict the effect of different control strategies. It extended the two-host model of Barbour [215] to allow for heterogeneity within human and bovine definitive hosts. It consists of a set of simultaneous equations which model rate of change in prevalence over time:

Prevalence in definitive host class i: $$\frac{dP_i}{dt} = g_i\left\{t_{ID_i}\,y(1-P_i)-P_i\right\}$$

Prevalence in intermediate host: $$\frac{dy}{dt} = \mu\left\{\sum\left(t_{DI_i}P_i\right)(1-y)-y\right\}$$

where $i = 1,2,\ldots n$

where t_{ID_i} and t_{DI_i} are composite transmission parameters for intermediate host → *i*th definitive host and *i*th definitive → intermediate host transmission, respectively, which depend upon duration of infection in respective hosts, snail and definitive host densities and force of infection per unit host [214]. The model is parameterized using data of *S. japonicum* epidemiology, including the distribution of endemic prevalences within host classes, and infection duration. Interventions can then be imposed on the system and equations solved numerically to predict the consequences for prevalence and incidence [42].

Simulation of transmission and control using this model has predicted that bovines are major reservoirs for human infection in the lake and marshland areas of China [185, 216], human mass chemotherapy alone is not sufficient for long-term sustainable control [186] and integrated approach, such as a combination of human chemotherapy and bovine vaccination, is required for long-term sustainable control in China [151, 185, 214]. With regard to the latter scenario, the model predicts that a hypothetical *S. japonicum* vaccine capable of reducing the faecal egg output of water buffaloes by 45% alone or in conjunction with PZQ treatment will lead to a significant reduction in transmission [214]. In fact, the two DNA plasmid vaccines, SjCTPI-Hsp70 and SjC23-Hsp70, developed and tested experimentally by Da'Dara et al. [151] both exceeded this hypothetical level. Indeed, mathematical modelling of SjCTPI-Hsp70 and SjC23-Hsp70 alone, and in combination with human chemotherapy, showed a significant reduction in transmission almost to the point of elimination (Fig. 9.5) [42].

9.7.3 Future Integrated Control

Whilst morbidity control is the strategy for the control of schistosomiasis recommended by WHO, providing fast gains in endemic communities, it is only effective in the short term. PZQ is highly effective in killing adult worms of all the human schistosome species [4, 86], and the drug controls morbidity well in infected persons who receive treatment. However, the PZQ-based control strategy has an intrinsic weakness in that the drug is unable to kill developing schistosomes and it does not prevent re-infection; therefore, PZQ has only a transient effect on transmission [91]. Re-infection can occur rapidly in endemic areas, returning prevalence to baseline levels within 18–24 months following treatment [184, 217]. Evidence also suggests that compliance is substantially reduced during prolonged chemotherapy campaigns, thus affecting the coverage of such programmes [218, 219]. Less well known, but highly significant for a control programme, is the evidence for severe 'rebound morbidity', particularly in high-transmission areas when chemotherapy campaigns are interrupted [184]. Recurrent aggressive inflammation following interrupted chemotherapy in 80% of children living in high-transmission areas requires frequent PZQ treatment to avoid making the situation worse than it would have been without any intervention at all [184, 220, 221].

The limitations of control programmes based primarily on mass PZQ treatment were highlighted in a recent study in Mali, where the prevalence of schistosomiasis returned to pre-intervention levels following almost a decade of mass chemotherapy [184, 217]. Likewise, evidence from Burkina Faso and Niger points to an unacceptably high prevalence in high-transmission areas despite extensive chemotherapy [222, 223].

The schistosomiasis control programme in China is one of the most successful globally with population-based PZQ treatment at its backbone, but the key to its success is the focus on transmission control rather than morbidity control. Augmenting human PZQ treatment are several other interventions including snail control, health education and bovine treatment or bovine replacement with mechanised tractors, which act upon the various transmission pathways [224]. The Chinese government has now subsequently moved from transmission control to elimination with the goal of eliminating *S. japonicum* from China by 2020.

Field trials are currently underway in China to test the effectiveness of multi-component integrated control strategies for schistosomiasis elimination, including the use of a vaccine targeting the bovine reservoir host (SjCTPI-Hsp70 DNA vaccine) and snail control. As we have indicated earlier, mathematical modelling has predicted that the SjCTPI-Hsp70 DNA vaccine in conjunction with human chemotherapy will lead to a significant reduction in schistosome transmission (Fig. 9.5). With additional controls measures, elimination could well be achieved.

The Chinese schistosomiasis control strategy is paving the way for future schistosomiasis control and should be used as the global model. Although a vaccine does not yet exist for the African schistosomes – research should continue – other control measures such as snail control, health education/promotion and improved sanitation should be added to the existing PZQ-based programmes, so that the global control strategy shifts back to transmission control. Further development of health services, particularly in Africa, will also be an important part of any future control programme [184]. Thus, the future of schistosomiasis control should:

1. Build on historical and current data and use case finding, GIS and RS tools to develop spatial models for the production of predictive maps allowing endemic areas and re-emerging pockets of transmission to be targeted.
2. Utilise transmission dynamics mathematical models to determine the most effective suite of integrated inventions for a particular endemic setting – validated empirically.
3. Initiate a multi-component integrated control programme that is sustainable – tailored to specific endemic settings – through developed national and local health services. Such a control programme would augment targeted chemotherapy with a combination of the following – determined by the models – snail control through molluscicising and/or environmental modification, health education/promotion, improved sanitation and, when vaccines are available, vaccination [184, 225].

Such an integrated control package will be needed to accelerate efforts to eliminate a disease that has existed for at least two millennia. This approach to control has the potential to improve the health of a billion of the world's poorest people, and its impact cannot and should not be underestimated.

Acknowledgements The authors' studies on schistosomiasis have received financial support from various sources including the UNICEF/UNDP/World Bank/WHO Special Program for Research and Training in Tropical Diseases (TDR), the National Health and Medical Research Council of Australia, the Wellcome Trust (UK), the Sandler Foundation (USA), the Dana Foundation (USA) and the National Institute of Allergy and Infectious Diseases (NIAID).

References

1. Steinmann P, Keiser J, Bos R, Tanner M, Utzinger J (2006) Schistosomiasis and water resources development: systematic review, meta-analysis, and estimates of people at risk. Lancet Infect Dis 6:411–425
2. Ross AG, Bartley PB, Sleigh AC et al (2002) Schistosomiasis. N Engl J Med 346: 1212–1219
3. Gryseels B, Polman K, Clerinx J, Kestens L (2006) Human schistosomiasis. Lancet 368:1106–1118
4. Gray DJ, Ross AG, Li YS, McManus DP (2011) Diagnosis and management of schistosomiasis. BMJ 342:d2651
5. King CH, Dickman K, Tisch DJ (2005) Reassessment of the cost of chronic helminthic infection: a meta-analysis of disability-related outcomes in endemic schistosomiasis. Lancet 365:561–569
6. King CH, Dangerfield-Cha M (2008) The unacknowledged impact of chronic schistosomiasis. Chronic Illn 4:65–79
7. Leshem E, Meltzer E, Marva E, Schwartz E (2009) Travel-related schistosomiasis acquired in Laos. Emerg Infect Dis 15:1823–1826
8. Mas-Coma S, Valero MA, Bargues MD (2009) Climate change effects on trematodiases, with emphasis on zoonotic fascioliasis and schistosomiasis. Vet Parasitol 163:264–280
9. Zhu HM, Xiang S, Yang K, Wu XH, Zhou XN (2008) Three Gorges Dam and its impact on the potential transmission of schistosomiasis in regions along the Yangtze River. Ecohealth 5:137–148
10. Ross AG, Vickers D, Olds GR, Shah SM, McManus DP (2007) Katayama syndrome. Lancet Infect Dis 7:218–224
11. Bottieau E, Clerinx J, De Vega MR et al (2006) Imported Katayama fever: clinical and biological features at presentation and during treatment. J Infect 52:339–345
12. Lambertucci JR (1993) Acute schistosomiasis: clinical, diagnostic and therapeutic features. Rev Inst Med Trop Sao Paulo 35:399–404
13. Rocha MO, Pedroso ER, Lambertucci JR et al (1995) Gastro-intestinal manifestations of the initial phase of schistosomiasis mansoni. Ann Trop Med Parasitol 89:271–278
14. Rocha MO, Rocha RL, Pedroso ER et al (1995) Pulmonary manifestations in the initial phase of schistosomiasis mansoni. Rev Inst Med Trop Sao Paulo 37:311–318
15. Wynn TA, Thompson RW, Cheever AW, Mentink-Kane MM (2004) Immunopathogenesis of schistosomiasis. Immunol Rev 201:156–167
16. Burke ML, Jones MK, Gobert GN, Li YS, Ellis MK, McManus DP (2009) Immunopathogenesis of human schistosomiasis. Parasite Immunol 31:163–176
17. Chen MG (1993) *Schistosoma japonicum and S japonicum*-like infections: epidemiology, clinical and pathological aspects. In: Jordan P, Webbe G, Sturrock FS (eds) Human schistosomiasis. CAB International, Wallingford, pp 237–270
18. Cheever AW, Hoffmann KF, Wynn TA (2000) Immunopathology of schistosomiasis mansoni in mice and men. Immunol Today 21:465–466

19. Abath FGC, Morais CNL, Montenegro CEL, Wynn TA, Montenegro SML (2006) Immunopathogenic mechanisms in schistosomiasis: what can be learnt from human studies? Trends Parasitol 22:85–91
20. Doenhoff MJ (1997) A role for granulomatous inflammation in the transmission of infectious disease: schistosomiasis and tuberculosis. Parasitology 115:S113–S125
21. Burke ML, McManus DP, Ramm GA et al (2010) Temporal expression of chemokines dictates the hepatic inflammatory infiltrate in a murine model of schistosomiasis. PLoS Negl Trop Dis 4:e598
22. Perry CR, Burke ML, Stenzel DJ, McManus DP, Ramm GA, Gobert GN (2011) Differential expression of chemokine and matrix re-modelling genes is associated with contrasting schistosome-induced hepatopathology in murine models. PLoS Negl Trop Dis 5:e1178
23. Ajanga A, Lwambo NJ, Blair L, Nyandindi U, Fenwick A, Brooker S (2006) *Schistosoma mansoni* in pregnancy and associations with anaemia in northwest Tanzania. Trans R Soc Trop Med Hyg 100:59–63
24. Cheever AW (1968) A quantitative post-mortem study of schistosomiasis mansoni in man. Am J Trop Med Hyg 17:38–64
25. Gryseels B, Polderman AM (1987) The morbidity of schistosomiasis mansoni in Maniema (Zaire). Trans R Soc Trop Med Hyg 81:202–209
26. Homeida M, Ahmed S, Dafalla A et al (1988) Morbidity associated with *Schistosoma mansoni* infection as determined by ultrasound: a study in Gezira, Sudan. Am J Trop Med Hyg 39:196–201
27. Kloetzel K (1967) Mortality in chronic splenomegaly due to schistosomiasis mansoni: follow-up study in a Brazilian population. Trans R Soc Trop Med Hyg 61:803–805
28. Ongom VL, Owor R, Grundy R, Bradley DJ (1972) The epidemiology and consequences of *Schistosoma mansoni* infection in West Nile, Uganda, II: hospital investigation of a sample from the Panyagoro community. Trans R Soc Trop Med Hyg 66:852–863
29. Hatz CF, Vennervald BJ, Nkulila T et al (1998) Evolution of *Schistosoma haematobium*-related pathology over 24 months after treatment with praziquantel among school children in southeastern Tanzania. Am J Trop Med Hyg 59:775–781
30. Elsebai I (1977) Parasites in the etiology of cancer – bilharziasis and bladder cancer. CA Cancer J Clin 27:100–106
31. Bedwani R, Renganathan E, El Kwhsky F et al (1998) Schistosomiasis and the risk of bladder cancer in Alexandria, Egypt. Br J Cancer 77:1186–1189
32. Cheever AW (1978) Schistosomiasis and neoplasia. J Natl Cancer Inst 61:13–18
33. Poggensee G, Feldmeier H (2001) Female genital schistosomiasis: facts and hypotheses. Acta Trop 79:193–210
34. IARC (1994) IARC Working Group on the evaluation of carcinogenic risks to humans. Schistosomes, liver flukes and *Helicobacter pylori*. In: IARC Monographs on the evaluation of carcinogenic risks to humans, vol 61. World Health Organisation, Geneva, pp 45–119
35. Koraitim MM, Metwalli NE, Atta MA, el Sadr AA (1995) Changing age incidence and pathological types of schistosoma-associated bladder carcinoma. J Urol 154:1714–1716
36. Nair SS, Bommana A, Bethony JM et al (2011) The metastasis-associated gene 1 encodes a host permissive factor for schistosomiasis, a leading global cause of inflammation and cancer. Hepatology 54:285–295. doi:10.1002/hep.24354
37. Goldsmith PC, Leslie TA, Sams V, Bryceson AD, Allason-Jones E, Dowd PM (1993) Lesions of schistosomiasis mimicking warts on the vulva. BMJ 307:556–557
38. Feldmeier H, Krantz I, Poggensee G (1995) Female genital schistosomiasis: a neglected risk factor for the transmission of HIV? Trans R Soc Trop Med Hyg 89:237
39. Carod-Artal FJ (2008) Neurological complications of *Schistosoma* infection. Trans R Soc Trop Med Hyg 102:107–116
40. Ferrari TC (2004) Involvement of the central nervous system in the schistosomiasis. Mem Inst Oswaldo Cruz 99:59–62
41. Lv S, Zhang Y, Steinmann P, Zhou XN, Utzinger J (2010) Helminth infections of the central nervous system occurring in Southeast Asia and the Far East. Adv Parasitol 72:351–408

42. McManus DP, Gray DJ, Li YS et al (2010) Schistosomiasis in the Peoples' Republic of China: the era of the Three Gorges Dam. Clin Microbiol Rev 23:442–466
43. Olds GR, Olveda R, Wu G, Weist P, McGarvey S, Aligui G et al (1996) Immunity and morbidity in schistosomiasis japonica infection. Am J Trop Med Hyg 55:S121–S126
44. McGarvey ST, Aligui G, Graham KK, Peters P, Olds GR, Olveda R (1996) Schistosomiasis japonica and childhood nutritional status in northeastern Leyte, the Philippines: a randomized trial of praziquantel versus placebo. Am J Trop Med Hyg 54:498–502
45. McGarvey ST, Wu G, Zhang S et al (1993) Child growth, nutritional status, and Schistosomiasis japonica in Jiangxi, People's Republic of China. Am J Trop Med Hyg 48:547–553
46. Nokes C, McGarvey ST, Shiue L et al (1999) Evidence for an improvement in cognitive function following treatment of *Schistosoma japonicum* infection in Chinese primary schoolchildren. Am J Trop Med Hyg 60:556–565
47. Lambertucci RL (1993) *Schistosoma mansoni*: pathological and clinical aspects. In: Jordan P, Webbe G, Sturrock FS (eds) Human schistosomiasis. CAB International, Wallingford, pp 195–235
48. Barsoum R (2004) The changing face of schistosomal glomerulopathy. Kidney Int 66:2472–2484
49. Jordan P, von Lichtenberg F, Goatly KD (1967) Experimental schistosomiasis in primates in Tanzania. Preliminary observations on the susceptibility of the baboon *Papio anubis* to *Schistosoma haematobium* and *Schistosoma mansoni*. Bull World Health Organ 37:393–403
50. Loker ES (1983) A comparative study of the life-histories of mammalian schistosomes. Parasitology 87:343–369
51. Sadun EH, Von Lichtenberg F, Cheever AW, Erickson DG, Hickman RL (1970) Experimental infection with *Schistosoma haematobium* in chimpanzees. Am J Trop Med Hyg 19:427–458
52. Standen OD (1949) Experimental schistosomiasis. II. Maintenance of *Schistosoma mansoni* in the laboratory, with some notes on experimental infection with *S. haematobium*. Ann Trop Med Parasitol 43:268–283
53. Taylor MG, Nelson GS, Smith M, Andrews BJ (1973) Comparison of the infectivity and pathogenicity of six species of African schistosomes and their hybrids. 2. Baboons. J Helminthol 47:455–485
54. Botros S, Pica-Mattoccia L, William S, El-Lakkani N, Cioli D (2005) Effect of praziquantel on the immature stages of *Schistosoma haematobium*. Int J Parasitol 35:1453–1457
55. Katz N, Chaves A, Pellegrino J (1972) A simple device for quantitative stool thick-smear technique for schistosomiasis mansoni. Rev Inst Med Trop Sao Paulo 14:397–400
56. Clerinx J, Van Gompel A (2011) Schistosomiasis in travellers and migrants. Travel Med Infect Dis 9:6–24
57. Rabello A (1999) Diagnosing schistosomiasis. Mem Inst Oswaldo Cruz 92:669–676
58. Ebrahim A, El-Morshedy H, Omer E, El-Daly S, Barakat R (1997) Evaluation of the kato-katz thick smear and formol ether sedimentation techniques for quantitative diagnosis of *Schistosoma mansoni* infection. Am J Trop Med Hyg 32:210–211
59. Ross AGP, Li Y, Sleigh AS et al (1997) Epidemiologic features of *Schistosoma japonicum* among fishermen and other occupational groups in the Dongting Lake region (Hunan Province) of China. Am J Trop Med Hyg 57:302–308
60. Kardorff R, Gabone RM, Mugashe C et al (1997) *Schistosoma mansoni* related morbidity on Ukerewe Island, Tanzania: clinical, ultrasonographical and biochemical parameters. Trop Med Int Health 2:230–239
61. Koukounari A, Webster JP, Donnelly CA et al (2009) Sensitivities and specificities of diagnostic tests and infection prevalence of *Schistosoma haematobium* estimated from data on adults in villages northwest of Accra, Ghana. Am J Trop Med Hyg 80:435–441
62. Lengeler C, Utzinger J, Tanner M (2002) Questionnaires for rapid screening of schistosomiasis in sub-Saharan Africa. Bull World Health Organ 80:235–242
63. Lengeler C, Utzinger J, Tanner M (2002) Screening for schistosomiasis with questionnaires. Trends Parasitol 18:375–377

64. Fagundes Teixeira C, Neuhauss E, Ben R, Romanzini J, Graeff-Teixeira C (2007) Detection of *Schistosoma mansoni* eggs in feces through their interaction with paramagnetic beads in a magnetic field. PLoS Negl Trop Dis 1:e73
65. Oliveira LM, Santos HL, Gonçalves MM, Barreto MG, Peralta JM (2010) Evaluation of polymerase chain reaction as an additional tool for the diagnosis of low-intensity *Schistosoma mansoni* infection. Diagn Microbiol Infect Dis 68:416–421
66. Wichmann D, Panning M, Quack T, Kramme S, Burchard GD, Grevelding C et al (2009) Diagnosing schistosomiasis by detection of cell-free parasite DNA in human plasma. PLoS Negl Trop Dis 3:e422
67. Gomes LI, Dos Santos Marques LH, Enk MJ, de Oliveira MC, Coelho PM, Rabello A (2010) Development and evaluation of a sensitive PCR-ELISA system for detection of *Schistosoma* infection in feces. PLoS Negl Trop Dis 4:e664
68. Ibironke OA, Phillips AE, Garba A, Lamine SM, Shiff C (2011) Diagnosis of *Schistosoma haematobium* by detection of specific DNA fragments from filtered urine samples. Am J Trop Med Hyg 84:998–1001
69. Xu J, Rong R, Zhang HQ, Shi CJ, Zhu XQ, Xia CM (2010) Sensitive and rapid detection of *Schistosoma japonicum* DNA by loop-mediated isothermal amplification (LAMP). Int J Parasitol 40:327–331
70. Wyler DJ, Talebian P (1997) A quantitative assay to detect circulating fibrosin and its application in experimental schistosomiasis. Am J Trop Med Hyg 56:66–70
71. Ellis MK, Li Y, Hou X, Chen H, McManus DP (2008) sTNFR-II and sICAM-1 are associated with acute disease and hepatic inflammation in schistosomiasis japonica. Int J Parasitol 38:717–723
72. Manivannan B, Rawson P, Jordan TW, Karanja DM, Mwinzi PN, Secor WE, La Flamme AC (2011) Identification of cytokeratin 18 as a biomarker of mouse and human hepatosplenic schistosomiasis. Infect Immun 79:2051–2058
73. Fabre V, Wu H, PondTor S et al (2011) Tissue inhibitor of matrix-metalloprotease-1 predicts risk of hepatic fibrosis in human *Schistosoma japonicum* infection. J Infect Dis 203:707–714
74. Hou XY, Ellis MK, McManus DP et al (2011) Diagnostic value of non-invasive bio-markers for stage-specific diagnosis of hepatic fibrosis in patients with advanced schistosomiasis japonica. Int J Parasitol 41:325–332
75. Bergquist R, Johansen MV, Utzinger J (2009) Diagnostic dilemmas in helminthology: what tools to use and when? Trends Parasitol 25:151–156
76. Tsang VC, Wilkins PP (1997) Immunodiagnosis of schistosomiasis. Immunol Invest 26: 175–188
77. Al-Sherbiny MM, Osman A, Hancock K, Deelder AM, Tsang VC (1999) Application of immunodiagnostic assays: detection of antibodies and circulating antigens in human schistosomiasis and correlation with clinical findings. Am J Trop Med Hyg 60:960–966
78. Xu J, Peeling RW, Chen JX et al (2011) Evaluation of immunoassays for the diagnosis of *Schistosoma japonicum* infection using archived sera. PLoS Negl Trop Dis 5:e949
79. Chand MA, Chiodini PL, Doenhoff MJ (2010) Development of a new assay for the diagnosis of schistosomiasis, using cercarial antigens. Trans R Soc Trop Med Hyg 104:255–258
80. Deelder AM, Qian ZL, Kremsner PG et al (1994) Quantitative diagnosis of *Schistosoma* infections by measurement of circulating antigens in serum and urine. Trop Geogr Med 46:233–238
81. Shane HL, Verani JR, Abudho B et al (2011) Evaluation of urine CCA assays for detection of *Schistosoma mansoni* infection in Western Kenya. PLoS Negl Trop Dis 5:e951
82. van Dam GJ, Wichers JH, Ferreira TM et al (2004) Diagnosis of schistosomiasis by reagent strip test for detection of circulating cathodic antigen. J Clin Microbiol 42:5458–5461
83. Midzi N, Butterworth AE, Mduluza T, Munyati S, Deelder AM, van Dam GJ (2009) Use of circulating cathodic antigen strips for the diagnosis of urinary schistosomiasis. Trans R Soc Trop Med Hyg 103:45–51
84. Standley CJ, Lwambo NJS, Lange CN et al (2010) Performance of circulating cathodic antigen (CCA) urine-dipsticks for rapid detection of intestinal schistosomiasis in schoolchildren from shoreline communities of Lake Victoria. Parasit Vectors 3:7

85. Cioli D, Pica-Mattoccia L (2003) Praziquantel. Parasitol Res 90:S3–S9
86. Doenhoff MJ, Cioli D, Utzinger J (2008) Praziquantel: mechanisms of action, resistance and new derivatives for schistosomiasis. Curr Opin Infect Dis 21:659–667
87. Mutapi F, Rujeni N, Bourke C et al (2011) *Schistosoma haematobium* treatment in 1–5 year old children: safety and efficacy of the antihelminthic drug praziquantel. PLoS Negl Trop Dis 5:e1143
88. Gönnert R, Andrews P (1977) Praziquantel, a new broad-spectrum antischistosomal agent. Z Parasitenkd 52:129–150
89. Kasinathan RS, Greenberg RM (2011) Pharmacology and potential physiological significance of schistosome multidrug resistance transporters. Exp Parasitol 8:548–558
90. Ismail M, Botros S, Metwally A et al (1999) Resistance to praziquantel: direct evidence from *Schistosoma mansoni* isolated from Egyptian villagers. Am J Trop Med Hyg 60:932–935
91. Doenhoff MJ, Hagan P, Cioli D et al (2009) Praziquantel: its use in control of schistosomiasis in sub-Saharan Africa and current research needs. Parasitology 136:1825–1835
92. Sayed AA, Simeonov A, Thomas CJ, Inglese J, Austin CP, Williams DL (2008) Identification of oxadiazoles as new drug leads for the control of schistosomiasis. Nat Med 14:407–412
93. Ray D, Williams DL (2011) Characterization of the phytochelatin synthase of *Schistosoma mansoni*. PLoS Negl Trop Dis 5:e1168
94. Dissous C, Grevelding CG (2011) Piggy-backing the concept of cancer drugs for schistosomiasis treatment: a tangible perspective? Trends Parasitol 27:59–66
95. Eissa MM, El-Azzouni MZ, Amer EI, Baddour NM (2011) Miltefosine, a promising novel agent for schistosomiasis mansoni. Int J Parasitol 41:235–242
96. Keiser J, Manneck T, Vargas M (2011) Interactions of mefloquine with praziquantel in the *Schistosoma mansoni* mouse model and in vitro. J Antimicrob Chemother 66:1791–1797
97. Li Y, Ross AG, Hou X, Lou Z, McManus DP (2011) Oriental schistosomiasis with neurological complications: case report. Ann Clin Microbiol Antimicrob 10:5
98. Utzinger J, Xiao SH, Tanner M, Keiser J (2007) Artemisinins for schistosomiasis and beyond. Curr Opin Investig Drugs 8:105–116
99. Xiao SH (2005) Development of antischistosomal drugs in China, with particular consideration to praziquantel and the artemisinins. Acta Trop 96:153–167
100. Hou XY, McManus DP, Gray DJ et al (2008) A randomized, double blind, placebo controlled trial of safety and efficacy of combined praziquantel and artemether treatment for acute schistosomiasis japonica in China. Bull World Health Organ 86:788–795
101. Obonyo CO, Muok EM, Mwinzi PN (2010) Efficacy of artesunate with sulfalene plus pyrimethamine versus praziquantel for treatment of *Schistosoma mansoni* in Kenyan children: an open-label randomised controlled trial. Lancet Infect Dis 10:603–611
102. Keiser J, N'Guessan NA, Adoubryn KD et al (2010) Efficacy and safety of mefloquine, artesunate, mefloquine-artesunate, and praziquantel against *Schistosoma haematobium*: randomized, exploratory open-label trial. Clin Infect Dis 50:1205–1213
103. Utzinger J, Tanner M, Keiser J (2010) ACTs for schistosomiasis: do they act? Lancet Infect Dis 10:579–581
104. Fenwick A, Webster JP, Bosque-Oliva E et al (2009) The Schistosomiasis Control Initiative (SCI): rationale, development and implementation from 2002–2008. Parasitology 136: 1719–1730
105. Lamb EW, Walls CD, Pesce JT et al (2010) Blood fluke exploitation of non-cognate CD4+ T cell help to facilitate parasite development. PLoS Pathog 6:e1000892
106. Maizels RM, Pearce EJ, Artis D, Yazdanbakhsh M, Wynn TA (2009) Regulation of pathogenesis and immunity in helminth infections. J Exp Med 206:2059–2066
107. Dewals B, Hoving JC, Horsnell WG, Brombacher F (2010) Control of *Schistosoma mansoni* egg- induced inflammation by IL-4-responsive CD4(+)CD25(−)CD103(+)Foxp3(−) cells is IL-10- dependent. Eur J Immunol 40:2837–2847
108. Phythian-Adams AT, Cook PC, Lundie RJ et al (2010) CD11c depletion severely disrupts Th2 induction and development in vivo. J Exp Med 207:2089–2096
109. Schramm G, Haas H (2010) Th2 immune response against *Schistosoma mansoni* infection. Microbes Infect 12:881–888

110. Anthony B, Allen JT, Li YS, McManus DP (2010) Hepatic stellate cells and parasite-induced liver fibrosis. Parasit Vectors 3:60
111. de Oliveira Fraga LA, Lamb EW et al (2010) Rapid induction of IgE responses to a worm cysteine protease during murine pre-patent schistosome infection. BMC Immunol 11:56
112. Allen JE, Maizels RM (2011) Diversity and dialogue in immunity to helminths. Nat Rev Immunol 11:375–388
113. McManus DP, Loukas A (2008) Current status of vaccines for schistosomiasis. Clin Microbiol Rev 21:225–242
114. Black CL, Mwinzi PN, Muok EM et al (2010) Influence of exposure history on the immunology and development of resistance to human schistosomiasis mansoni. PLoS Negl Trop Dis 4:e637
115. Black CL, Muok EM, Mwinzi PN, Carter JM, Karanja DM, Secor WE et al (2010) Increases in levels of schistosome-specific immunoglobulin E and CD23(+) B cells in a cohort of Kenyan children undergoing repeated treatment and reinfection with *Schistosoma mansoni*. J Infect Dis 202:399–405
116. Mutapi F, Bourke C, Harcus Y et al (2011) Differential recognition patterns of *Schistosoma haematobium* adult worm antigens by the human antibodies IgA, IgE, IgG1 and IgG4. Parasite Immunol 33:181–192
117. Nausch N, Midzi N, Mduluza T, Maizels RM, Mutapi F (2011) Regulatory and activated T cells in human *Schistosoma haematobium* infections. PLoS One 6:e16860
118. Pinot de Moira A, Fulford AJ, Kabatereine NB, Ouma JH, Booth M, Dunne DW (2010) Analysis of complex patterns of human exposure and immunity to schistosomiasis mansoni: the influence of age, sex, ethnicity and IgE. PLoS Negl Trop Dis 4:e820
119. McManus DP, Li Y, Gray DJ, Ross AG (2009) Conquering 'snail fever': schistosomiasis and its control in China. Expert Rev Anti Infect Ther 7:473–485
120. Hotez PJ, Bethony JM, Diemert DJ, Pearson M, Loukas A (2010) Developing vaccines to combat hookworm infection and intestinal schistosomiasis. Nat Rev Microbiol 8:814–826
121. Bethony JM, Cole RN, Guo X et al (2011) Vaccines to combat the neglected tropical diseases. Immunol Rev 239:237–270
122. Capron A, Riveau G, Capron M, Trottein F (2005) Schistosomes: the road from host–parasite interactions to vaccines in clinical trials. Trends Parasitol 21:143–149
123. Tendler M, Simpson AJ (2008) The biotechnology-value chain: development of Sm14 as a schistosomiasis vaccine. Acta Trop 108:263–266
124. Ramos CR, Spisni A, Oyama S Jr et al (2009) Stability improvement of the fatty acid binding protein Sm14 from *S. mansoni* by Cys replacement: structural and functional characterization of a vaccine candidate. Biochim Biophys Acta 1794:655–662
125. Ahmad G, Torben W, Zhang W, Wyatt M, Siddiqui AA (2009) Sm-p80-based DNA vaccine formulation induces potent protective immunity against *Schistosoma mansoni*. Parasite Immunol 31:156–161
126. Zhang W, Ahmad G, Torben W et al (2010) Sm-p80-based DNA vaccine provides baboons with levels of protection against *Schistosoma mansoni* infection comparable to those achieved by the irradiated cercarial vaccine. J Infect Dis 201:1105–1112
127. Zhang W, Ahmad G, Torben W, Siddiqui AA (2011) *Schistosoma mansoni* antigen Sm-p80: Prophylactic efficacy of a vaccine formulated in human approved plasmid vector and adjuvant (VR 1020 and alum). Acta Trop 118:142–151
128. Torben W, Ahmad G, Zhang W, Siddiqui AA (2011) Role of antibodies in Sm-p80-mediated protection against *Schistosoma mansoni* challenge infection in murine and nonhuman primate models. Vaccine 29:2262–2271
129. Tran MH, Pearson MS, Bethony JM et al (2006) Tetraspanins on the surface of *Schistosoma mansoni* are protective antigens against schistosomiasis. Nat Med 12:835–840
130. Tran MH, Freitas TC, Cooper L, Gaze S, Gatton ML, Jones MK et al (2010) Suppression of mRNAs encoding tegument tetraspanins from *Schistosoma mansoni* results in impaired tegument turnover. PLoS Pathog 6:e1000840

131. Don TA, Bethony JM, Loukas A (2008) Saposin-like proteins are expressed in the gastrodermis of *Schistosoma mansoni* and are immunogenic in natural infections. Int J Infect Dis 12:e39–e47
132. Marques HH, Zouain CS, Torres CB, Oliveira JS, Alves JB, Goes AM (2008) Protective effect and granuloma down-modulation promoted by RP44 antigen a fructose 1,6 bisphosphate aldolase of *Schistosoma mansoni*. Immunobiology 213:437–446
133. Cardoso FC, Macedo GC, Gava E et al (2008) *Schistosoma mansoni* tegument protein Sm29 is able to induce a Th1-type of immune response and protection against parasite infection. PLoS Negl Trop Dis 2:e308
134. Githui EK, Damian RT, Aman RA, Ali MA, Kamau JM (2009) *Schistosoma spp.*: isolation of microtubule associated proteins in the tegument and the definition of dynein light chains components. Exp Parasitol 121:96–104
135. Lopes DO, Paiva LF, Martins MA et al (2009) Sm21.6 a novel EF-hand family protein member located on the surface of *Schistosoma mansoni* adult worm that failed to induce protection against challenge infection but reduced liver pathology. Vaccine 27:4127–4135
136. Pinho JM, Cardoso FC, Lopes DO et al (2010) Immunization with SmIg, a novel tegument protein from *Schistosoma mansoni*, fails to induce protection in mice but reduces liver pathology. Parasitology 137:1079–1088
137. Tararam CA, Farias LP, Wilson RA, Leite LC (2010) *Schistosoma mansoni* Annexin 2: molecular characterization and immunolocalization. Exp Parasitol 126:146–155
138. Hofmann A, Osman A, Leow CY, Driguez P, McManus DP, Jones MK (2010) Parasite annexins– new molecules with potential for drug and vaccine development. Bioessays 32:967–976
139. Farias LP, Cardoso FC, Miyasato PA et al (2010) *Schistosoma mansoni* stomatin like protein-2 is located in the tegument and induces partial protection against challenge infection. PLoS Negl Trop Dis 4:e597
140. Peng J, Han H, Hong Y, Fu Z, Liu J, Lin J (2010) Molecular cloning and characterization of a gene encoding methionine aminopeptidase 2 of *Schistosoma japonicum*. Parasitol Res 107:939–946
141. Hong Y, Han H, Peng J, Li Y, Shi Y, Fu Z et al (2010) *Schistosoma japonicum*: cloning, expression and characterization of a gene encoding the α5-subunit of the proteasome. Exp Parasitol 126:517–525
142. Kumagai T, Osada Y, Ohta N, Kanazawa T (2009) Peroxiredoxin-1 from *Schistosoma japonicum* functions as a scavenger against hydrogen peroxide but not nitric oxide. Mol Biochem Parasitol 164:26–31
143. Lv ZY, Yang LL, Hu SM et al (2009) Expression profile, localization of an 8-kDa calcium-binding protein from *Schistosoma japonicum* (SjCa8), and vaccine potential of recombinant SjCa8 (rSjCa8) against infections in mice. Parasitol Res 104:733–743
144. You H, Zhang W, Jones MK et al (2010) Cloning and characterisation of *Schistosoma japonicum* insulin receptors. PLoS One 5:e9868
145. You H, Gobert GN, Jones MK, Zhang W, McManus DP (2011) Signalling pathways and the host- parasite relationship: putative targets for control interventions against schistosomiasis: signalling pathways and future anti-schistosome therapies. Bioessays 33:203–214
146. Cai P, Bu L, Wang J, Wang Z, Zhong X, Wang H (2008) Molecular characterization of *Schistosoma japonicum* tegument protein tetraspanin-2: sequence variation and possible implications for immune evasion. Biochem Biophys Res Commun 372:197–202
147. Yuan C, Fu YJ, Li J et al (2010) *Schistosoma japonicum*: efficient and rapid purification of the tetraspanin extracellular loop 2, a potential protective antigen against schistosomiasis in mammalian. Exp Parasitol 126:456–461
148. Zhang W, Li J, Duke M et al (2011) Inconsistent protective efficacy and marked polymorphism limits the value of *Schistosoma japonicum* tetraspanin-2 as a vaccine target. PLoS Negl Trop Dis 5:e1166
149. Wu W, Cai P, Chen Q, Wang H (2011) Identification of novel antigens within the *Schistosoma japonicum* tetraspanin family based on molecular characterization. Acta Trop 117:216–224

150. Wu XH, Wang XH, Utzinger J et al (2007) Spatio-temporal correlation between human and bovine schistosomiasis in China: insight from three nationwide surveys. Geospat Health 2:75–84
151. Da'dara AA, Li YS, Xiong T et al (2008) DNA-based vaccines protect against zoonotic schistosomiasis in water buffalo. Vaccine 26:3617–3625
152. Schistosoma japonicum Genome Sequencing and Functional Analysis Consortium (2009) The *Schistosoma japonicum* genome reveals features of host-parasite interplay. Nature 460:345–351
153. Berriman M, Haas BJ, LoVerde PT et al (2009) The genome of the blood fluke *Schistosoma mansoni*. Nature 460:352–358
154. Han ZG, Brindley PJ, Wang SY, Chen Z (2009) *Schistosoma* genomics: new perspectives on schistosome biology and host-parasite interaction. Annu Rev Genomics Hum Genet 10:211–240
155. Fitzpatrick JM, Peak E, Perally S et al (2009) Anti-schistosomal intervention targets identified by lifecycle transcriptomic analyses. PLoS Negl Trop Dis 3:e543
156. Farias LP, Tararam CA, Miyasato PA et al (2011) Screening the *Schistosoma mansoni* transcriptome for genes differentially expressed in the schistosomulum stage in search for vaccine candidates. Parasitol Res 108:123–135
157. Chuan J, Feng Z, Brindley PJ et al (2010) Our wormy world genomics, proteomics and transcriptomics in East and southeast Asia. Adv Parasitol 73:327–371
158. Gobert GN (2010) Better understanding of anti-schistosomal strategies through microarray analysis. Infect Disord Drug Targets 10:251–257
159. Gobert GN, McManus DP, Nawaratna S, Moertel L, Mulvenna J, Jones MK (2009) Tissue specific profiling of females of *Schistosoma japonicum* by integrated laser microdissection microscopy and microarray analysis. PLoS Negl Trop Dis 3:e469
160. Gobert GN, Moertel L, Brindley PJ, McManus DP (2009) Developmental gene expression profiles of the human pathogen *Schistosoma japonicum*. BMC Genomics 10:128
161. Nawaratna SS, McManus DP, Moertel L, Gobert GN, Jones MK (2011) Gene atlasing of digestive and reproductive tissues in *Schistosoma mansoni*. PLoS Negl Trop Dis 5:e1043
162. DeMarco R, Verjovski-Almeida S (2009) Schistosomes–proteomics studies for potential novel vaccines and drug targets. Drug Discov Today 14:472–478
163. Mulvenna J, Moertel L, Jones MK et al (2010) Exposed proteins of the *Schistosoma japonicum* tegument. Int J Parasitol 40:543–554
164. Liu F, Cui SJ, Hu W, Feng Z, Wang ZQ, Han ZG (2009) Excretory/secretory proteome of the adult developmental stage of human blood fluke, *Schistosoma japonicum*. Mol Cell Proteomics 8:1236–1251
165. Yang LL, Lv ZY, Hu SM et al (2009) *Schistosoma japonicum*: proteomics analysis of differentially expressed proteins from ultraviolet-attenuated cercariae compared to normal cercariae. Parasitol Res 105:237–248
166. Abdel-Hafeez EH, Kikuchi M, Watanabe KI et al (2009) Proteome approach for identification of schistosomiasis japonica vaccine candidate antigen. Parasitol Int 58:36–44
167. Castro-Borges W, Dowle A, Curwen RS, Thomas-Oates J, Wilson RA (2011) Enzymatic shaving of the tegument surface of live schistosomes for proteomic analysis: a rational approach to select vaccine candidates. PLoS Negl Trop Dis 5:e993
168. Hokke CH, Deelder AM, Hoffmann KF, Wuhrer M (2007) Glycomics-driven discoveries in schistosome research. Exp Parasitol 117:275–283
169. de Boer AR, Hokke CH, Deelder AM, Wuhrer M (2008) Serum antibody screening by surface plasmon resonance using a natural glycan microarray. Glycoconj J 25:75–84
170. Wang Y, Li JV, Saric J, Keiser J, Wu J, Utzinger J, Holmes E (2010) Advances in metabolic profiling of experimental nematode and trematode infections. Adv Parasitol 73:373–404
171. Driguez P, Doolan DL, Loukas A, Felgner PL, McManus DP (2010) Schistosomiasis vaccine discovery using immunomics. Parasit Vectors 3:4
172. Cogswell AA, Collins JJ 3rd, Newmark PA, Williams DL (2011) Whole mount in situ hybridization methodology for *Schistosoma mansoni*. Mol Biochem Parasitol 178:46–50

173. Tchoubrieva E, Kalinna B (2010) Advances in mRNA silencing and transgene expression: a gateway to functional genomics in schistosomes. Biotechnol Genet Eng Rev 26:261–280
174. Mann VH, Morales ME, Rinaldi G, Brindley PJ (2010) Culture for genetic manipulation of developmental stages of *Schistosoma mansoni*. Parasitology 137:451–462
175. Yang S, Brindley PJ, Zeng Q et al (2010) Transduction of *Schistosoma japonicum* schistosomules with vesicular stomatitis virus glycoprotein pseudotyped murine leukemia retrovirus and expression of reporter human telomerase reverse transcriptase in the transgenic schistosomes. Mol Biochem Parasitol 174:109–116
176. Xu X, Zhang D, Sun W et al (2009) A *Schistosoma japonicum* chimeric protein with a novel adjuvant induced a polarized Th1 immune response and protection against liver egg burdens. BMC Infect Dis 9:54
177. Wei F, Zhai Y, Jin H et al (2010) Development and immunogenicity of a recombinant pseudorabies virus expressing Sj26GST and SjFABP from *Schistosoma japonicum*. Vaccine 28:5161–5166
178. Wei F, Liu Q, Zhai Y et al (2009) IL-18 enhances protective effect in mice immunized with a *Schistosoma japonicum* FABP DNA vaccine. Acta Trop 111:284–288
179. Li L, Hu X, Wu Z et al (2009) Immunogenicity of self-adjuvanticity oral vaccine candidate based on use of Bacillus subtilis spore displaying *Schistosoma japonicum* 26 KDa GST protein. Parasitol Res 105:1643–1651
180. Zhu Y, Lu F, Dai Y et al (2010) Synergistic enhancement of immunogenicity and protection in mice against *Schistosoma japonicum* with codon optimization and electroporation delivery of SjTPI DNA vaccines. Vaccine 28:5347–5355
181. Tao FF, Yang YF, Wang H et al (2009) Th1-type epitopes-based cocktail PDDV attenuates hepatic fibrosis in C57BL/6 mice with chronic *Schistosoma japonicum* infection. Vaccine 27:4110–4117
182. Dai Y, Zhu Y, Harn DA et al (2009) DNA vaccination by electroporation and boosting with recombinant proteins enhances the efficacy of DNA vaccines for schistosomiasis japonica. Clin Vaccine Immunol 16:1796–1803
183. Zhu L, Liu HF, Lu MB, Long QK, Shi YE, Yu LJ (2011) Construction, purification, and evaluation of multivalent DNA vaccine against *Schistosoma japonicum*. Parasitol Res 108:115–121
184. Gray DJ, McManus DP, Li YS, Williams GM, Bergquist R, Ross AG (2010) Schistosomiasis elimination: lessons from the past guide the future. Lancet Infect Dis 10:733–736
185. Gray DJ, Williams GM, Li YS, McManus DP (2008) Transmission dynamics of *Schistosoma japonicum* in the Lake and Marshlands region of China. PLoS One 3:e4058
186. Gray DJ, Williams GM, Li Y et al (2009) A cluster-randomised intervention trial against *Schistosoma japonicum* in the Peoples' Republic of China: bovine and human transmission. PLoS One 4:e5900
187. Urbani C, Sinoun M, Socheat D et al (2002) Epidemiology and control of mekongi schistosomiasis. Acta Trop 82:157–168
188. WHO (2006) Preventive chemotherapy in human helminthiasis – coordinated use of anthelmintic drugs in control interventions: a manual for health professionals and program managers. WHO, Geneva
189. Utzinger J, Raso G, Brooker S et al (2009) Schistosomiasis and neglected tropical diseases: towards integrated and sustainable control and a word of caution. Parasitology 136: 1859–1874
190. Utzinger J, Bergquist R, Shu-Hua X et al (2003) Sustainable schistosomiasis control - the way forward. Lancet 362:1932–1934
191. WHO (2011) Schistosomiasis: number of people treated, 2009. WHO – Weekly Epidemiological Record 86:73–80
192. Brooker S, Clements A (2009) Spatial heterogeneity of parasite co-infection: Determinants and geostatistical prediction at regional scales. Int J Parasitol 39:591–597
193. Raso G, Matthys B, N'Goran EK, Tanner M, Vounatsou P, Utzinger J (2005) Spatial risk prediction and mapping of *Schistosoma mansoni* infections among schoolchildren living in western Côte d'Ivoire. Parasitology 131:97–108

194. Guo J, Vounatsou P, Cao CL et al (2005) A geographic information and remote sensing-based model for prediction of *Oncomelania hupensis* habitats in the Poyang Lake area, China. Acta Trop 96:213–222
195. Clements A, Lwambo N, Blair L et al (2006) Bayesian spatial analysis and disease mapping: tools to enhance planning and implementation of a schistosomiasis control programme in Tanzania. Trop Med Int Health 11:490–503
196. Clements ACA, Firth S, Dembelé R et al (2009) Use of Bayesian geostatistical prediction to estimate local variations in *Schistosoma haematobium* infection in West Africa. Bull World Health Organ 87:921–929
197. Yang K, Zhou XN, Wu XH et al (2009) Landscape pattern analysis and Bayesian modeling for predicting *Oncomelania hupensis* distribution in Eryuan County, People's Republic of China. Am J Trop Med Hyg 81:416–423
198. Clements A, Garba A, Sacko M et al (2008) Mapping the probability of schistosomiasis and associated uncertainty, West Africa. Emerg Infect Dis 14:1629–1632
199. Yang GJ, Vounatsou P, Tanner M, Zhou XN, Utzinger J (2006) Remote sensing for predicting potential habitats of Oncomelania hupensis in Hongze, Baima and Gaoyou lakes in Jiangsu province, China. Geospat Health 1:85–92
200. Hairston NG (1962) On the mathematical analysis of schistosome populations. Bull World Health Organ 33:45–62
201. Macdonald G (1965) The dynamics of helminth infections, with special reference to schistosomes. Trans R Soc Trop Med Hyg 59:489–506
202. Carabin H, Guyatt HL, Engels D (2000) A comparative analysis of the cost-effectiveness of treatment based on parasitological and symptomatic screening for *Schistosoma mansoni* in Burundi. Trop Med Int Health 5:192–202
203. Carabin H, Chan MS, Guyatt HL (2000) A population dynamic approach to evaluating the impact of school attendance on the unit cost and effectiveness of school based schistosomiasis chemotherapy programmes. Parasitology 121:171–183
204. Chan MS, Bundy DAP (1997) Modelling the dynamic effects of community chemotherapy on the patterns of morbidity due to *Schistosoma mansoni*. Trans R Soc Trop Med Hyg 91:216–220
205. Guyatt HL, Tanner M (1996) Different approaches to modeling the cost-effectiveness of schistosomiasis control. Am J Trop Med Hyg 55:159–164
206. Medley GF, Bundy DAP (1996) Dynamic modeling of epidemiologic patterns of schistosomiasis morbidity. Am J Trop Med Hyg 55:149–158
207. Woolhouse MEJ (1991) On the application of mathematical models of schistosome transmission dynamics I. Natural transmission. Acta Trop 49:241–270
208. Woolhouse MEJ (1992) On the application of mathematical models of schistosome transmission dynamics II. Control. Acta Trop 50:189–204
209. Woolhouse MEJ (1996) Mathematical models of transmission dynamics and control of schistosomiasis. Am J Trop Med Hyg 55:144–148
210. Liang S, Seto E, Remais JV et al (2007) Environmental effects on parasitic disease transmission exemplified by schistosomiasis in western China. Proc Nat Acad Sci U S A 104: 7110–7115
211. Liang S, Spear RC, Seto E, Hubbard A, Qiu D (2005) A multi-group model of *Schistosoma japonicum* transmission dynamics and control: model calibration and control prediction. Trop Med Int Health 10:263–278
212. Spear RC, Hubbard A, Liang S, Seto E (2002) Disease transmission models for public health decision making: toward an approach for designing intervention strategies for schistosomiasis japonica. Environ Health Perspect 110:907–915
213. Riley S, Carabin H, Belisle P et al (2008) Multi-host transmission dynamics of *Schistosoma japonicum* in Samar Province, the Philippines. PLoS Med 5:e18
214. Williams GM, Sleigh AC, Li Y et al (2002) Mathematical modelling of schistosomiasis japonica: comparison of control strategies in the Peoples' Republic of China. Acta Trop 82:253–262

215. Barbour AD (1996) Modeling the transmission of schistosomiasis: an introductory view. Am J Trop Med Hyg 55:135–143
216. Guo J, Li Y, Gray DJ et al (2006) A drug-based intervention study on the importance of buffaloes for human *Schistosoma japonicum* infection around Poyang Lake, People's Republic of China. Am J Trop Med Hyg 74:335–341
217. Clements AC, Bosqué-Oliva E, Sacko M et al (2009) A comparative study of the spatial distribution of schistosomiasis in Mali in 1984–1989 and 2004–2006. PLoS Negl Trop Dis 3:e431
218. Tallo VL, Carabin H, Alday PP et al (2008) Is mass treatment the appropriate schistosomiasis elimination strategy? Bull World Health Organ 86:765–771
219. Parker M, Allen T (2011) Does mass drug administration for the integrated treatment of neglected tropical diseases really work? Assessing evidence for the control of schistosomiasis and soil-transmitted helminths in Uganda. Health Res Policy Syst 9:3
220. Olveda RM, Daniel BL, Ramirez BD et al (1996) Schistosomiasis japonica in the Philippines: the long-term impact of population-based chemotherapy on infection, transmission, and morbidity. J Infect Dis 174:163–172
221. Reimert CM, Tukahebwa EM, Kabatereine NB, Dunne DW, Vennervald BJ (2008) Assessment of *Schistosoma mansoni* induced intestinal inflammation by means of eosinophil cationic protein, eosinophil protein X and myeloperoxidase before and after treatment with praziquantel. Acta Trop 105:253–259
222. Garba A, Touré S, Dembelé R, Bosque-Oliva E, Fenwick A (2006) Implementation of national schistosomiasis control programmes in West Africa. Trends Parasitol 22:322–326
223. Garba A, Touré S, Dembelé R et al (2009) Present and future schistosomiasis control activities with support from the Schistosomiasis Control Initiative in West Africa. Parasitology 136:1731–1737
224. Wang LD, Chen HG, Guo JG et al (2009) A strategy to control transmission of *Schistosoma japonicum* in China. N Eng J Med 360:121–128
225. Bergquist R, Utzinger J, McManus DP (2008) Trick or treat: the role of vaccines in integrated schistosomiasis control. PLoS Negl Trop Dis 2:e244

Chapter 10
Dengue Infections

Annelies Wilder-Smith

10.1 Introduction

The dengue viruses are among the most widespread geographically of the arboviruses and are found in tropical and subtropical areas where 2.5–3 billion people are at risk of infection [1]. Each year, an estimated 50–100 million dengue infections occur, with several hundred thousand cases of dengue hemorrhagic fever (DHF), and about 20,000 deaths [2]. Global deaths from DHF already rank with yellow fever in exceeding combined deaths from all other viral hemorrhagic fevers, including Ebola, Marburg, Lassa, and Crimean-Congo. The past two decades saw an unprecedented geographic expansion of dengue.

10.2 The Virus

Dengue viruses belong to the family of Flaviviridae (single-stranded, non-segmented RNA viruses); there are four serologically distinct dengue virus serotypes (DENV-1, DENV-2, DENV-3, DENV-4). Infection with one serotype confers long-term immunity to that serotype but not to the other types. Dengue virus infection of all four virus serotypes causes a spectrum of illness ranging from asymptomatic or mild febrile illness to classical dengue fever (DF) and to severe and fatal hemorrhagic disease.

The evolution of dengue viruses has had a major impact on their virulence for humans and on the epidemiology of dengue disease around the world [3]. The RNA genome of the virus is susceptible to random mutations due to the lack of proofreading

A. Wilder-Smith, M.D., Ph.D., M.I.H. (✉)
Institute of Public Health, University of Heidelberg,
Im Neuenheimer Feld 365, 69120 Heidelberg, Germany
e-mail: Wilder-Smith@uni-heidelberg.de

I.W. Fong (ed.), *Challenges in Infectious Diseases*, Emerging Infectious Diseases of the 21st Century 502, DOI 10.1007/978-1-4614-4496-1_10,

capacity of the RNA-dependent RNA polymerase, which could thus give rise to more virulent strains following increased levels of infection in a population [4]. Although antigenic and genetic differences in virus strains have become evident, the lack of animal models for severe dengue has made it difficult to study variation in virulence among dengue viruses. However, phylogenetic studies of many different dengue virus samples have led to the association between specific subtypes (within serotypes) and the presentation of more or less severe disease [3]. Currently, dengue viruses can be classified as being of epidemiologically low, medium, or high impact [3]. Subtypes within the American genotype of DENV-2 and genotype IV of DENV-3, for example, are less virulent with a reduced ability to grow in cell cultures and mosquitoes compared to the Asian genotypes of DENV-2 and DENV-3. Phylogenetic and epidemiological analyses suggest that the genotypes and subtypes with greater epidemic potential are now displacing those that have lower epidemiological impact [1].

10.3 The Vector

Dengue viruses are transmitted by mosquitoes of the genus *Aedes*, subgenus *stegomyia* (such as *Aedes aegypti* and *albopictus*) [2]. *Aedes aegypti* is well established in much of the tropical and subtropical world. It is the principal vector and is an efficient epidemic vector for several reasons: it is highly susceptible to dengue virus, feeds preferentially on human blood, is a daytime feeder, has an almost imperceptible bite, and is capable of biting several people in a short period for one blood meal [2, 5]. As a peri-domicillary mosquito, it is well adapted to urban life as it typically breeds in clean stagnant water in a wide variety of man-made containers such as tires, tin cans, pots, and buckets that collect rainwater. The alternative dengue vector, *Aedes albopictus*, is continuing its geographic expansion into both tropical and temperate climates, but this has had little impact on epidemic dengue transmission [6].

Epidemic dengue was effectively controlled in most of tropical America in the 1950s and the 1960s as a side benefit of malaria and yellow fever control programs [2]. Disruption of vector control programs, be it for reasons of political and social unrest or scientific reservations about the safety of DDT, has contributed to the resurgence of dengue around the world. Lack of political will or complacency concerning vector-borne diseases is another factor. Few new and effective mosquito control methods have been developed in the past 30 years [7].

10.4 Epidemiology of Dengue

At the beginning of the twenty-first century, dengue is the most important arboviral disease of humans [8]. More than 100 tropical countries now have endemic dengue virus infections, and DHF has been documented in >60 of these countries [2]. Global reports of DHF have increased on average by fivefold in the past 20 years [2]

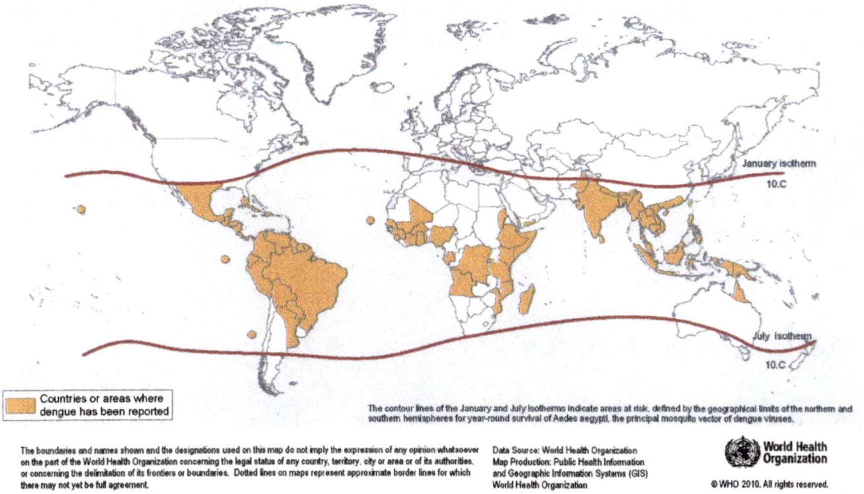

Fig. 10.1 Countries and areas at risk of dengue, 2010 (NB: Reproduced with the permission of the WHO)

(Fig 10.1). Dengue epidemics vary greatly in magnitude and severity. In 1998, the largest epidemics in history occurred throughout Asia and the Americas, with >1.2 million cases of DF/DHF reported to the WHO. The reasons for the resurgence of dengue are complex. It is impossible to determine the extent that single factors such as climate change, virus evolution, deteriorating vector control, and societal changes play in the expansion of dengue. Population growth associated with rapid uncontrolled urbanization is likely the main factor that has driven the rapid amplification of dengue in the past decades. But the main factors responsible for the geographic spread are movements of populations or individuals via travel [1, 9, 10].

The factors responsible for periodic epidemics in an area are not well understood. They are likely a combination of the increased movement of viruses in people among countries and regions, the level of herd immunity to specific virus serotypes in human population, and genetic changes in circulating or introduced viruses that give them greater epidemic potential [10].

The World Health Organization (WHO) states that the Southeast Asian and Western Pacific Regions bear nearly 75 % of the current global disease burden of dengue [11]. Dengue inflicts a significant health, economic, and social burden on the populations of endemic areas. Globally, the number of disability-adjusted life years (DALYs) per million population lost to dengue is estimated to be between 528 and 621 per million population [11]. Dengue imposes substantial costs on both the health sector and the overall economy.

The number of cases reported annually to WHO ranged from 0.4 to 1.3 million in the decade 1996–2005 [11]. The number of cases varies substantially from year to year, with epidemics occurring every 3–5 years. The underlying reason for this cyclical trend is poorly understood but is perhaps best explained by demographic, immunologic, and environmental changes combined with globalization and ineffective public health measures [1, 12–14]. Climatic influences, such as the El Nino Southern Oscillation (ENSO) and global warming, have been suggested as other factors contributing to the cyclical pattern of dengue activity [7, 15]. Furthermore, dengue activity is seasonal within a year in most endemic countries [12, 16, 17]. The greatest burden of dengue in endemic countries is in children. However, there has been an increasing trend of adult infection in certain countries [18, 19]. Most travelers with dengue have been adults [9].

10.4.1 Risk for Travelers

The chance of contracting DF is determined by several factors including travel destination, length of exposure in endemic areas, the intensity of dengue transmission, and the season of travel. Risk is thought to be higher during periods of intense mosquito feeding activity 2–3 h after dawn and during the early evening.

The GeoSentinel [20] global network of travel and tropical medicine clinics reported on illness in returned travelers and determined that the regions at highest risk for dengue were SE Asia and the Caribbean [16]. The true incidence of dengue fever in travelers is probably underestimated because in many countries reporting is not obligatory, and, due to its nonspecific symptoms, it is probably underdiagnosed [9].

10.5 Pathogenesis, Clinical Manifestations, Diagnosis and Differential Diagnosis, and Clinical Management

Dengue fever is most often a self-limiting disease with a low case fatality rate. Often presenting as nonspecific febrile illness, its differential diagnosis is broad, thereby posing diagnostic challenges. In the absence of specific antiviral therapy, the clinical management of dengue is supportive.

10.5.1 Pathogenesis

After the bite of an infected mosquito, the virus replicates in regional lymph nodes and is disseminated via the lymph and blood to other tissues [21]. Replication in the reticuloendothelial system and skin produces a viremia [21]. The incubation period is 3–14 days. Dengue virus infection of all four virus serotypes causes a spectrum of illness ranging from asymptomatic or mild febrile illness to severe and fatal hemorrhagic disease, depending largely on age and immunologic condition [5]. Although the mechanisms for developing severe hemorrhagic disease are not fully understood, the majority view is that secondary infection is the main risk factor for dengue hemorrhagic fever (DHF) and dengue shock syndrome (DSS) [22, 23]. Secondary infection with a different serotype may result in complexes between heterotypic antibodies and dengue viruses, a phenomenon that has been called antibody-dependent enhancement [24–26]. Severity of disease also depends on the strain and serotype of the infecting virus, age and genetic background of the patient [23, 27, 28], and the degree of viremia [29].

The primary pathophysiological abnormality in DHF and DSS is an acute increase in vascular permeability that leads to leakage of plasma into the extravascular compartment, resulting in hemoconcentration and decreased blood pressure [28]. Plasma volume studies have shown a reduction of more than 20 % in severe cases [30].

10.5.2 Clinical Manifestations

10.5.2.1 Asymptomatic Infections

The vast majority of dengue infection in endemic areas are asymptomatic or subclinical (mild febrile illness), particularly among young children [5, 31].

10.5.2.2 Classic Dengue Fever (DF)

Classic dengue fever is characterized by a sudden onset of fever, accompanied by a significant headache (usually frontal), retro-orbital pain and fatigue, and often associated with severe myalgia and arthralgia ("breakbone disease") and gastrointestinal and respiratory symptoms [32]. The conjunctivae may be injected and the pharynx inflamed. Lymphadenopathy is common. Rash is variable and may not occur in 50 % of patients [33–35]. Transient flushing (which can be differentiated from a sunburn in a traveler by its blanching) or erythematous mottling may be present during the first 24–48 h. Fever usually lasts 5–7 days. A second rash, varying from scarlatiniform to maculopapular, may appear at the time of defervescence, often lasts for 2–3 days and may be accompanied by scaling and pruritus [32]. Hemorrhagic manifestations in dengue fever patients may occur with skin hemorrhages being the most frequent (petechia and purpura) [21]. The tourniquet test (a simple bedside test that reflects capillary fragility) may be positive. Gum bleeding, epistaxis, menorrhagia, and gastrointestinal hemorrhage may also occur, but are less common. Very rare complications of dengue fever include myocarditis, hepatitis [36], and neurological abnormalities such as encephalopathy and neuropathies [32, 37]. Convalescence may be prolonged for weeks with asthenia and depression [38].

Laboratory findings commonly associated with dengue fever include thrombocytopenia, leucopenia with lymphopenia, mild to moderately elevated liver transaminases and lactate dehydrogenase, and hyponatremia [5, 33, 39].

10.5.2.3 Dengue Hemorrhagic Fever (DHF) and Dengue Shock Syndrome (DSS)

The hallmark of this syndrome is a capillary leakage syndrome, accompanied by hemorrhagic manifestations. Patients present in the first days similarly to DF, but then plasma leakage develops at the time of defervescence around 5–7 days after onset of symptoms. Abdominal pain and vomiting, restlessness, change in level of consciousness, and a sudden change from fever to hypothermia may be the first clinical warning signs, associated with a significant decrease in platelets [5].

The diagnosis of DHF is made based on the combination of hemorrhagic manifestations, platelet count <100,000/mm^3, and objective evidence of plasma leakage shown by either fluctuation of packed cell volume >20 % during the course of illness or clinical signs of plasma leakage such as pleural effusion, ascites, or hypoproteinemia. Hemorrhagic manifestations without capillary leakage do not constitute DHF. A positive tourniquet test differentiates poorly between DF and DHF and seems to be not very specific [40]. Mortality of DHF can be up to 10–20 %, but it is as low as 0.2 % in hospitals with staff experienced in the management of the disease [5, 28, 41]. The criteria for dengue shock syndrome are those for DHF plus either a narrowing pulse pressure <20 mmHg or hypotension (defined as systolic pressure <80 mmHg for those aged <5 years or <90 mmHg for those ≥5). DSS is associated with a mortality up to 40 % [5].

10.5.3 New Case Definition

The World Health Organization (WHO) has outlined in its new global dengue guidelines a revised classification into levels of severity: dengue fever with an intermediary group of "dengue fever with warning sings," and severe dengue [11]. The revised dengue classification has a high potential for facilitating dengue case management and surveillance [42].

10.5.4 Diagnosis and Differential Diagnosis of Dengue Fever

Nonspecific fever with or without a rash, in particular if associated with thrombocytopenia and leukopenia, should alert the clinician to the possibility of dengue fever and should initiate laboratory confirmation. Probable diagnosis of dengue infection is made based on a supportive serology on a single serum sample of a positive IgM antibody test or a titer ≥1,280 with the hemagglutination inhibition test [5]. Confirmed diagnosis of dengue requires at least one of the following: fourfold or greater rise in serum IgG titers (by hemagglutination inhibition test) specific to dengue virus between acute and convalescent serum; detection of dengue virus in serum, tissue, or autopsy samples; and detection of dengue virus genomic sequences by reverse transcription-polymerase chain reaction (RT-PCR) [5].

During the first 5 days of illness, the most sensitive test is virus isolation (i.e., PCR), but these tests may not be available in many settings. The more commonly available IgM capture enzyme-linked immunosorbent assay is negative early in the illness and should only be done at least 5 days after onset of symptoms [43]. Cross-reactivity exists between Dengue ELISA IgG and other flaviviruses, such as Japanese encephalitis (JE), yellow fever (YF), and West Nile virus, but far less so for dengue IgM [21, 44, 45]. The ELISA IgG test is therefore of limited use in JE or YF vaccinated travelers to differentiate between primary and secondary dengue and to determine seroconversion rates [43].

As a diagnosis of dengue is often hard to make in a timely manner, the diagnosis of dengue is initially only clinical, based on the development of clinical manifestations and laboratory features over time, while excluding other potentially life-threatening diagnoses such as malaria.

The differential diagnosis of dengue is extensive and includes malaria, measles, rubella, influenza, typhoid, leptospirosis, Epstein-Barr virus infection, Chikungunya, viral hemorrhagic fevers and rickettsial diseases, and any other diseases that may present in the acute phase as an undifferentiated febrile syndrome.

10.5.5 Clinical Management

There is no specific antiviral drug yet developed against dengue. Treatment is therefore symptomatic and supportive, with the primary aim to prevent mortality from severe DHF/DSS. Classic dengue is treated with antipyretics (i.e., paracetamol), bed rest, and oral (rarely parenteral) fluid replacement, and most cases can be managed on an outpatient basis. Aspirin and nonsteroidal anti-inflammatory drugs are contraindicated as they may increase bleeding tendencies. Intramuscular injections are contraindicated as they may cause massive hematomas. Patients should be advised to repeat platelet and hematocrit determinations every 24 h [30]. Prompt and correct institution of fluid replacement is thought to reduce mortality due to DHF/DSS [46]. The critical period is usually on the day of defervescence, typically 4–7 days after onset of the illness. A decrease in the platelet count which usually precedes the rise in hematocrit is of diagnostic and prognostic value [30]. A rise in hematocrit of 20 % indicates significant plasma loss, and prompt institution of intravenous fluid replacement is indicated, with normal saline or lactated Ringer's solution [46, 47]. In continued shock, plasma or other colloid may be added [21, 46]. If there is evidence of bleeding or disseminated intravascular coagulation, fresh blood or fresh frozen plasma/platelets should be administered. Once the capillary leakage stops and resorption of extravasated fluid begins, care must be taken not to induce fluid overload and pulmonary edema [21].

10.6 Prevention and Control

Dengue control follows three main strategies: source reduction (location and destruction of mosquitoes, breeding sites), use of larvicides, and use of ultralow-volume aerosolised adulticides. The first two strategies have been used with varying success. However, the efficacy of current methods to control adult mosquitoes is controversial. *Aedes aegypti* had been highly susceptible to DDT, with DDT-based control strategies resulting in the eradication of *A. aegypti* from 22 countries in the Americas in 1962 and from all countries in the Mediterranean region in 1972 [48]. Since DDT was abandoned, the control of dengue has shifted to source reduction and use of larvicides and adulticides from other chemical classes. Biological control of larvae in the form of larvivorous fish and/or predatory copepods – small freshwater crustaceans – has proved effective in operational contexts in specific container habitats, but has not yet been used on a large scale. The willingness of local communities to accept the introduction of organisms into water containers is essential to make biological control agents such as mesocyclops successful. Vector control should be integrated and include a combined vertical and horizontal approach that depends on community participation [49].

Personal protection against dengue is difficult to implement on a long-term basis as it requires daily protective measures with insect repellents, applied throughout the day as Aedes mosquitoes are day-biting mosquitoes. Bed-nets therefore have only very limited or no benefit, in contrast to malaria.

10.6.1 Dengue Vaccines

Vector control is currently the mainstay for the control of dengue, but it is not sufficient. Several models have shown that vaccination against dengue would be the most cost-effective strategy. However, development of a safe and effective vaccine against a disease with such strong immunological ramifications poses considerable challenges [50]. A dengue vaccine has to protect reliably and long-term against all four serotypes for two reasons: first, to protect the individual against disease resulting from any serotype and second, to preclude the development of immune-mediated severe disease. Weak immune responses that wane below protective levels over time are not acceptable because of the severe consequences seen during secondary DENV infections [51]. The lack of an animal model, limited understanding of immune correlates of protection, and the difficulty of distinguishing cross-reactions from the development of type-specific antibodies create further challenges [50].

Nevertheless, the development of dengue vaccines has seen significant progress in recent years, and the pace toward clinical efficacy trials has accelerated substantially. The vaccine pipeline is now sufficiently advanced for it to be possible to have a first-generation dengue vaccine licensed within the next 5–7 years. In addition, a number of diverse candidates are at earlier stages of evaluation and could become second-generation vaccines [52].

The vaccine in furthest development is the chimeric tetravalent vaccine (developed by Sanofi Pasteur). For this vaccine, the structural genes (prM and E) of each of the four dengue viruses were inserted individually to replace those of yellow fever virus in the backbone of the yellow fever 17D vaccine [10]. This vaccine is currently in phase 3 trials. Other vaccines in development are the live attenuated vaccines, subunit vaccines, recombinant vaccines, DNA vaccines, and vector-based vaccines [10].

More work is required to bring a vaccine from licensing to programmatic use in dengue endemic areas. Depending on cost-effectiveness and national epidemiology, countries may decide to introduce dengue vaccines into the national immunization programs for routine administration. If the vaccine is to be used for infants, the dengue vaccination will need to be carried out on a schedule compatible with other vaccines, and absence of interference with other childhood vaccines need to be shown. Post-marketing surveillance is paramount to identify rare serious adverse events that were not picked up during phase 1–3 trials.

10.7 Conclusions

Due to the expanding geographical distribution of both the virus and the mosquito vector, increased frequency of epidemics, co-circulation of multiple virus serotypes, and the emergence of DHF in new areas, WHO classifies dengue as a major international public health concern [2, 5]. The reasons for this resurgence are complex and include unprecedented urbanization with substandard living conditions, lack of vector control, virus evolution, and international travel [1, 5, 23]. Of all these factors, urbanization has probably had the most impact on the amplification of dengue within a given country, and travel had the most impact for the spread of dengue from country to country and continent to continent. Modern rapid intercontinental transportation has had a major influence on the distribution and transmission dynamics of dengue. The development of dengue vaccines has seen significant progress in recent years.

References

1. Wilder-Smith A, Gubler DJ (2008) Geographic expansion of dengue: the impact of international travel. Med Clin North Am 92(6):1377–1390, x
2. Gubler DJ (2002) The global emergence/resurgence of arboviral diseases as public health problems. Arch Med Res 33(4):330–342
3. Rico-Hesse R (2003) Microevolution and virulence of dengue viruses. Adv Virus Res 59:315–341
4. Gubler DJ, Trent DW (1993) Emergence of epidemic dengue/dengue hemorrhagic fever as a public health problem in the Americas. Infect Agents Dis 2(6):383–393
5. Gibbons RV, Vaughn DW (2002) Dengue: an escalating problem. BMJ 324(7353):1563–1566

6. Gubler DJ (2003) Aedes albopictus in Africa. Lancet Infect Dis 3(12):751–752
7. Gubler DJ (2004) The changing epidemiology of yellow fever and dengue, 1900 to 2003: full circle? Comp Immunol Microbiol Infect Dis 27(5):319–330
8. Gubler DJ (2002) Epidemic dengue/dengue hemorrhagic fever as a public health, social and economic problem in the 21st century. Trends Microbiol 10(2):100–103
9. Wilder-Smith A, Schwartz E (2005) Dengue in travelers. N Engl J Med 353(9):924–932
10. Wilder-Smith A, Ooi EE, Vasudevan SG, Gubler DJ (2010) Update on dengue: epidemiology, virus evolution, antiviral drugs, and vaccine development. Curr Infect Dis Rep 12(3):157–164
11. World Health Organization (WHO) (2009) Dengue: guidelines for diagnosis, treatment, prevention and control. World Health Organization, Geneva
12. Ooi E, Gubler D (2009) Global spread of epidemic dengue: the influence of environmental change. Future Virol 4:571–580
13. Cheng S, Kalkstein LS, Focks DA, Nnaji A (1998) New procedures to estimate water temperatures and water depths for application in climate-dengue modeling. J Med Entomol 35(5):646–652
14. Egger JR, Ooi EE, Kelly DW, Woolhouse ME, Davies CR, Coleman PG (2008) Reconstructing historical changes in the force of infection of dengue fever in Singapore: implications for surveillance and control. Bull World Health Organ 86(3):187–196
15. Hales S, Weinstein P, Souares Y, Woodward A (1999) El Nino and the dynamics of vectorborne disease transmission. Environ Health Perspect 107(2):99–102
16. Schwartz E, Weld LH, Wilder-Smith A, von Sonnenburg F, Keystone JS, Kain KC et al (2008) Seasonality, annual trends, and characteristics of dengue among ill returned travelers, 1997-2006. Emerg Infect Dis 14(7):1081–1088
17. Bartley LM, Donnelly CA, Garnett GP (2002) The seasonal pattern of dengue in endemic areas: mathematical models of mechanisms. Trans R Soc Trop Med Hyg 96(4):387–397
18. Ooi EE, Goh KT, Gubler DJ (2006) Dengue prevention and 35 years of vector control in Singapore. Emerg Infect Dis 12(6):887–893
19. Cummings DA, Iamsirithaworn S, Lessler JT, McDermott A, Prasanthong R, Nisalak A et al (2009) The impact of the demographic transition on dengue in Thailand: insights from a statistical analysis and mathematical modeling. PLoS Med 6(9):e1000139
20. Freedman DO, Kozarsky PE, Weld LH, Cetron MS (1999) GeoSentinel: the global emerging infections sentinel network of the International Society of Travel Medicine. J Travel Med 6(2):94–98
21. Vaughn DW, Green S (2000) Dengue and dengue hemorrhagic fever. In: Strickland GT (ed) Hunter's Tropical medicine and emerging infectious diseases, 8th edn. W.B. Saunders, Philadelphia, pp 240–241
22. Gubler DJ (1998) The global pandemic of dengue/dengue haemorrhagic fever: current status and prospects for the future. Ann Acad Med Singapore 27(2):227–234
23. Guzman MG, Kouri G (2002) Dengue: an update. Lancet Infect Dis 2(1):33–42
24. Halstead SB, O'Rourke EJ (1977) Dengue viruses and mononuclear phagocytes. I. Infection enhancement by non-neutralizing antibody. J Exp Med 146(1):201–217
25. Halstead SB (1979) In vivo enhancement of dengue virus infection in rhesus monkeys by passively transferred antibody. J Infect Dis 140(4):527–533
26. Halstead SB (1982) Immune enhancement of viral infection. Prog Allergy 31:301–364
27. Rosen L (1977) The emperor's new clothes revisited, or reflections on the pathogenesis of dengue hemorrhagic fever. Am J Trop Med Hyg 26(3):337–343
28. Gubler DJ (1998) Dengue and dengue hemorrhagic fever. Clin Microbiol Rev 11(3):480–496
29. Vaughn DW, Green S, Kalayanarooj S, Innis BL, Nimmannitya S, Suntayakorn S et al (2000) Dengue viremia titer, antibody response pattern, and virus serotype correlate with disease severity. J Infect Dis 181(1):2–9
30. Gubler D (2001) Dengue and dengue hemorrhagic fever. In: Guerrant RL, Walker DH, Weller PF (eds) Essentials of tropical infectious diseases. Churchill Livingstone, Philadelphia, pp 580–583

31. Wilder-Smith A, Foo W, Earnest A, Sremulanathan S, Paton NI (2004) Seroepidemiology of dengue in the adult population of Singapore. Trop Med Int Health 9(2):305–308
32. Oh H (1998) Clinical manifestations and management of dengue in Singapore. In: Goh KT (ed) Dengue in Singapore. Ministry of the Environment, Singapore, pp 73–79
33. Schwartz E, Mendelson E, Sidi Y (1996) Dengue fever among travelers. Am J Med 101(5):516–520
34. Jelinek T, Muhlberger N, Harms G, Corachan M, Grobusch MP, Knobloch J et al (2002) Epidemiology and clinical features of imported dengue fever in Europe: sentinel surveillance data from TropNetEurop. Clin Infect Dis 35(9):1047–1052
35. Watt G, Jongsakul K, Chouriyagune C, Paris R (2003) Differentiating dengue virus infection from scrub typhus in Thai adults with fever. Am J Trop Med Hyg 68(5):536–538
36. Lum LC, Lam SK, George R, Devi S (1993) Fulminant hepatitis in dengue infection. Southeast Asian J Trop Med Public Health 24(3):467–471
37. Sumarmo HW, Wulur H, Jahja E, Gubler DJ, Sutomenggolo TS, Saroso JS (1978) Encephalopathy associated with dengue infection. Lancet 1(8061):449–450
38. Jensenius M, Gundersen SG, Vene S, Bruu AL (1997) Dengue fever imported to Norway. Serologically confirmed cases 1991–96. Tidsskr Nor Laegeforen 117(29):4230–4233
39. Chadwick D, Arch B, Wilder-Smith A, Paton N (2006) Distinguishing dengue fever from other infections on the basis of simple clinical and laboratory features: application of logistic regression analysis. J Clin Virol 35(2):147–153
40. Phuong CX, Nhan NT, Kneen R, Thuy PT, van Thien C, Nga NT et al (2004) Clinical diagnosis and assessment of severity of confirmed dengue infections in Vietnamese children: is the world health organization classification system helpful? Am J Trop Med Hyg 70(2):172–179
41. Rigau-Perez JG (1997) Clinical manifestations of dengue hemorrhagic fever in Puerto Rico, 1990–1991. Puerto Rico Association of Epidemiologists. Rev Panam Salud Publica 1(5):381–388
42. Kularatne SA, Walathara C, Mahindawansa SI, Wijesinghe S, Pathirage MM, Kumarasiri PV et al (2009) Efficacy of low dose dexamethasone in severe thrombocytopenia caused by dengue fever: a placebo controlled study. Postgrad Med J 85(1008):525–529
43. Schwartz E, Mileguir F, Grossman Z, Mendelson E (2000) Evaluation of ELISA-based serodiagnosis of dengue fever in travelers. J Clin Virol 19(3):169 173
44. Cobelens FGJ, Groen J, Osterhaus ADME, Leentvaar-Kuipers A, Wertheim-van Dillen PME, Kager PA (2002) Incidence and risk factors of probable dengue virus infection among Dutch travellers to Asia. Trop Med Int Health 7(4):331–338
45. Rigau-Perez JG, Clark GG, Gubler DJ, Reiter P, Sanders EJ, Vorndam AV (1998) Dengue and dengue haemorrhagic fever. Lancet 352(9132):971–977
46. Dung NM, Day NP, Tam DT, Loan HT, Chau HT, Minh LN et al (1999) Fluid replacement in dengue shock syndrome: a randomized, double-blind comparison of four intravenous-fluid regimens. Clin Infect Dis 29(4):787–794
47. Nimmannitya S (1987) Clinical spectrum and management of dengue haemorrhagic fever. Southeast Asian J Trop Med Public Health 20:320–330
48. Massad E, Coutinho FA (2011) The cost of dengue control. Lancet 377(9778):1630–1631
49. Kay B, Vu SN (2005) New strategy against *Aedes aegypti* in Vietnam. Lancet 365(9459): 613–617
50. Monath TP (2007) Dengue and yellow fever–challenges for the development and use of vaccines. N Engl J Med 357(22):2222–2225
51. Whitehead SS, Blaney JE, Durbin AP, Murphy BR (2007) Prospects for a dengue virus vaccine. Nat Rev Microbiol 5(7):518–528

Index

I.W. Fong (ed.), *Challenges in Infectious Diseases*, Emerging Infectious Diseases of the 21st Century 502, DOI 10.1007/978-1-4614-4496-1,

GPSR Compliance

The European Union's (EU) General Product Safety Regulation (GPSR) is a set of rules that requires consumer products to be safe and our obligations to ensure this.

If you have any concerns about our products, you can contact us on ProductSafety@springernature.com

In case Publisher is established outside the EU, the EU authorized representative is:

Springer Nature Customer Service Center GmbH
Europaplatz 3
69115 Heidelberg, Germany

Batch number: 10620084

Printed by Printforce, the Netherlands